Sociolegal Control of Homosexuality

A Multi-Nation Comparison

PERSPECTIVES IN SEXUALITY
Behavior, Research, and Therapy

Series Editor: RICHARD GREEN

University of Cambridge
Cambridge, England, United Kingdom and
Gender Identity Clinic
Charing Cross Hospital
London, England, United Kingdom

Sociolegal Control of Homosexuality

A Multi-Nation Comparison

Edited by

Donald J. West

University of Cambridge
Cambridge, England, United Kingdom

and

Richard Green

University of Cambridge
Cambridge, England, United Kingdom and
Gender Identity Clinic
Charing Cross Hospital
London, England, United Kingdom

PLENUM PRESS • NEW YORK AND LONDON

Library of Congress Cataloging-in-Publication Data

Sociolegal control of homosexuality : a multi-nation comparison /
  edited by Donald J. West and Richard Green.
       p.   cm. -- (Perspectives in sexuality)
    Includes bibliographical references and index.
    ISBN 0-306-45532-3
    1. Homosexuality--Cross-cultural studies. 2. Homosexuality--Law
and legislation--Cross-cultural studies. 3. Gay men--Legal status,
laws, etc. 4. Gay men--Mental health. 5. Lesbians--Legal status,
laws, etc. 6. Lesbians--Mental health.   I. West, D. J. (Donald
James), 1924-   . II. Green, Richard, 1936-   . III. Series.
HQ76.25.S65 1997
306.76'6--dc21   97-20368
                                                           CIP

ISBN 0-306-45532-3

© 1997 Plenum Press, New York
A Division of Plenum Publishing Corporation
233 Spring Street, New York, N. Y. 10013

http://www.plenum.com

10 9 8 7 6 5 4 3 2 1

Printed in the United States of America

Contributors

PAUL R. ABRAMSON • Department of Psychology, University of California–Los Angeles, Los Angeles, California 90024

PETER AVERY • Kings College, Cambridge CB2 1ST, England, United Kingdom

HOWARD BARBAREE • Clarke Institute of Psychiatry, and University of Toronto, Toronto, Ontario M5T 1R8, Canada

KEVAN BOTHA • National Coalition for Gay and Lesbian Equality, Johannesburg, Republic of South Africa, 2000

CHRISTINE BROWN • Clarke Institute of Psychiatry, and University of Toronto, Toronto, Ontario M5T 1R8, Canada

EDWIN CAMERON • The High Court of South Africa, Johannesburg, Republic of South Africa, 2000

HELMUT GRAUPNER • Rechtskomitee LAMBDA, Austrian Sexological Society, Linke Wienzeille, 102, A-1060 Vienna, Austria

RICHARD GREEN • Institute of Criminology, University of Cambridge, Cambridge, CB3 9DT, England, United Kingdom; and Gender Identity Clinic, Charing Cross Hospital, London W6 8RF, England, United Kingdom

ALEXANDER GREER • Clarke Institute of Psychiatry, and University of Toronto, Toronto, Ontario M5T 1R8, Canada

RAINER HOFFMANN • Department of Gay and Lesbian Studies Fachbereich 8, University of Bremen, D-28334 Bremen, Germany

JÖRG HUTTER • Department of Gay and Lesbian Studies Fachbereich 8, University of Bremen, D-28334 Bremen, Germany

JUAN LUIS ÁLAVAREZ-GAYOU JURGENSON • Mexican Institute of Sexology, Del. Cuauhtémoc, Mexico, D.F. CP. 06760, Mexico

BADRUDDIN KHAN • El Instituto Obregón, San Francisco, California 94107-3239

IGOR S. KON • Institute of Ethnology and Anthropology, Russian Academy of Sciences, Moscow 117334, Russia

RÜDIGER LAUTMANN • Department of Gay and Lesbian Studies Fachbereich 8, University of Bremen, D-28334 Bremen, Germany

LAURENCE WAI-TENG LEONG • Department of Sociology, National University of Singapore, Singapore 119260, Singapore

STEPHEN O. MURRAY • El Instituto Obregón, San Francisco, California 94107-3239

MARTIN MOERINGS • Institute for Criminal Sciences, University of Utrecht, Utrecht 3512 BM, The Netherlands

OLIVER PHILLIPS • Institute of Criminology, University of Cambridge, Cambridge CB3 9DT, England, United Kingdom

STEVEN D. PINKERTON • Department of Psychiatry and Behavioral Medicine, Center for AIDS Intervention Research, Medical College of Wisconsin, Milwaukee, Wisconsin 53226

IVO PROCHÁZKA • Institute of Sexology, Charles University, Prague 120 00, Czech Republic

ALAN REEKIE • International Gay and Lesbian Association, Brussels B-1000, Belgium

FANG-FU RUAN • The Institute for Advanced Study of Human Sexuality, San Francisco, California 94109

DONALD J. WEST • Institute of Criminology, University of Cambridge, Cambridge CB3 9DT, England, United Kingdom

ANDREA WÖELKE • Solicitor, Anthony, Gold, Lerman and Muirhead, London SE1, England, United Kingdom

RICHARD WRIGHT • Department of Criminology and Criminal Justice, University of Missouri–St. Louis, St. Louis, Missouri 63121

TIMOTHY WRIGHT • Formerly of Collaborative Program for the Prevention and Control of STDs and AIDS, Santa Cruz, Bolivia

PREFACE

In this volume, we record and compare diverse national systems of sociolegal regulation of homosexual behavior. Controls can be embodied in criminal law or, equally powerfully, enshrined in the traditional norms and dominant attitudes and beliefs of a society.

Chapters have been written by authorities who know well the countries they describe. This is important because what is critical is not the content of formal regulations or official pronouncements, but whether and how these are enforced and whether they have public support.

Chapters adhere to no standard format. Each reflects the issues uppermost in a particular country. Apart from the obvious issues that arise when homosexual behaviors are criminalized, many aspects of life are affected by an individual's sexuality, including housing, partnership arrangements, parenting, employment, health, and military service. Some or all of these issues feature in the chapters that follow.

Only in recent years, and mostly in the industrialized West, has homosexual behavior emerged as a prominent civil rights concern. Following recognition of the rights of racial minorities and the rights of women to gender equality, the homosexual minority has become increasingly visible and active in demanding similar respect for their social dignity and freedom from discrimination. Whereas varying degrees of corresponding legal reform have taken place in Europe and North America, in many other parts of the world the concept of civil rights remains undeveloped and the homosexual minority is oppressed or ignored, or its existence is denied. Yet, with the advent of the "global village," with mass media, mass tourism, and international business spreading Western ideas, the beginnings of change can be seen worldwide.

Contributions are included from cultures that are often omitted or given only passing reference when social control of homosexuality is discussed in English-language publications. Thus, there are chapters about countries in Africa, Asia, Latin America, and the Far East. Practical considerations of book length and availability of information necessarily limit coverage, but the diversity of cultures that has been included makes for an innovative enterprise.

The penultimate chapter gives a brief overview of contemporary academic thinking and research on the origins of homosexual behaviors and the implications for social control. The final chapter examines emerging trends, as well as inconsistencies, across nations, including some areas not previously covered. Although the information presented by contributors defies easy integration, the conclusion attempts to provide an overview of the current state of sociolegal control of homosexuality.

ACKNOWLEDGMENTS

Particular thanks are due to Andrea Wöelke for help in the editing of some European contributions, to Alan Reekie for contacts and information via the Internet, and to Patrick Sweeney for solving computer problems.

CONTENTS

Chapter 6

Chapter 7

Chapter 8

Chapter 9

SINGAPORE 127

Laurence Wai-Teng Leong

Chapter 10

THE UNITED STATES 145

Richard Green

Chapter 11

CANADA 169

Alexander Greer, Howard Barbaree, and Christine Brown

Chapter 15

THE CZECH AND SLOVAK REPUBLICS 243

Ivo Procházka

Chapter 16

GERMANY 255

Rainer Hoffmann, Jörg Hutter, and Rüdiger Lautmann

Chapter 17

AUSTRIA 269

Helmut Graupner

Chapter 18

BELGIUM 289

Alan Reekie

Chapter 19

THE NETHERLANDS 299

Martin Moerings

Chapter 20

Donald J. West

Donald J. West and Richard Green

INTRODUCTION

DONALD J. WEST AND RICHARD GREEN

HOMOSEXUAL RELATIONS: A HUMAN RIGHT?

Freedom to engage in consensual homosexual relations is felt by some to be as important to them as freedom to express heterosexuality is to others. In recent decades it has come to be argued by Western liberals that this freedom is a basic human right deserving protection by international law (Wintemute, 1995).

The notion of natural "rights" goes back a long way. Ancient Greek and Roman authors discussed it. Philosophers of the eighteenth-century "Enlightenment" expressed an ideology of personal freedom in the American Declaration of Independence (1776) and in the French Declaration of the Rights of Man and of the Citizen (1789). The latter embodied the then revolutionary assertions that all men are born free and equal in their rights to liberty, property, and inviolability of the person and that all citizens should be equal before the law and should enjoy freedom of speech and religion. Similar ideas were promulgated in the American Bill of Rights (1791).

In modern times the United Nations has laid down standards to which all its member states should conform. The principles were first set out in the Universal Declaration of Human Rights proclaimed by the General Assembly of the United Nations on December 10, 1948. Particularly relevant is Article 2 of the Declaration, which provides that "Everyone is entitled to the rights and freedoms set forth in this Declaration, without distinction of any kind, such as race, color, sex, language, religion, political or other opinion, national or social origin, property, birth or other status."

These principles were reinforced and amplified in the International Covenant on Civil and Political Rights, which came into effect in 1976, taking the form of a treaty binding the nations that ratified it. Article 2 states, "Each state party to the present Covenant undertakes to respect and to ensure to all individuals within its territory and subject to its jurisdiction the rights recognized in the present Covenant without distinction of any kind, such as race, color, sex, language, religion, political or other opinion, national origin, property, birth or other status." Article 17 reads, "(1) No one shall be subjected to arbitrary or unlawful interference with his privacy, family, home or correspondence, nor to unlawful attacks on his honour and reputation. (2) Everyone has the right to the protection of the law against such intereference or attacks."

DONALD J. WEST • Institute of Criminology, University of Cambridge, Cambridge CB3 9DT, England, United Kingdom.   RICHARD GREEN • Institute of Criminology, University of Cambridge, Cambridge CB3 9DT, England, United Kingdom; and Gender Identity Clinic, Charing Cross Hospital, London W6 8RF, England, United Kingdom.

Sociolegal Control of Homosexuality, edited by West and Green, Plenum Press, New York, 1997.

1

Application to Homosexual Conduct

In their decision in the case of *Toonen v. Australia* (1994) the United Nations Human Rights Committee found that the Tasmanian law criminalizing all intermale sexual activity violated the right to privacy outlined in Article 17 of the United Nations International Covenant on Civil and Political Rights, which by that time had been ratified by 128 countries. This decision, the first of its kind, does not rule out other forms of discrimination based on sexual orientation, but it paves the way for other appeals on related grounds.

Protagonists of gay rights press for much more. Besides arguing that the terms "sex" or "other status" in the U.N. Covenant should encompass "sexual orientation," they want all legal freedoms and restrictions to apply equally to homosexual and heterosexual behavior. For example, in Britain, Liberty (the National Council for Civil Liberties), arguing the case for recognition of sexual orientation as a relevant "status," asserted, "Sexual orientation is an immutable part of every person, like their race and gender,... the expression of sexual orientation entails the exercise of other fundamental human rights, such as privacy, freedom of expression and freedom of association;" and "lesbians, gays and bisexuals form a recognized and distinct group within society and they are entitled to protection from discrimination" (Liberty, 1994).

Condemnatory laws are generally directed toward specific behaviors, regardless of motivation or whether the conduct is sporadic, situational, or the habitual expression of sexuality by individuals self-identifying as gay, lesbian, or bisexual and organizing their whole lives and sociosexual relationships accordingly.

Some countries have taken up the United Nations human rights principles and expanded them for incorporation into their own laws. In the new South African constitution, exceptional for a national constitution, equal rights for homosexual men and women have been explicitly included. Discrimination on grounds of sexual orientation is expressly prohibited in a number of provincial constitutions, such as those in Brandenburg and Thuringia in Germany and in many regional legislations within Canada, Australia, and the United States (see Wintemute, 1995, Appendix II). The European Union and the Council of Europe have condemned criminalization of consensual homosexual behavior and have gone some way toward protecting homosexuals from any form of discrimination, but not all member states have incorporated European directives into their domestic laws.

Violations of Human Rights

The U.N. standards, to whatever categories of person they may apply, operate in many places more as a moral statement than a practical reality. The most basic tenets of the 1948 Declaration, such as the bans on slavery and torture or the guarantees of "security of the person" and a fair, public trial of any charge of crime, are all widely flouted. When the press is full of stories of genocide and "ethnic cleansing" and Amnesty International publishes endless lists of "prisoners of conscience," it is all too clear that the United Nations' power to impose respect for their own principles and treaty obligations upon its member states is severely limited.

The *World Human Rights Guide* (Humana, 1992) contains maps showing a substantial portion of the world marked in black, signifying areas where "most human rights are denied." China is an example of a country in which state torture, extra-judicial killings or "disappearances," indefinite detention without trial, censorship of mail and personal correspondence, and the compulsory teaching of state ideology in schools are reported. The *Guide* lists similar phenomena in other countries, such as Libya, Sudan, and Iran. In all these places homosexuality is severely repressed.

Many governments simply issue bland denials of their violations; others seek to invoke Article 2(7) of the U.N. Charter, which exempts from intervention "matters which are essentially within the jurisdiction of any state."

Where such gross violations are endemic, homosexuals are particularly liable to be treated as outcasts, and their concerns are unlikely to be heeded. A report by Amnesty International (1994) points out that there are many places where homosexuals, along with other vulnerable citizens, live in constant fear of detention without charge; police intimidation, extortion, and torture; and semi-official "death squads" and resultant "disappearance." In other places lesbian women and gay men face more subtle forms of everyday hostility and discrimination in their contact with government agencies.

In those countries where civil liberties have taken root, mainly in the West, discrimination against homosexuals has become a subject of lively political debate and almost obsessive public concern. Homosexuals have won greater recognition, but even in the most tolerant countries, sections of the population, most notably the religious fundamentalists, decry that fact. They are implacably opposed to further concessions, and a backlash threatens further accommodation.

CITED CASES

Toonen v Australia, 50th session, UN Human Rights Committee, Doc. No. CCPR/C/50/ D/488/1992, 1, I.H.R.R. 97 (March 31, 1994).

REFERENCES

Amnesty International. (1994). *Breaking the silence: Human rights violations based on sexual orientation.* New York: Author.
Humana, C. (1992). *World human rights guide* (3rd. ed.). Oxford: Oxford University Press.
Liberty. (1994). *Sexuality and the state. Report no. 6.* London: National Council for Civil Liberties.
Wintemute, R. (1995). *Sexual orientation and human rights.* Oxford: Clarendon Press.

South Africa

KEVAN BOTHA AND EDWIN CAMERON

Introduction

The establishment of the Union of South Africa in 1910[1] purportedly ended the domination of colonial power. But union signified a process of progressive exclusion — reduction of direct foreign legislative and executive control, the entrenchment of white economic and political privilege (to the exclusion of the majority), and civil rights oppression of the majority of South Africa's population. Against this background, the African National Congress was established in 1913.

At the time of the Union, South African law criminalizing sexual conduct was not wholly uniform between the former colonial regions. However, in its varied forms, the law against same-sex conduct had the principal aim to stigmatize, punish, and exclude (Cameron, 1993). The systems of law the colonial powers (both Dutch and later English) introduced significantly influenced the customary law of the African communities they subjugated.

The Cape of Good Hope was colonized in 1652 as a provisions station for ships of the Dutch East India Company. The territory received the Roman Dutch common law of the States General of Holland. This incorporated the prohibitions against same-sex conduct of the ancient *lex Sca(n)tinia*,[2] the *lex Julia*, the medieval canon law, and the Placaat of July 1730 [the latter being promulgated upon a perceived outbreak of sodomy in Holland in 1730 (van der Keessel, 1809)]. When disgruntled burghers trekked northward from the Cape colony in the 1830s, they took with them the Roman-Dutch common law. In 1859 they adopted the Dutch scholar van der Linden's *Koopmans Handboek* as the definitive exposition of the common law (Hosten, Edwards, Nathan, & Bosman, 1983). The *Handboek* specifically criminalized acts of *sodomie* and *onnatuurlijke ontucht* ("unnatural immorality"). As punishments, it prescribed public execution by hanging and immediate burning of the body.

The British took occupation of the Cape Colony in 1803. By a twist of history, this prevented the adoption at the Cape of the Napoleonic Code, which after 1810 decriminalized same-sex activity in Holland. The subsequent British occupation influenced the

---

[1]Established by the Union of South Africa Act 1909, 9 Edw VII c9.

[2]Boswell (1980) dates this law to around 226 BC, noting that it is uncertain precisely what it regulated. He suggests that it protected minor and infant males from involuntary prostitution or castration rather than homosexual behaviour. Accordingly, the assertion by van der Keessel that criminality attached to same-sex conduct in pre-Republic Rome on the authority of this law should be treated with caution.

KEVAN BOTHA • National Coalition for Gay and Lesbian Equality, Johannesburg, Republic of South Africa, 2000. EDWIN CAMERON • The High Court of South Africa, Johannesburg, Republic of South Africa, 2000.

Sociolegal Control of Homosexuality, edited by West and Green, Plenum Press, New York, 1997.

nature of punishments inflicted for same-sex offenses. The British also entrenched legal restrictions on homosexuality, intruded on indigenous practices, and reinforced reactionary attitudes toward sexuality. Unlike the attitudes espoused by scholars of the enlightenment, British attitudes were conservative and slow to reform (Dynes, 1989).

Parallelling the position in the United Kingdom itself, pre-Union South African law contained no legislated prohibitions against lesbian sexual expression. The colony of Natal had enacted a law prohibiting "indecent assault and conduct" (Natal Criminal Act, s. 10) and the Transkei prohibited "unnatural sexual offences," including any "carnal intercourse" outside marriage (Transkei Penal Code, s. 121). The Roman-Dutch common law in addition criminalized acts of "sodomy" and "unnatural sexual offences."

Union made this disapproving common law uniformly applicable throughout South Africa.

PRESERVING ANCIENT LAWS AGAINST SAME-SEX CONDUCT

Sodomy

Early Roman-Dutch common law branded almost every form of nonconformist sexual behavior as "sodomy." Sodomy was regarded as the most outrageous of all crimes of the flesh, a precursor to plague, famine, pestilence, and earthquakes. Many early writers included sodomy, bestiality, self-masturbation, oral intercourse, and lesbian acts collectively as 'sodomy' (Carpzovius, 1752; Damhouder, 1656; Matthaeus, 1661; van der Linden, 1806; van Leeuwen, 1662). Some early jurists regarded heterosexual intercourse between a Jew and a Christian as sodomy (Hunt, 1982; Snyman, 1992; S v. C, 1988). However, by the early part of the twentieth century sodomy in South Africa had come to signify "that particular kind of unnatural offence where there is penetration *per anum*" (R v. Gough & Narroway, 1926, p. 163; S v. M, 1979a, p. 168). (See also De Wet & Swanepoel, 1975; Gardiner & Lansdown, 1926; Hunt, 1982; Snyman, 1992). The punishment was usually extreme. Unlike other common law crimes where penal enforcement lapsed after 5 years, the crime of sodomy lapsed only after 30 years (van der Keessel, 1809).

Unnatural Sexual Offenses

In addition to sodomy, Roman-Dutch common law penalized bestiality, as well as a third, broad category of sexual acts, classified broadly as "unnatural sexual offences"[3] or *venus monstrosa* (unnatural sexual love). Under the common law unnatural offenses comprised a punishable misuse of the organs of procreation (Quistorp, 1770). One reason given for punishing unnatural acts was that possible procreation of children was defeated (Carpzovius, 1752; Kersteman, 1768, *s.v. sodomie*; Menochius, 1583). This rationale embraced the prohibition of lesbian acts (Carpzovius, 1752; Criminal Ordinance, 1544, Art. 116; Matthaeus, 1661). It has never been possible to determine the ambit of this crime precisely. However, the common law condemned "whatsoever substitutes for the male or the female" as unnatural lust, specifically mentioning "pederasts, catamites,

---

[3]These offenses were usually grouped together under the generic title of *venus monstrosa, onkuysheyd tegens de natuur, onnatuurlijke ontucht,* or sodomy in its broad connotation.

masturbators, and those that practise fellatio, obscenities," bestiality, and necrophilia. These were all capital offenses (Matthaeus, 1661, par. 48.3.6.8.).

A discernable trend among judges has been to refer to these offenses in euphemisms. The Dutch jurist van der Keessel stated in 1806, "the turpitude of this unspeakable crime is so great that it ought, it seems, to be passed over in silence rather than to be expounded to the ears of the chaste, and hence many commentators on the criminal law too have merely touched on it with very few words" (van der Keessel, 1809, p. 857; see also Carpzovius, 1752; Matthaeus, 1661). This reluctance is illustrated by Chief Justice Solomon in R v. Baxter & Another (1928): "the acts of indecency complained of … are of so disgusting a nature that I refrain from repeating them, and in respect of which it is sufficient to state that the appellants are alleged to be the active agents … in the acts of indecency charged" (p. 431).

This coy refusal to be explicit has compounded the uncertain scope of the crime. In addition, it has perpetuated in the public mind images of depravity and perversion that persist in modern discussion. In eighteenth-century cases at the Cape, the crime of sodomy was used primarily to prosecute cases of bestiality. One of the earliest recorded cases was that of Jan Pietersen from Vlieland who appeared before the Court of Justice at the Castle in January 1757. A convict on Robben Island, he was accused of carnal intercourse with certain pigs in his care. The case has two noteworthy aspects. First, the sources used to justify the prosecution included the law of Moses and the writings of Damhouder, Van Leewen, and Carpzovius as well as the Placaat of the States-General of the Netherlands of 21 July 1730 (Hosten et al., 1983). Secondly, an extremely harsh sentence was imposed, on pigs and perpetrator. The pigs were ordered to be shot and buried on Robben Island. Pietersen was ordered to be bound and drowned at sea. The first attempt was defeated by a raging southeasterly wind and was carried out only 2 days later (Court of Justice, 1652–1827, vol. CJ3683). The categorization of same-sex conduct with bestiality still informs the debate.

In the twentieth century, South African judges adopted with zeal the ample and unrestricted ambit of the common law definitions so as to criminalize conduct the status of which was at least open to interpretation as uncertain. Rubbing a penis between the thighs of another male, resulting in the emission of semen, was in 1926 held criminal (R v. Gough & Narroway, 1926). The appeal judges justified their stand on the basis of public opinion, which, they said, had not changed to regard such conduct as otherwise than abhorrent. This reasoning was used only months later in a decision that further extended common law concepts by holding mutual masturbation between two males criminal. The judge reasoned that "there can be no distinction between the case where sexual gratification is obtained by friction between the legs of another person, and the case where it is obtained by friction against another's hand" (R v. Curtis, 1926, p. 386). Under Roman-Dutch law self-masturbation (to which Curtis still referred as a "disgusting act against himself") was considered criminal, although by the mid-1600s the death penalty was already disapproved "because the high frequency [of masturbation makes it] difficult and almost impossible to enforce the penalty" (Matthaeus, 1661, par. 48.3.6.8.). In S v. V (1967) mutual masturbation between consenting male adults was still considered criminal, the judge denying that "the present outlook has developed to the stage of regarding such conduct as not constituting an unnatural offence." The attorney general of the Cape (the region's chief law enforcement officer) in 1968 expressed the view that two men sitting next to each other kissing with their hands on each others legs were committing an indecent and unnatural offense (Select Committee, 1968; cf. *R v. S*, 1950, where it was held that a male merely touching with his hand the private parts of another male does not commit an unnatural offense). More permissively, the Transvaal attorney general noted that "the police mention [men] dancing together and kissing. I am afraid that I cannot agree that that is an indecent act.... Lots of fathers kiss their sons" (Select Committee, 1968, p. 333).

Distinguishing natural from unnatural acts was, like so much else in South African history, overlain with considerations of race. The insertion of a white penis between the legs of another white male was considered an unnatural sexual offence. Similar activity between black heterosexuals was ruled not unnatural. Judge Pittman in *R v. K & F* (1932) noted that "no one, who has taken part in the administration of criminal justice among the natives, can have failed to become impressed with the general prevalence of their practice of *metsha*, in which sexual gratification is afforded as a result of the male organ being inserted between the female's thighs, and yet despite this notoriety ... the conduct itself is never questioned, [and] is definitely outside the range of criminal responsibility" (p. 73). The custom of *metsha* is widely practiced in Africa as an acceptable form of intercourse primarily between young unmarried men and women. McLean and Ngcobo (1994) explain that a "despoiled" bride, if she were to marry at all, would fetch a low *lobola* (or bride price) for her parents. Thigh sex was accordingly an acceptable alternative.

Such cultural pragmatism toward premarital intercourse should be contrasted with the criminal prohibition the Transkei Penal Code (s. 121) imposed by providing that carnal intercourse outside marriage constitutes an unnatural sexual offense. Ritual fertility rites and dances, known as *intonjane*, were specifically outlawed in the same code. Even so, South African courts have excluded the custom of *metsha* from the broad ambit of this code because of the "general prevalence of the practice." Judge Munnik in *S v. M* (1977) held that "it cannot be contended with any justification that in a penal code enacted especially for the 'Transkeian Territories' it was intended to legislate against a *generally accepted* and *relatively innocuous* custom extant among the peoples of those territories" (p. 358) However the practice of *metsha* was not confined only to the Transkeian territories. The practice is referred to as *hlobongo* by the Zulus and *gangisa* among the Southern Mozambicans. Other documented cases are found among the Tsonga-speaking Shangaan (Moodie, 1994).

The sharply contrasting values and moral worth that custom and the legal system place on the practice of *metsha* are revealing in the context of homosexuality. While prevalent among heterosexual youth, the practice took on a wider application in same-sex mine hostels where migrant workers were separated from their families for lengthy periods. Caution should obviously be exercised in labelling same-sex conduct in this environment as a manifestation of "gay" identity in any essentialist sense. Moodie (1994) cautions that in the case of black miners, sensible discussion of sexuality cannot take place "outside the context of power relations, both power structures on the mines and the power of men in marriage" (p. 119). Moodie suggests that homosexual relationships were used as resources in the long-standing resistance by migrant workers to proletarianization. For present purposes, it is enough to note that same-sex relationships among mine workers were a reality — and that, in addition to domestic support services, they included sexual intimacy.

Moodie (1994) records that in 1907, as a result of reports by missionaries of endemic "unnatural vice," H. M. Taberer from the Transvaal Native Affairs Department conducted an investigation. The report concluded that sexual activity between miners did not involve penetration but took place externally by "action between the thighs" (Taberer, 1902–1934, 1907). Mine managements turned a blind eye to this activity. It was the Transkeian Territories General Council in 1928 that sent a delegation of senior counselors to the mines to lecture mine workers on the "immoral practices obtaining among labourers working on the mines" (Moodie, p. 123). Even so, the director of native labor, H. S. Cooke, told the council that the immorality complained of, "except that the subject is male and not female, took the form of what is known among Transkeian Natives as *ukumetsha* which, when girls were concerned, was to some extent condoned by Native Custom." Moodie continues, "Ukumetsha was consistently condemned by Christian missionaries, however, and among the urban African elite its extension to men was quite repugnant." For instance, when one of the Commissioners on the Native Economic Commission asked A. W. G. Champion "whether this bad practice amounts to *hlobongo* between man and man," he answered in the affirmative. However, when the questioner implied that it was thus not sodomy in the European sense, Champion was indignant: "I do not know what is used among Europeans; all I know is that this thing is very low among the natives — it is unspeakable" (Moodie, p. 123). Within the miners' communities themselves, however, notwithstanding moralistic censure by their white bosses, the practice was not only condoned, but customary rules also regulated the relationships of the men with the boys known as the "wives of the mine."

Despite the reactionary views of missionaries, who frowned even on the custom of heterosexual *metsha*, judges condoned the practice as natural and an accepted custom. A similarly pragmatic view was taken of same-sex *metsha* by mine workers themselves, including the practical recognition of these relationships, the self-regulation of their patrimonial and social consequences, and the noninterference of mine managements. However, state agencies and the law viewed the conduct as criminal simply because it was committed between two males. Conduct considered "relatively innocuous" in S v. M (1977) or "outside the range of criminal responsibility" in R v. K & F (1932) when heterosexual, was considered as "more abhorrent than adultery" (*Cunningham v. Cunningham*, 1952, p. 170) or as being an act of a "horrible nature" and entirely "unnatural" when homosexual (R v. *Taylor*, 1927, p. 19). The uneven attitude judges evinced in foregoing censure of customary practices when they accorded with perceptions of social tolerance, while deferring to prejudices when same-sex conduct was at issue, is notable.

Heterosexual conduct has accordingly been treated with greater leniency and acceptance than same-sex conduct. Although Carpzovius regarded many heterosexual acts as also unnatural, by 1931 heterosexual fellatio was no longer regarded as criminal (*R v. K & F*, 1932). Similarly it was determined in 1961 that heterosexual sodomy no longer constituted a criminal offense in South Africa (Joubert, 1981; R v. H, 1962; R v. M, 1969; R v. N, 1961; S v. M, 1979b; van der Linden, 1806; van Leeuwen, 1662). By the middle of this century the only acts still regarded by South African law as "unnatural" were between men.

Pervasive Consequences of the Criminal Law

Under South African law a police officer or a private person is authorized to arrest without a warrant any person *suspected* of having committed various offenses, such as murder, rape, and robbery. The schedule creating this list includes the offense of sodomy [Criminal Procedure Act, Schedule 1, read with ss. 40(1)(b), 42(1)(a)]. Further statutory authority permits the killing of a person reasonably suspected of having committed sodomy when such a person cannot otherwise be arrested or prevented from fleeing [s. 49(2)].[4] Persons convicted of sodomy are further, by reference back to the schedule, prohibited from registering as security officers [Security Officers Act, s. 12(1)(b)]. The same mechanism permits the interception of postal articles and communications [Interception and Monitoring Prohibition Act, ss. 1, 3(1)(b)].

Retribution: Eliminating All Trace of the Offense

Perhaps the most startling aspect of the criminalization of same-sex activity has been the severity of punishment. Under the *lex Julia* sodomy was a capital offense. The appropriate means of execution was death by the sword (Carpzovius, 1752; Institutes, n.d., par. 4.18.4). This extreme penalty was justified by scholars on the basis of both civil and divine law (van der Keessel, 1809). The only discretion allowed a judicial officer was to determine the manner in which the capital punishment was to be imposed (*R v. Taleke*, 1886). In earlier periods the execution was carried out secretly in prisons "so that the public should not indulge in any conversation about such great turpitude" (van der Keessel, 1809, p. 859). However, in 1730 the offense supposedly became common in the states of Holland (Huussen, 1989);[5] more extreme measures were accordingly enacted. The *Placaat* of July 21, 1730, provided specifically that execution should take place in public, so as to act as an example to others. These public executions were carried out with great cruelty depending on the circumstances of the crime. Carpzovius (1752) regarded burning sodomites alive as a suitable punishment to prevent contagion and to "obliterate the crime from the face of the earth" (par. 69.6). Where more than one instance of sodomy was involved, the penalty was preceded by torture.

Groenewegen (1669), in his treatise on the abrogation of Roman law in Holland, notes the disparity in criminal sanction in the states of Holland: In some, burning alive was reported; others reported hanging together with burning, or simply hanging or beheading. Groenewegen (1669) specifically requires the punishment to be appropriate in its severity in order that "all memory of such dishonourable lust be erased from the minds of men" (par. 4.14). However, the British governor, the Earl of Macartney, in 1797 abolished the use of torture at the Cape (Theale, 1905). Van der Linden (1806), writing in the early nineteenth century, required execution by hanging and the immediate burning of the condemned with the ashes being thrown into the sea or publicly displayed.

Under the later common law, provision was also made for solitary confinement in prison for cases not warranting execution, principally because sodomy was considered as a very serious and contagious crime (van der Keessel, 1809). Permanent banishment was also permitted under the Criminal Ordinance (Articles 326–328) (alongside the "damaging of dykes"). According to Carpzovius (1752), banishment was a suitable punishment for self-masturbation and acts with an inanimate instrument, which fell short of sodomy with another human or animal.

---

[4]This section of the Criminal Procedure Act is currently the subject of a constitutional challenge under the interim constitution, although not in relation to sodomy.

[5]Huussen's analysis of the incidence of sodomy cases in the States General of Holland indicates that 65 percent of all sodomy cases between 1730 and 1810 took place in 1730 and 1731 in the Provincial Court of Frisia (8), the Provincial Court of Holland (52), the Town Court of Leiden (21), and the Town Court of Amsterdam (13).

The first record of this punishment being inflicted at the Cape was the case of private Hugh Robertson, a soldier in the 98th Regiment sentenced in the Court of Justice on March 9, 1827. Late on a certain evening in January of that year a fellow soldier, John Brown, was allegedly lying "dead drunk and totally insensible." Robertson, with his "generative member in a state of excessive erection," is alleged to have attempted sodomy on Brown, but "prior to consummation was prevented from accomplishing it." The fiscal called for public punishment "next unto that of death," and Robertson was duly found guilty of sodomy, discharged, and banished to New South Wales for 14 years (Court of Justice, Vol. CJ 3624).

By the early nineteenth century, Enlightenment scholars of Europe had started to question the criminality of unnatural offenses, particularly the penalties inflicted. Van der Linden, however, pertinently rejected the contention of the French scholar Montesquieu[6] that sodomy should not be regarded as a capital offense. As already mentioned, van der Linden's definition of sodomy was regarded as the definitive exposition of the common law. Accordingly, sodomy remained a capital offense, with executions carried out in the cases of Jan Ruijter (1826) and the slave Fortuin (1831). The latter involved a case of double misfortune. Fortuin was a slave of Hendrik van der Merwe, a farmer at Uitvlygt in the district of Graaff Reinet. In June 1830 he stole two canisters, a tea pot and a sugar pot with a collective value of 5 shillings. For this he was sentenced to 45 lashes. While in prison awaiting trial he met another slave prisoner by the name of Frederik. Chained together, sharing the same blanket and sleeping pallet, the two prisoners engaged in sodomy. The matter came to a head when a fellow prisoner, Klaus Valentyn, laid a complaint with the authorities following a quarrel over the blanket. In his testimony, Frederik stated that Fortuin "used me nearly every night, [and] I push him away from me as soon as I awake." However, the affair had been going on for months without complaint from Frederick. The element of consent was not argued before the circuit court, and Fortuin was eventually executed in Cape Town in 1831.

A commission of enquiry by John Bigge, William Colebrooke, and W. Blair into criminal law and jurisprudence at the Cape reported in 1827 that "crimes against nature" were still punishable by death (Theale, 1905, p. 6). The same report records that "it has fallen within the power of the supreme authority to mitigate ... the spirit of a Statute which punishes with death the intercourse (altho' unattended by violence) of a Heathen, Moham-medan, or slave with a Christian woman" (p. 9), acts that were regarded as unnatural offenses under the common law. The death penalty at that time was effected by hanging in the case of men and strangulation in the case of women. Bigge's report records two cases of "unnatural crime" heard by the Court of Justice in the period between 1814 and 1825. In both these cases — one involving a free person, the other a Hottentot — the death penalty was approved by "fiat" of the governor (Theale, 1905). Although the exposition by van der Linden was adopted as the law in the Transvaal Republic in 1857, there appear to be no recorded cases of execution for sodomy in the Transvaal.

By 1883 the capital nature of "unnatural" crimes, at least at the Cape, was under review. In R v. Taleke (1886), Judge President Barry (in a case dealing with bestiality) noted

[6]In his Spirit of Laws, Montesquieu stated, "It is very odd that the crimes of magic, heresy, and that against nature, should be punished with fire," ventures to affirm that the crime against nature would never make progress but for certain customs that he suggests should be abandoned, and evidently condemns the severity of the sentence. (See translation by Jefferson, T., Philadelphia, 1811.)

that "it has been constant practice of our courts to punish this offence otherwise than capitally ... it may be contended that death is with us almost obsolete for such an offence" (p. 182). This attitude appears to have been influenced by British penal reforms and particularly English criminal statutes (24 and 25 Victoria, chap. 100, s. 61), which altered the punishment for buggery to penal servitude for life, with a minimum of 10 years. At about the same time the British conducted a lengthy commission of inquiry into customary law of Africans[7] resident along the southeastern coastline and noted that "many punishments known to the Roman-Dutch law are too cruel to be enforced" (Transkei Report, 1883, p. 25). The commissioners recommended that flogging with a maximum of 50 strokes be retained *only in cases of unnatural offenses*, together with a discretionary 5 years imprisonment, whipping, or a fine.

Between 1883 and the turn of the century the influence of British criminal law is apparent. Both the Cape and Natal acts are almost identical to the comparable British statute (48 and 49 Victoria, 1885, chap. 69, s. 11; R v. V, 1953).

In general, sentencing has followed several patterns. In the case of consenting adults the trend has been decidedly reformist. In the early part of this century custodial sentences of an average of 6 months with hard labor and corporal punishment were usual. By the mid-1950s corporal punishment was no longer regarded as a suitable punishment (R v. C, 1959; R v. M, 1958). However, incarceration was considered mandatory. This is demonstrated in the comments of Judge Bresler in R v. S (1956): "whilst appreciating the great importance of reformative measures in this and similar types of cases,... persons who have been guilty of depraved practices ... should not escape gaol sentences" (p. 650H). During the 1980s custodial sentences were reduced to periods averaging 2 months imprisonment and later to noncustodial sentences but with the imposition of a fine (R v. Mateba, 1950; R v. Serei, 1951; S v. R, 1992). The diminution of punishment reached its culmination in 1993, when two Cape judges decided that custodial sentences were inappropriate in such cases and substituted the most lenient sentence known to the criminal law, a caution and discharge (S v. H, 1993).

PROSECUTIONS, LEGAL ATTITUDES, AND GOVERNMENTAL REGULATION

Application of the Sexual Offenses Laws

Control of homosexuality through the law has been an important aspect of the sexual–ideological aims of those in power, from colonialism through apartheid. Mischke (1995) alludes to the dilemma all law faces: "When it is expected of the law to deal with matters relating to sexuality, the moral content and underlying structures of the law reveal themselves in dizzying moments of vertiginous horror, as the legal process breaks through the constraints of legality to disclose its morality, those powerful but hidden structures, those norms termed 'common sense,' *boni mores*, that which is decent and proper" (p. 34). Perceptions of sexual propriety in South Africa have thus depended significantly on dominant political and legal ideology. Sociolegal control of homosexuality has accordingly

[7]Following the incorporation of the area then known as British Kaffraria with the Cape Colony by Act 3 of 1865. The aim of the commission was essentially the codification of local customary law into a written form in compliance with the reforms of the British criminal system earlier in the century.

been influenced by a complex of interrelated interests. Exclusivist definitions of human identity, European constructions of morality, preconceived perceptions of what is considered "natural" and ideological stereotypes of race, class, and ethnography have been primary among these.

Criminalizing Same-Sex Conduct: Imposing a Eurocentric Value System

Moshesh, a Chief of the Basotho, testified in 1883 that "unnatural crimes" among the African people of Basutoland were a rare occurrence and that there was no punishment for such conduct under customary law (Transkei Report, 1883). The commissioners had initially committed themselves to the notion "that in legislating for natives we should not innovate unless innovation is a necessity … unless its recognition clearly perpetuates evils which could not be tolerated" (Transkei Report, 1883, p. 21). The commissioners, however, disregarded the evidence of Moshesh. In order to justify their inclusion of this new category of unnatural crimes into the customary law of the indigenous people of the Transkei, they noted in their draft penal code that some tribes regarded same-sex conduct as the work of a wizard or a witch. In the same report they recommended the criminalization of acts of witchcraft.

Historical reports of same-sex activity among indigenous African people are overlain by Eurocentric notions of what constituted "unnatural" activity. Theale (1887) alludes to "certain horrible customs" that took place during initiation rites (p. 17). Bleys (1996) notes that Theale does not explicitly state whether he is referring to mutual masturbation or intracrural or anal intercourse. However, he does contend that the reports indicate with great probability acts of homoerotic tenor. Such reports have tended to color the historical record of same-sex activity in precolonial regions. The records inflict Western condemnation on conduct that drew no criminal sanction in the customary practices of indigenous populations. As Bleys' analysis illuminates, this pitted Western notions of superior "civilization" against the

> savages, [who] within this diachronic model were seen not as inferior offshoots of the human race, but rather as the contemporary, living witnesses of humanity's pristine moral state. Ethnographic observation of living primitive people would thus allow for restructuring evolutionary processes, that eventually made the white European into the most adapted and developed subspecies of all. He had placed reason above the animistic religion of primitive folk, civilization above anarchy and violence, control above instinct. (p. 160)

The Impact of Apartheid and Preoccupation with Race

In addition to the disparities between the laws regarding heterosexual versus homosexual conduct, the application of these laws has been biased and racially motivated.

A striking feature of colonial statutes regulating sexual behavior is a frenetic preoccupation with race. The Transvaal Immorality Ordinance 46 of 1903 (s. 19) made it a criminal offense for any white woman to voluntarily permit a black man to have unlawful carnal connection with her and vice versa. This provision effectively prohibited any cohabitation or intimate association between black and white in the Transvaal. It was the precursor to section 16 of the Immorality Act, which notoriously prohibited intercourse between white and black persons (Bunting, 1986).[8] The fervor with which these early proscriptions were enacted is instructive. In the debates on the Criminal Amendment Act in the Transvaal Legislative Council on July 22, 1908, Colonel Dalrymple told the house "that no nation could tolerate such intercourse between diverse races" (Council Debates, 1908, p. 238). The debate in the Legislative Assembly on August 7 brought far worse. Mr. De Waal, the member for Wolmaransstad, claimed "he had never met a young Boer who had immoral relations with a Kafir girl" (Assembly Debates, 1908, p. 1445). The paradox that the legislature should have found it necessary to enact such prohibitions appears to have gone unnoticed. However, this new provision prohibiting interracial sex acts amended a 1903 law outlawing any soliciting or importuning for immoral purposes by any male [Criminal Amendment Act (Transvaal), s. 5, repealing the Transvaal Immorality Ordinance, s. 21(1)].

Racial and ideological themes in the control of sexual behavior find sharp focus in a 1954 appeal (R v. C, 1954). The accused had been convicted of both receptive and insertive sodomy with a black man ("a native") who proved to be a police agent provocateur (p. 52). Two further convictions were upheld in respect of juveniles referred to as "boys." In his judgment Judge Ramsbottom stated,

> On the first count the person incited was a native. That person had been sent by the police to watch the accused.... He says that the accused made some overture towards him and he then went away and consulted the police, and it is admitted that, according to the expression used in evidence "he was given permission to perform indecent acts with the accused." ... It is to me a most shocking thing that a native should be "given permission" to perform indecent acts in order to secure the conviction of the person suspected of an aberration of this kind. (p. 54)

In a brief concurring statement, Judge Clayden reiterates this position: "I do wish, however, to associate myself with the expression of disapproval of the fact that a native constable was allowed ... to continue and subject himself to the possibility of further such acts" (p. 55). The comments indicate two competing points of censure: that a "native" should have been used to procure the conviction of the accused and that a police officer should have been permitted to "subject himself" to homosexual conduct.

In a contrasting case, a white policeman from a farming town in Natal, nearing 50 and with 27 years' service in the South African police, had a fallout with his wife. She threatened to leave him. He took off in his car on an alcoholic binge. On the outskirts of Pietermaritzburg he drove up to a group of black men. He told them he wanted a woman. One of the men, a youngster of 15 or 16, then got into the car with him. The policeman undid his fly buttons and lay on top of the boy. He put his penis between the boy's legs and was later seen, as the court put it, "going through the motions of sexual intercourse." He was arrested and arraigned in court. He lost his job and his pension. His wife started divorce proceedings against him. A magistrate sent him to jail. Two Supreme Court judges suspended the jail sentence. The fact that the young boy was black was specifically noted as not being additionally aggravating. They saw grounds to be merciful. The policeman did "not

---

[8]Bunting notes that "no Act has done more to injure the reputation of South Africa in the eyes of the world, for thousands of people ... have fallen foul of its provisions and been sent to jail. Over 6000 people have been convicted under this Act between 1950 and June 1966.... No reasonable system of morality, can tolerate the ethics of the Immorality Act, which condones immorality between people of the same race, but converts it into a criminal offence from the moment that the race groups are different."

normally behave in this way." He did not set out to pervert the morals of a young person. It did not appear from the evidence that he had a "tendency to perversion." What happened was "a temporary aberration," and all the "quite appalling consequences which have resulted" were enough of a deterrent against future repetition (S v. S, 1965, p. 409).

In another case, a 52-year-old white man was charged with having a "veneral affair against the order of nature" (although the facts of the case indicated that a sexual assault had taken place) with an "African male" who was 21 years old. After initially placing his hands on the victim's private parts, the accused stopped his motor vehicle at a lonely spot and led the young man to a spot behind a bush. There he told him to kneel down and remove his trousers, whereafter he committed sodomy on him. He then gave the complainant 50 cents. In the appeal the judge considered the fact that the defendant was a "European of some 52 years of age" to have been an important element in view of the fact that the complainant was a "humble African domestic servant of 21 years of age, the sort of man who would be likely to yield easily to persuasion of this sort" (S v. K, 1973, p. 88). Here the hierarchies flowing from class and racial subordination are invoked to underscore the exploitative nature of the accused's conduct.

During the apartheid era, key moments of political crisis have coincided with incidents of repression against nonconformist sexuality. Retief (1993a) notes that "at these moments, repression of nonconformist sexuality has been seen by the state to be necessary in order to keep the white nation morally pure so that it could resist the 'black communist onslaught'" (p. 17). He draws attention to the influence of Christian Nationalist ideology and the role of the Calvinist churches, the military, and the police in the subsequent repression.

An example of the link between military patriotism, religious fundamentalism, and racism is illustrated by the experience of Dr. Ivan Toms, an openly gay anti-apartheid activist who was jailed for 18 months for refusing to complete his compulsory military service. Toms (1994) describes the disinformation and dirty tricks campaign waged against him by covert military intelligence:

> The first volleys in the disinformation campaign against me and the End Conscription Campaign (ECC) were amateurish enough. Yellow posters saying "Ivan Toms is a fairy?," part of a batch of homophobic posters with declarations like "ECC does it from behind" and "The ECC believes in fairy tales." Then the graffiti. "Ivan Toms fucks young boys" in the University of Cape Town subway; "Toms is a moffie pig" spray-painted on my house and car. Other slogans sprayed on the walls in Mowbray and Observatory included "Toms does it rectally," "ECC homo perverts" and rather bluntly, "Hang Toms." ... Along with these were the usual death threats, the advertising of my car for sale at a ridiculously low price, the delivery of a load of pig manure, and black condoms sent with obscene messages that linked anti-gay and anti-black prejudice. (p. 258)

This harassment continued for 5 years between 1983 and 1988. Abel (1995) comments on the strategy employed by prosecutors to discredit and expose flaws in defendants' characters in military resistance cases:

> What prosecutors could not prove they insinuated—political radicalism, communism, ANC sympathies, homosexuality—particularly damning charges in South Africa. The SADF broadcast homophobic slurs against Ivan Toms; the prosecutor reiterated them at

trial; Charles Bester, David Bruce, and the entire [ECC] were taunted as gay; homosexual attacks on Toms and Bester in prison may have been orchestrated.... By publicizing
Toms's gay activism the prosecutor sought to convince the court that he was not an
exemplary Christian. (p. 120)

Invoking public prejudices about the sexual orientation and conduct of political
activists was not confined only to the ECC. The apartheid regime repeatedly exploited the
social opprobrium then still attached to homosexuality to stigmatize political opponents.
This had an effect also on activists' views on homosexuality. Patrick ("Terror") Lekota, a
fellow trialist of Simon Nkoli in the Delmas Treason Trial (Lekota is now speaker in the
National Council of Provinces) accused of holding anti-gay views, explained instead that
during the trial one of the accused was "interacting with criminal prisoners with a view to
this type of liaison.... This was a security matter for us, not just an idle debate. Those of us
returning to jail for the second time knew that security police had used complicity in
[homosexuality], drug abuse and other things to compromise and/or demoralize freedom
fighters" ("Gays not rejected," 1996). Ultimately the oppressive aspects of the state campaign were recognized by many activists. They gave an important impetus to the willingness of the African National Congress (ANC) to embrace protection from discrimination
on the grounds of sexual orientation in the constitution.

Prosecutions for Sodomy

Religious attitudes to contraception have also been blamed as a cause for sodomy,
particularly as practiced by heterosexuals. A medical doctor testified before the 1968
parliamentary committee that heterosexual sodomy used as a contraceptive method "often
seems to confuse their whole sexual approach and they afterwards prefer the rectum to the
vagina for sexual purposes" (Select Committee, 1968, p. 293). Probed further whether
heterosexual men then practice this with other people, Dr. Fourie unhesitatingly confirmed that "yes, they often use anybody's rectum and, of course, can try to purchase the
right from younger people." While similar generalizations have been used to justify
criminalization of same-sex conduct, heterosexual sodomy has long not been a crime.

There is of course a wide difference between legal enactments and legal enforcement.
The conduct of the police in enforcing criminal sanctions is dependent upon (1) the
individual officer's attitudes and interpretations of his or her role; (2) the varying community pressures from time to time for the police to "do something" about the "homosexual
problem"; and (3) the organization of the police department (Helm, 1973). Retief (1993)
points out that concerted attacks against gays and lesbians date from the premiership of
Hendrik Verwoerd, the architect of grand apartheid, in the mid 1960s. The police had
previously dealt with "various forms of homosexuality,... however [homosexuality] was
regarded as isolated" (Select Committee, 1968, p. 11).

Prosecutions and convictions for sodomy reflect key moments of political and moral
crisis. Figure 1 compares the frequency of convictions (between 1921 and 1994) and
prosecutions (between 1963 and 1994) for black and white men as a proportion of the black
and white male population. Although the statistics here require detailed sociological
deliberation, they nonetheless suggest interesting features in the application of the sodomy
laws. It appears that black men were three to four times more likely to be convicted than

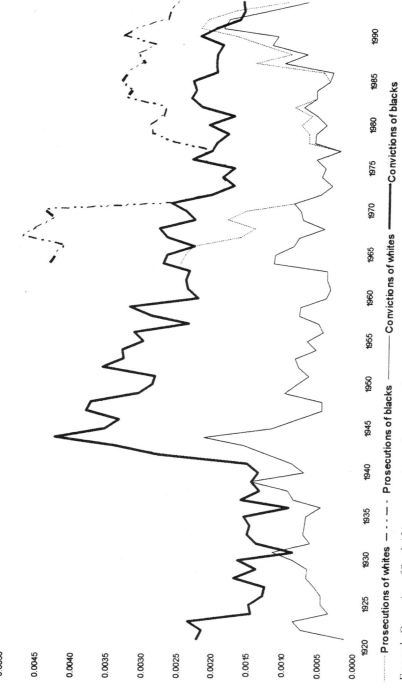

FIGURE 1. Comparison of South African prosecutions and convictions for sodomy indicating distinction between races, 1920–1994. Source: Republic of South Africa (1962–1994); Union of South Africa (1923–1947).

whites. The only periods during which there was a relatively similar correlation between the incidence of conviction is in the years between 1924 and 1940 and in 1990. Following the World War II and the homosexual panic campaigns from 1945 throughout the Verwoerdian period, blacks appear to have been targeted to a much greater degree than whites. During the period of the Forest Town raid in 1966–1970, prosecutions far outweighed convictions. This may suggest a high level of harassment. Finally, between 1975 and 1994 there is a disparity between the number of prosecutions and convictions between black and white men. Black men were nearly ten times more likely to be prosecuted for sodomy, again an indication of possible harassment or prosecutions based on tenuous evidence or spurious complaints.

Prosecutions for sodomy also appear to be enforced selectively between different races (Botha & Cameron, 1994). Table 1 illustrates that, of the 396 prosecutions for sodomy in 1993, 357 were of acts committed between persons classified by the compilers as "non-whites." Of those finally convicted, 88 percent were classified as "non-white." The overall statistics are roughly proportionate to broad demographic distributions. But on closer examination they seem to indicate that selective criteria are employed in launching prosecutions. The statistics for 1993 reveal that the "success rate" for sodomy prosecutions involving a "white" accused is between 74 and 75 percent, while the success rate for "non-white" prosecutions is only 64 percent. A non-white male prosecuted for sodomy is thus less likely to be convicted than a white counterpart. This raises difficult questions about race and class, many of which are beyond the scope of this chapter. Figure 1 and Table 1 may suggest the possibility that sodomy prosecutions involving whites are selected with greater circumspection and therefore achieve a greater success rate. The disparity may also indicate a greater component of harassment experienced by "non-white" men or that the

TABLE 1. South African Sodomy Prosecutions, 1978–1992

Year	Prosecutions	Convictions	Convictions[a]
1978	266	207	106
1979	289	186	108
1980	317	226	108
1981	304	197	101
1982	313	257	157
1983	376	275	148
1984	b	b	b
1985	398	283	173
1986	400	275	145
1987	406	275	184
1988	414	270	169
1989	401	279	164
1990	479	323	186
1991	476	324	194
1992	428	283	195
1993	396	266	145

[a]Convictions involving juveniles under the age of 20 have been excluded.
[b]Statistics not released.

TABLE 2. South African Sodomy Convictions per Province, 1987–1993

Province	1987	1988	1989	1990	1991	1992	1993
Cape							
Urban	140	152	147	144	135	111	137
Rural	42	43	70	91	75	65	31
% of total	66.2	72.2	77.8	72.8	64.8	62.2	66.9
Natal							
Urban	14	15	12	16	22	9	14
Rural	2	1	3	3	1	7	3
% of total	5.8	5.9	5.4	5.9	7.1	5.7	6.4
Transvaal							
Urban	40	27	29	44	58	56	49
Rural	16	7	7	16	15	10	18
% of total	20.4	12.6	12.9	18.6	22.5	23.3	25.2
Orange Free State							
Urban	6	12	8	8	17	23	4
Rural	15	13	3	1	1	2	0
% of total	7.6	9.3	3.9	2.8	5.6	8.8	1.5
Total	275	270	279	323	324	283	266

police or prosecuting authorities rely on more tenuous evidence in these cases. Alternatively, prosecutors in the period in question may have pursued convictions against white accused with more fervor than against black men.

Perhaps the most disturbing inference from the statistics in Table 2 is that enforcement of these laws is dependent on the vicissitudes of local law enforcement agencies. A geographical analysis of the application of the sodomy laws — in 1993 the then Cape Province accounted for 67 percent (1992, 62 percent) of sodomy convictions; Natal, 6 percent (1992, 6 percent); the then Transvaal (with very nearly half of the country's total population), 25 percent (1992, 23 percent); and the Orange Free State, 2 percent (1992, 9 percent) — indicates that government agencies in certain regions are consistently and disproportionately disposed to prosecute such cases.

The conviction "success rate" reflects the same trend: In 1993, 67 percent of the convictions occurred in the Cape Province. Of the 178 convictions in the Cape Province, 29 occurred in the Cape peninsula, 10 in the Eastern Cape, 98 in other urban areas, and 41 in rural areas. The rural incidence in the Cape must be contrasted against other rural areas — Natal (3), Transvaal (16), and the Orange Free State (0).

These convictions are in conflict with the stated policy that attorneys general are reluctant to prosecute in the case of adult, private, consensual activity.[9] Particularly in the lower courts, judicial pronouncements have been made and harsher sentences imposed as

[9]Isaacs & McKendrick (1992) refer to personal correspondence with the Cape attorney general, indicating "that since 1972, no case of sodomy between consenting adults in private has been prosecuted, and that it is not policy to do so" (p. 153). Isaacs & McKendrik also cite research in Cape Town that both the Cape Town Regional Magistrate's Court and the Wynberg District Magistrate's Court apparently have no records of any prosecutions of the conduct of consenting adults in private. The statistics for prosecutions for sodomy [Republic of South Africa (1980–1990)] and the circumstances of the consenting adult conduct reported in S v. H [1993, (2) SACR 545 (C)] bring these contentions into question.

a supposed deterrent to the claim that these offenses have become "more prevalent." Such an approach was criticized by two judges in the Eastern Cape in S v. M (1990). Considering that only 12 cases of sodomy had been recorded in the Eastern Cape in 1989, the appeal judges were correct in asserting that the regional magistrate had misdirected himself by not "stating the source of his knowledge" that "sodomy is on the increase in the Eastern Cape and in particular in the Grahamstown area" (p. 512f). This case clearly illustrates how law enforcement officers use unsubstantiated and subjective claims to bolster the notion of rampant outbreaks of nonconformist sex.

Censorship

In South Africa the notion of public indecency has not been confined to acts alone. Publications or even newspaper reports dealing with obscenity have been held to constitute public indecency (R v. Hardy, 1905). In 1956 the Cronje Commission published a detailed report on "indecent, offensive and harmful literature" (par. 1.4). The report concluded that there should be a prohibition on any material that

> describes, depicts, represents or portrays one or more of the following in an indecent, offensive, or harmful manner: ... sexual intercourse, prostitution, promiscuity, white-slavery, licentiousness, lust, passionate love scenes, homosexuality, sexual assault, rape, sodomy, masochism, sexual bestiality, abortion, change of sex, night life, physical poses, nudity, scantily or inadequately dressed persons, divorce, marital infidelity, adultery, illegitimacy, human or social deviation or degeneracy, or any other similar related phenomenon. [par. 5:93(2)(d)]

The result was the enactment of the Publications and Entertainment Act in 1963. With the addition of sadism, this statute adopted the Cronje Commission (1956) definition of "matter harmful to public morals" (s. 1). This 1963 act was supplemented in 1967 with the Obscene Photographic Matter Act, which prohibited the possession of photographic matter "depicting, displaying, exhibiting, manifesting, portraying or representing sexual intercourse, licentiousness, lust, homosexuality, Lesbianism, masturbation, sexual assault, rape, sodomy, masochism, sadism, sexual bestiality or anything of a like nature" (s. 1). The 1963 act was repealed in 1974 and replaced by the Publications Act, which prohibited the production, importation, and distribution of material deemed "indecent or obscene or harmful to public morals" [s. 47(2)].

A singular feature of these three statutes is their pervasive reach. However, all three have their origins in the period of moralistic conservatism (represented in America by the McCarthy era and in South Africa by Verwoerdian apartheid). In parliament, as statutory apartheid became more rigorously enforced, the minister of justice attributed the 1963 act to the need to prevent moral subversion of "a Christian, civilised country such as the one in which we are living" (Hansard, 1967, p. 2659).

At the height of apartheid control of what citizens were allowed to read, see, or know, the Publications Control Board regularly imposed censorship of literature about homosexuality. Link/Skakel, the precursor of the gay newspaper Exit was frequently banned in 1984 (Davidson & Neiro, 1994). The Publications Control Board justified the banning because the newspaper was "offensive and harmful to public morals" and was "calculated to promote homosexuality which, in the view of South African citizens is an offensive and immoral form of sexual activity" (p. 226). American gay interest publications such as the *Advocate* were banned on the basis that they encouraged the view that homosexuality is an alternative lifestyle. Retief (1993) records the banning of videos promoting safe sex practices, "the most sensible and practical erotic productions, gay news magazines and theoretical writings on sexuality" (p. 21).

In the first case of censorship to come before the new Constitutional Court, the 1967 act was struck down as unconstitutional. One member of the Court, Justice Mokgoro, used an overbreadth argument to overturn the statute, invoking homosexuality sympathetically in a series of examples:

> As the definition stands it could be read to classify a virtually limitless range of expressions, from ubiquitous and mundane manifestations like commercial advertising to the most exalted artistic expressions as *indecent or obscene*, simply because they contain oblique, isolated to arcane references to matters sexual, or deal frankly with a variety of social problems. Thus a television documentary treating safe sex and the causes of AIDS may be construed as a *manifestation of licentiousness*. Cinematic versions of the works of South Africa's most acclaimed playwrights and novelists may be labelled *exhibitions or portrayals of lust, masochism or sadism*. An illustrated public service brochure dealing with the incidents of sexual assault on women could potentially be outlawed as a *depiction of rape*. A photograph of persons of the same gender in tender embrace could fairly be construed as *manifesting homosexuality or lesbianism*. (*Case v. The Minister of Safety and Security*, par. 59)

Regulating Social Spaces

Despite the harsh criminal laws that have existed, urban communities have always attracted, and created a safe space for, gay and lesbian people. Following the diamond and gold rushes of the late nineteenth century, bars and public entertainments attracted a gay clientele. A gay bar existed in Johannesburg on the corner of Commissioner and Troye streets in the early 1900s before roads were tarred. Low-key surveillance and policing of gay venues commenced in the 1940s, and raids of these venues proved a favored method of controlling gay activities in the 1960s through the 1980s. In Johannesburg during the 1940s, a club referred to colloquially as the "Red and Green" flourished in a quaint Victorian building on Noord Street. Patrons would arrive in mixed groups, and, while the red light shone, gay and lesbian couples would dance together and party. Regular police raids were signalled by the advent of a green light, and mixed couples would suddenly emerge on the dance floor. The original venue of the "Red and Green" is now the local community center for the Gay and Lesbian Organisation of the Witwatersrand (GLOW). Retief (1993) describes the actions of the police in raids on gay or lesbian venues:

> Anecdotal accounts of gay life … paint a picture of constant police harassment and surveillance. Police would allegedly raid a bar, grab people who were kissing or dancing together, and bundle them into a police van. [Police] photographers would line people up against the wall and snap pictures of as many faces as possible while police officers took down the [registration] numbers of the cars parked outside. A serious threat was that one's name and picture would appear in the daily newspapers. In the puritanical social climate of the time, exposure as a "homosexual" could have meant total social ostracisation. (p. 20)

However, many of these venues did not attract an exclusively gay clientele. Gays and lesbians were regarded as "bohemian" and were the subject of fascinating intrigue by other patrons (Wasserfall & Anderson, 1996).

The open existence of gay meeting places played a significant role in the opinion of Judge Jansen in S v. M (1990), where he commented, "It is common knowledge that so-called gay clubs are formed, where homosexuals openly meet and have social intercourse. If that is accepted by society, even with reluctance or distaste, it is also a factor to be taken into account by the courts" (p. 5146).

Eliminating Lesbianism by Prohibiting Ownership of Dildos

The use of any inanimate instrument for masturbation was regarded as sodomy by Carpzovius (1752). No prosecutions were recorded in South Africa for using any instrument for "unnatural" purposes. However, in 1968 the issue was raised by the South African police as one of major importance to law and order. Whereas the principal intention of the Parliamentary Select Committee investigation was to stamp out homosexual gatherings, the intention of prohibiting possession of dildos was expressly to stamp out lesbian activity (van Niekerk, 1970).

A police raid on a party in Forest Town in 1966 (see the next section) was against a party of men. There is no record of lesbians attending the party, and the police acknowledged that they had never before received any complaint about lesbian activity (Select Committee, 1968). Nevertheless, the police used the opportunity to introduce to parliamentarians the "disturbing" subject of dildo usage by lesbians. Police testified that lesbians "range in age from 16–45" and obtain sexual gratification "either by way of artificial apparatus or by means of physical contact" (p. 24). Dildos, they noted, were very sought after because of their scarcity and were being smuggled into the country by air stewardesses. As lesbian acts were not an offense under South African law, this focus on lesbian activity was unusual. The Transvaal attorney general, Advocate Rein, gave evidence that he had never prosecuted a woman for lesbianism. But he noted "of course, it goes on, but I think it is done very discreetly. Nor have I ever heard of a woman importuning or soliciting another woman in the street" (p. 331).

The Department of Justice urged it absolutely necessary that a prohibition on ownership of dildos be hastily legislated. During the proceedings a revealing exchange took place between the committee and Mr. van Vuuren:

DR. RADFORD: Do you think that the police brought this [prohibition] in with the idea that there should be a prosecution of lesbianism? — I suppose so, because apparently this particular type of article can only be used by women, and I think that that amounts to lesbianism, does it not?

DR. FISHER: Not really. I would say that the article can be used by a single woman for masturbation? — But it is not intended for that purpose ... As far as I know the main object for which this thing is intended is for lesbianism....

Mr. le Grange (a future Minister of Police) appeared incredulous. He observed that these objects can be easily obtained in hairdressing salons. Mr van Vuuren persisted:

MR. VAN VUUREN: [Translated] This article really is used for lesbianism; it is used by women and young girls are misled into doing the deed.... The entire idea [behind this prohibition] was actually to stop lesbianism (p. 6).

The committee was anxious to test this theory. When the first lesbian (Miss B) testified, she was promptly asked if she knew anything about the use of instruments for lovemaking among women. She denied any knowledge of such instruments. The committee persisted: "Do you achieve an orgasm in this sexual urge that you practice?" (p. 239).

Advocate Rein was concerned about terminology. "In the police memorandum they call it a 'dilder.' I am no expert, but I think it should be called a 'diddler.' I think in English 'to diddle' means 'to mislead'; so it is more apt to call it a diddler than a dilder, but that is just by the way" (p. 331).

The result was the enactment of a provision outlawing the "manufacture, sale or supply of any article which is intended to be used to perform an unnatural sexual act" (Immorality Amendment Act, s. 2).

1968 Inquiry and Further Amendments to the Sexual Offences Act

The 1968 hearings by a parliamentary select committee were the result of a raid in January 1966 on a homosexual party in the affluent Johannesburg suburb of Forest Town. The police reported that a party "the likes of which has seldom been seen in the Republic" was in progress. "[A]pproximately 300 male persons [were] present." All of them were "obviously homosexuals." The main complaint was that "males were dancing with males to the strains of music, kissing and cuddling each other in the most vulgar fashion imaginable,... continuing their love making in the garden and in motor cars in the streets, engaging in the most indecent acts imaginable." The police noted that the events "filled even hardened members of the Criminal Investigation Department with disgust and revulsion" (Select Committee, 1968, p. 11). This description is telling for its portrayal of same-sex activity as worse than any other social evil and of police officers, hardened by exposure to the darker elements of human behavior, as recoiling in horror from what they saw. The police at all events purported to regard this organized manifestation of homosexual activity as "constituting a threat to the moral basis of the populace" (Select Committee, 1968, p. 11). Within 3 weeks of the raid, police wrote to the Minister of Justice complaining that "stringent measures cannot be taken against homosexuals in terms of existing legislation" (Select Committee, 1968, p. 18). A sense of moral mission is usually manifest in police culture (Burke, 1992, p. 33; Swerling, 1978). But the level of panic that followed the Forest Town raid suggests that police officers saw it as morally imperative to curtail the threat to the predominance of white heterosexual males. Underlying their revulsion and disgust was perhaps a threat to their own masculinity and macho image. After all, "the police do have something of a masculinity complex and [homosexual activity] may be the conceptual key that unlocks the door to their personality dynamics" (Adlam, 1981, p. 161). During the course of later police testimony, Major van Zyl was asked how activity that takes place in private could possibly affect police duties. He replied: "the mere fact that people are complaining about something which *we* regard as not being right, as being a deviation from the norm [was a] threat to the maintenance of law and order" (Select Committee, 1968, p. 32).

Further raids took place on private homes in Pretoria and Johannesburg and on gay clubs in Johannesburg and Durban. In all cases the conclusion was the same: "All levels of society practise homosexuality on a scale which was hitherto considered unthinkable." Evidence indicated that "schools, universities, cultural bodies and a host of other fields formerly regarded as pure and unsullied" were being infiltrated and corrupted, particularly to "influence young boys" (Select Committee, 1968, p. 12).

Gay men were of course, regarded as "unapprehended felons" by attributing criminal predispositions to them. But police reports went further to describe an insidious form of conspiracy or deliberate subversion. "Investigations revealed that many business concerns are owned by homosexuals and that preference in regard to employment there is given to homosexuals, other homosexuals make their purchases there at a considerable reduction and they often commit fraud to help each other" (Select Committee, 1968 p. 23). Asked by a member of the committee whether homosexuals could be placed in the same class as people who rob and steal, Major van Zyl explained: "These people will really stop at nothing if their life partner is affected" (p. 44). Furthermore, "it is universally recognised that homosexuals drink excessively" and "become estranged from the church and religion," the police continued. Their "addiction to habit forming drugs" results in them "becoming physically and spiritually weak and consequently causes loss of productivity" (p. 24). As if these findings were not enough to stigmatize homosexuals, they were portrayed as an "unpredictable pestilence." The warning was clear: "as with every virulent infection, it spreads …" (p. 26).

The Christian Nationalist preoccupations of the time were evident. Godless, non-Christian religious sentiment was portrayed as "condoning, enjoying, and even encouraging vice and vileness" (Select Committee, 1968, p. 28).

Racial concerns predictably also emerged in the proceedings. Dr. Radford, a member of the select committee, was concerned that homosexual activity was taking place "across the colour bar." He wanted to know whether the police could deal with this aspect adequately. Surprisingly, the police admitted that they had never conducted a survey along these lines, although some clubs in Johannesburg had patrons who could "definitely be regarded as coloured." The police in Johannesburg were concerned that environmental circumstances exacerbated the incidence of homosexuality, particularly "Bantu compounds [which] are known to be a breeding ground for homosexuality as is life in prisons" (Select Committee, 1968, p. 25). But these concerns did not lead to any recommendation to eliminate the single-sex hostel system.

The committee equally showed no concern for the security and safety of gay men and lesbians. The police led with extensive evidence on the brutal murders of numerous gays and lesbians. They expressed concern that they were vulnerable to extortion and blackmail. However, the members of the committee expressed no concern at this and no recommendation was made to address homophobia (Select Committee, 1968). This is hardly surprising, since the police were themselves using blackmail and entrapment against gays and lesbians.

The Department of Justice and the police saw the elimination of every expression of homosexuality as the only solution. Consideration was given to outlawing homosexuality itself, not just the expression of homosexual conduct.

In addition, an amendment to the Immorality Act was proposed to impose a presumption that any masseur not registered under the Medical, Dental and Pharmacy Act was keeping a brothel.[10] There is little indication of any massage activity taking place during

---

[10]The Department of Justice proposed amending Section 3 of the Immorality Act (1957) with the insertion of a paragraph reading: "(h) any person who for or in expectation of any consideration for himself or herself or

the early 1960s, and the subject was not canvassed during the select committee hearings. Twenty years later, advertisements were appearing openly in the classified sections of newspapers in large cities for "massage" services. There is no record of any prosecution of these informal businesses, although police raids have been reported from time to time.

Men at a Party

The result of the select committee investigation was the introduction into South African law of a unique criminal provision. A male person who commits with another male person at a party *any act* that is calculated to stimulate sexual passion or to give sexual gratification is guilty of an offense. "A party" is defined as "any occasion where more than two persons are present" (Sexual Offences Act, s. 20A, inserted by s. 3 of Act 57 of 1969).

The enforcement of this provision has not been without comedy. Its jurisprudence includes a solemn decision by two judges of the Supreme Court that "a party" did not come about when a police major, visiting a well known gay sauna in Johannesburg for entrapment purposes, barged in on a cubicle where two men were engaging in sexual acts and turned on the light. The court held — in a liberal decision — that the two men's jumping apart when the major switched on the light prevented a three-person "party" from being constituted (*S v. C*, 1987).

Age of Consent: 1968 and 1988

Another object of the select committee's interest, which had no foundation in the facts of the Forest Town party, was the supposed protection of minors against the influence of homosexual men. Before 1968 South African statute law provided for a uniform age of consent at 16 years. While this did not detract from the common law prohibition against *all* sexual contact between men, it did at least mean that homosexuals and heterosexuals were treated alike in statutory prosecutions for underage sex. The stated reason for the 1968 investigation was to contain homosexual parties. But, no doubt predictably, in parliamentary debates "protecting the youth" became the rationale for the legislation. The Minister of Justice stated, "with this amendment homosexuals are being unequivocally informed that rather than relaxing existing measures we are going to take stricter steps for the protection of our youth" (Hansard, 1969, p. 4800).

The committee recommended imposing a differential statutory age of consent for acts between males. Any immoral or indecent act committed by a male with a boy under 19 became a separate statutory offense, subject to imprisonment for a period not exceeding 6 years with or without a fine not exceeding 12,000 Rand in addition to such imprisonment [Sexual Offences Act, ss. 14(1)(b), 22(f)].

In 1985 the President's Council [an apartheid legislative body consisting of whites, "coloureds" (persons of mixed-race descent), and Indians] embarked on an investigation to determine whether the existing laws against homosexuality were sufficient and satisfactory to curb the practice. This paralleled investigations by the council into factors influencing "the youth" detrimentally. Following the report of the President's Council, the Sexual

---

any other person practises massage or physiotherapy and who is not a holder of the registration certificate referred to in section 30 of the Medical, Dental and Pharmacy Act, 1928 (Act 13 of 1928)" shall be deemed to be keeping a brothel.

Offences Act was amended in 1988. Parliament broadened the ambit of statutory underage offenses. It now became an offense for any woman to commit an immoral or indecent act with a girl under 19 [s. 14(3)(b)]. This is the only reference to lesbian conduct in modern South African law.

Other Public Panic Campaigns

Police methods of control have frequently included blackmail and fear. Following the van Dyne scandal in the mid 1940s, which involved an alleged male prostitute ring, gay men generally became the targets of police action in assuaging public panic. Known gay men were rounded up and threatened with public exposure unless they named friends and gay acquaintances. Those who resisted had their names and occupations published in the print media. Criminal prosecutions escalated. This coercive climate generated fear and panic, which abated only after an eminent mayor of Johannesburg and a member of the cabinet were named as homosexual (Wasserfall & Anderson, 1996).

A similar panic was generated in the late days of the apartheid government in 1988. The apartheid government faced mounting domestic resistance and international condemnation over the thousands of children detained under the various states of emergency. The role of the police in enforcing apartheid repression was increasingly attacked. In response, a homosexual "child sex scandal" was created. Groups of men were rounded up and accused of running organized child sex rings. Retief (1993) describes the police action:

> In the three months between June and August 1988, detectives from the Child Protection Unit (CPU) arrested more than sixty adult men and teenage boys in what quickly came to be seen by the media as a "countrywide net against child abuse" and a fight against the "alarming rise in child violations" (*The Star*, 21 Aug 1988). Thick front page headlines in the daily newspapers proclaimed "Child Sex Rife in City" (*Argus*, 18 June 1988) and "Jong Seuns in Seksnet" ["*Young Boys in Sex Net*"] (*Rapport*, 14 July 1988). Media hysteria mounted, fed by police claims that they were uncovering "child sex rings" and that the arrests represented only the "tip of the iceberg" (*Argus*, 16 Aug 1988). Sensational reports of the discovery of more "victims" broke one after the other in waves, confirming the perception that South Africa was facing a surging tide of immorality and perversion. (p. 22)

Media coverage fueled considerable hysteria and panic. Reports failed to reveal that most of the "children" involved were older than 16 and thus, by statutory heterosexual standards, hardly "defenceless."[11] In some cases the relationships had been consenting and nonexploitative. The police action also displayed a selective bias as heterosexual child abuse cases were ignored. The news media indulged in a frenzied stereotype of the teenagers as "victims" and their older partners as "monsters" (Retief, 1993, p. 23). The existence of organized rings was never proved. A senior official of the respected National Institute for Prevention of Crime and Rehabilitation of Offenders (NICRO), Heather Regenass, reflected later on this late-apartheid episode: "I have no doubt that the whole scare was an exaggeration, if not a complete fabrication. At the time the [police's] image

[11]Cf. the finding in S v. R 1993, (1) SACR 209 (A), where it was held that "the victim was not a defenceless child but a boy of 15 for whom masturbation was no shocking revelation." See also S v. E 1992 (2) SACR 625 (A) where it was held that complainants between ages 14 and 17 "were not so young."

had been harmed by revelations of abuses under the emergency regulations. Gay men were easy targets; the police could arrest 'child molesters' and appear the heroes of the community instead of the villains" (Retief, 1993, p. 24).

An Increasing Trend toward Judicial Reform

In judgments in South African courts over the past decade there has been a consistent trend toward reform and tolerance of same-sex conduct. The first relatively reformist trend emerged in the early 1960s with judicial acceptance of a medical model of homosexuality, despite the expression in these early cases of repugnance for same-sex conduct. *Baptie v. The State* (1963), a case involving two consenting adults, is a good instance: "it is now well understood as a result of the recent advances of medical knowledge that offences of this kind, involving perversity, are offences which have a background in the disordered mental condition of the perpetrators and that they can usually be cured by psychiatric treatment" (p. H96).

S v. Matsemela (1988) was the first judicial decision that expressed frank skepticism about the alleged "unnaturalness" of homosexual acts. With characteristic forthrightness, Judge Kriegler condemned the uncritical adoption of medieval prejudices. In *S v. M* (1990) Judges Jansen and Cooper refused to broaden the scope of the crime of sodomy. In wide-ranging comments, they called for judicial notice to be taken of social acceptance of homosexuality. They stated,

> It must be accepted that times have changed.... We cannot close our eyes ... to the fact that society accepts that there are individuals who have homosexual tendencies and who form intimate relationships with those of their own sex. It has to be taken into account that homosexuality is more openly discussed and written about. It is common knowledge that so-called gay clubs are formed, where homosexuals openly meet and have social intercourse. If that is accepted by society, even with reluctance or distaste, it is also a factor to be taken into account by the courts. (p. 514b)

The most uncompromisingly reformist judgment is that by Judges Ackermann and Tebbutt in *S v. H* (1993). The case approvingly refers to recent understanding of homosexuality as a natural variant in sexuality. Although sodomy was then, preconstitutionally, still an offense, the judges held that where committed consensually in private between adults it "can rarely, if ever, justify a custodial sentence" (p. 549). They expressed the view that labelling homosexuality as abnormal in *S v. M* (1990) was unfortunate, "as it might suggest a prejudgment of much current psychological and sociological opinion which is critical of various contentions and assumptions regarding human sexuality" (p. 550).

Discriminatory Family Law

Under South African family law gay and lesbian relationships are not prohibited by statute (Boberg, 1977). The Marriage Act makes no express mention that solemnization can take place only between a man and a woman. However, in *W v. W* (1976) (a case where a transgendered plaintiff sought a divorce) the court refused to recognize the plaintiff's gender change and ruled that at common law persons of the same sex cannot marry each other, and any attempt to conclude such a ceremony would be null and void because marriage is "the union of a man and a woman" (Cronje, 1994, p. 163; *Seedat's Executors v. The Master Natal*, 1917). Before 1984, sodomy was a ground for divorce or separation (*Croft v. Croft*, 1923; *Cunningham v. Cunningham*, 1952; *McGill v. McGill*, 1926).

There have been numerous calls for the law to be altered to allow recognition for permanent gay and lesbian partnerships (Cameron, 1993; Costa, 1994; Mischke, 1995). Costa notes that the Constitutional Court "will require new thinking as it will be a radical break from white colonial Christian teachings and culture which have found their way into our law relating to family and personal relationships.... Why should homosexuals not be permitted to marry each other? It is no answer to say that it is because it is against religious teachings or offensive to some members of society" (p. 916).

The right to custody of biological children has been impeached in at least one decision of the South African courts. In *van Rooyen v. van Rooyen* (1994) a lesbian mother applied for a declaratory order defining her access rights to her two biological children (ages 11 and 9) after a divorce. Custody of the children had been awarded to the father. She was at the time of her application living with her lesbian partner in a stable and loving relationship. The father contested her suitability to have access to the children on the grounds of her lesbianism. Judge Flemming ordered that she could have access to the children every second weekend, provided that the children were not allowed to sleep over if the mother shared the bedroom with her partner. During alternate school holidays with the children her partner would not be allowed to sleep under the same roof. The order required that the mother "take all reasonable steps and do all things necessary in order to prevent the children being exposed to lesbianism or to have access to all videos, photographs, articles and personal clothing, including male clothing, which may connote homosexuality or approval of lesbianism" (p. 332D). The case reflects a reflexive condemnation of homosexuals and has elicited a torrent of unfavorable analysis. A telling example of the court's approach is the fact that the judge seemed to assume, without evidence, that the mother, simply because she was a lesbian, would wear male garments (Bonthuys, 1994): "Nowhere does the court refer to any evidence that the applicant was indeed in the habit of wearing male apparel. Similarly, no facts were stated which justify the fear that the applicant would expose or had in the past exposed the children to homosexual video or photographic material.... [These comments] serve no purpose other than to reflect the ignorance and homophobia of society" (p. 303).

A conspicuous feature of the judgment is the absence of scientific or social authority, or indeed judicial precedent, for its findings and assumptions. "The wrong signals are given when, if it is true, the applicant wears male underclothes, apart from male apparel. The signals come when there are signs of emotional attachment, not only by kissing and hugging as counsel argues, but by the way of speaking, the words of endearment used, the manner in which there is a glance" (*van Rooyen v. van Rooyen*, 1994, p. 330B). This judgment predates the interim constitution and is unlikely to survive the deluge of unfavorable academic attention it has attracted (Bonthuys, 1994; Brits, 1994; de Vos, 1994; Mischke, 1995; Singh, 1995). Singh sums up the response to the sentiments expressed in the judgment:

> Homosexuality in a democratic and open society requires acceptance and understand-
> ing, not judgment, censure and condemnation. Intolerance under the apartheid regime
> had become the cornerstone of the South African ethos. Now, rather than seeking to

perpetuate this evil, our courts should strive to alleviate it. It is incumbent on the legal system to remove barriers to full participation by all people. The legal recognition of homosexual equality in matters of family would, ideally, confirm South Africa's commitment to full and equal justice for all people. (p. 575)

Democracy, Tolerance, Equality, and Opportunity

South Africa's transition to democracy has presented new opportunities for a reevaluation of the law and the role of the state in fostering a system based on equality, individual dignity, and a commitment to human rights. While colonial and modern South African history has been characterized by exclusion and the highlighting of difference, the new constitutional state promises inclusivity and appreciation of diversity. That commitment has extended to the gay and lesbian community (Botha, 1995).

The political impetus for protecting gays and lesbians from discrimination was initiated in the principled stand of the ANC. The policy of the ANC was endorsed by its policy conferences in both 1993 and 1995 (African National Congress, 1995).

By April 1996 every political party — with the exception of the minority African Christian Democratic Party (ACDP) — had stated their support for protecting gays and lesbians from discrimination in the constitution ("Most Parties State Backing," 1996), and the final constitution, adopted in the Constitutional Assembly on May 8, 1996, emphatically embraced protection from discrimination on the ground of sexual orientation.

Rejecting the Myth that Homosexuality Is "UnAfrican"

The interim constitution created, by contract in the negotiation process during 1993, a series of entrenched "constitutional principles" that formed the basis for the final constitutional text. Among these is principle III, which provides that a future constitution must prohibit all forms of discrimination. Early in the constitution-making process ACDP leader Rev. Kenneth Meshoe gave notice that he intended to amend this principle:

> Although ... constitutional principles cannot be amended, the ACDP would like to see an amendment made to the set of 34 Constitutional Principles which the Constitutional Assembly has to abide by during the process of drafting the final constitution of this nation. Principle III of Schedule 4, which refers to all other forms of discrimination, should not include sexual orientation as we have it under chapter 3, section 8(2) of the present Constitution. This section promotes homosexuality, which is against family values, African culture and biblical teachings. (Hansard, 1995, 30–32)

He invoked the traditional biblical arguments together with the controversial averment that homosexuality is "unAfrican."

This claim was first recorded in 1987 when ANC national executive member Ruth Mompati, in an unreflective and unrepresentative outburst, told the British publication *Capital Gay*, "I cannot even understand why people want gay rights. The gays have no problems. They have nice houses and plenty to eat. No-one is persecuting them" (quoted in Gevisser, 1994, p. 70). Gevisser notes her assumption that homosexuality was an essentially white phenomenon, foreign to the experiences and oppression of black people. In 1991 Strini Moodley, a leader of the Azanian Peoples' Organisation (Azapo) stated "at this time

Azapo does not consider homosexuality a priority. It seems to us that this phenomenon is largely affecting the more affluent sections of the community" (Gevisser, 1994, p. 70). In 1992 the secretary general of the Pan-Africanist Congress, Benny Alexander (who later changed his name to Khoisan !X), stated that "homosexuality is unAfrican. It is part of the spin-off of the capitalist system. We should not take the European Leftist position on the matter. It should be looked at in its total perspective from our Afrocentric position" (Gevisser, p. 70). Gevisser describes this position as an attempt to equate homosexuality with the exploitation of black people through the migrant labor and hostel system.

In her trial for kidnapping and assault in 1991, Winnie Mandela relied on a defense that she was in fact "saving" the youngsters kidnapped from the homosexual advances of a white clergyman, Paul Verryn. A banner outside the court proclaimed "Homosex is not in African Culture." Gevisser (1994) makes the point that "according to this particular strain of nationalism, homosexuality has been imported into black communities by inhuman labour systems, perverse priests, and white gay activists looking to expand their constituency and the validity of their cause. This ideology has its roots in the patriarchal notion that colonialism emasculated and feminised the black man" (p. 69).

Picking up on this theme, Kenneth Meshoe invoked a familiar North American cliché in his address to the Constitutional Assembly: "I wish to remind those who have forgotten that in the beginning God created Adam and Eve, and not Adam and Steve. To build a family, Adam needed Eve and not Steve. Even today, Eve needs Adam not Madam, to build a family. Nation-building cannot be possible while we try to legally destroy family values and the moral fibre of our society with clauses in the Constitution that promote a lifestyle that is an embarrassment even to our ancestors." A persistent theme was the notion of uncontaminated and pure roots, ancestral blessing for a heterosexual world view, and the demonization of gays and lesbians by demeaning epithets: "Not a single person in this house, including the one on the floor, is a product of homosexuality, therefore it cannot be right" (Debates of the Constitutional Assembly, 1995, p. 31).

The ACDP had polled only a tiny proportion of the total votes in the 1994 democratic elections, giving it two seats in the 400-seat National Assembly. Meshoe claimed that "statistics have proven that most South Africans are religious people. Their voices must be heard and listened to. On the question of this sexual orientation clause in our interim Constitution, I am speaking on behalf not only of millions of Christians, but also Muslims, Jews, Hindus other religions of significance, and Africans who still believe in moral values. True sons and daughters of the soil who have not forgotten their roots agree with me on this issue" (Debates of the Constitutional Assembly, 1995, p. 31).

This use of the "unAfrican" argument to appeal to patriotism and [black] identity evokes historical ironies. A decade earlier F. W. de Klerk (then Transvaal leader of the National Party and Minister of National Education and subsequently State President) told *Exit* newspaper that political questions about gay identity were "foreign to [white] South African political culture" ("De Klerk," 1987, p. 2). The attempt by the ACDP to "purify" African culture by denying the existence of homosexuality has resonances with the racial and moral purity sought to be attained under apartheid.

A significant feature contributing to the successful fight for the retention of the sexual orientation clause in the final constitution was the open support of influential clergy with a proven history in the struggle for human rights. Mmutlanyane Mogoba, Presiding Bishop of the Methodist Church, in a submission to the Constitutional Assembly (June 8,

1995) stated that "the ACDP does not represent all Christian viewpoints in South Africa and in this matter especially, I must dissociate the Methodist Church of Southern Africa[12] from their stance." Bishop Mogoba praised the principle of inclusivity when he concluded, "I appeal to you to resist any attempt to limit the recognition of the rights of all people, which is the genius of the proposed Constitution, and to retain the 'sexual orientation' clause." Archbishop Desmond Tutu (Constitutional Assembly, 1995) also supported constitutional protection for gays and lesbians. He said, "it is indisputable that people's sexual nature is fundamental to their humanity." In terms going beyond mere nondiscrimination, he challenged the lawmakers to respond to the laws making gays and lesbians social outcasts and criminals in the land of their birth: "It would be a sad day for South Africa if any individual or group of law-abiding citizens in South Africa were to find that the final constitution did not guarantee their fundamental human right to a sexual life, whether heterosexual or homosexual." The Southern African Catholic Bishops Conference, commenting on the draft of the equality clause, which included sexual orientation, noted that "given our history it is important to acknowledge that a large proportion of our population were unfairly discriminated against in the past. Therefore, the inclusion of such people in the equality clause is justifiable" (Constitutional Assembly, 1996).

The South African Police Service (SAPS)

Under apartheid, the police were the state agency most prominently engaged in repressive and discriminatory attitudes toward gay and lesbian people. The role of the police in a democratic system has been a major debate in the transition period. Commendably, there have been indications of an improved attitude recently toward the gay and lesbian community.

In June 1993 the then commissioner of police, General Johann van der Merwe, wrote that the police strongly reject "homosexualism, lesbianism and indecent behaviour, loose living, relationships outside marriage and live-in arrangements."[13] However, a year later, after the first democratic elections, the commissioner of the Johannesburg North District, Brigadier de Vries, by special invitation attended the opening of the gay and lesbian film festival. He later wrote to GLOW that the police were there to serve the entire community, including gays and lesbians.[14]

In 1994 a group of gay and lesbian organizations responded to an invitation by the new minister for safety and security to make submissions on the manner in which human rights issues should be addressed within the police service (Submission, 1994). In 1995 the minister of safety and security endorsed the submission by the gay community, writing to the national commissioner, "I trust that the Secretariat and the Police Service will work together to ensure that these important aspects of human rights and equality are taken up

---

[12]The Methodist Church of Southern Africa reaffirmed its support for the inclusion of sexual orientation in the constitution on February 16, 1996 (Constitutional Assembly, 1996).

[13]The original letter, dated June 16, 1993, under reference 4/8/5/1 (13/93)(k) read, "Die Suid-Afrikaanse Polisie keur egter homoseksualisme, lesbianisme, sowel as onsedelike gedrag, losbandigheid, buite-egtelike verhoudings en saamblyverhoudings ten sterkste af." ["The South African Police absolutely discourage homosexualism, lesbianism as well as immoral behaviour, loose living, extra-marital relationships and live-in relationships outside of marriage."]

[14]Letter dated June 2, 1994, under reference 2/11/3.

wholeheartedly by the Department of Safety and Security."[15] By November 1995 the national commissioner had issued a press statement announcing that the police "would address discrimination on the grounds of sexual orientation."[16] In December the police issued a new policy directive on gay and lesbian police officers, noting that the SAPS recognized the right to equality in any appointment, promotion, or transfer and that the police service "does not equate the ability, competence or potential of an individual in terms of their particular sexual orientation." The policy notes that gay and lesbian persons are afforded equal rights in the SAPS, that "no discrimination in terms of their sexual orientation shall be tolerated," and that no private prejudice would be allowed to compromise the relationship between the police and the gay community. Any discrimination or prejudice would be regarded as "misconduct against duty and discipline" (Police Policy, 1995).

The eradication of prejudice and institutionalized homophobia will undoubtedly take some time. The SAPS has engaged the gay and lesbian community in developing a training course on heterosexism, which will be compulsory for all police officers. Technikon South Africa provides tertiary education for police officers; courses offered on community policing include modules and assignments on provision of policing services to the gay and lesbian community.

In February 1996 police reservists (part-time officers) passing by Pandora's Box, a gay bar in Johannesburg, became engaged in an altercation with patrons. In the course of the exchanges, they hurled homophobic epithets at the crowd gathered outside. The crowd became restless when the police officers arrested the owner and a patron, allegedly for assaulting a police officer and damaging a police vehicle. After members of the crowd pelted the police vehicles with beer cans, the police called in reinforcements. Later it appeared that the reservists had targeted the establishment on spurious charges. The commissioner of police has agreed to establish a police liaison committee with the gay and lesbian community.

The South African National Defence Force

The debate about gays and lesbians serving in the armed forces is necessarily ambivalent, since many groups committed to equality have a tradition of nonmilitarism. In a nonpacifist society, however, including gays and lesbians in military service is an important test of the state's commitment to equality and human rights. In South Africa the debate has taken on an added significance in being one of the first issues to determine the extent of constitutional protection. Abel (1995) notes that it is ironic that "liberal" America continued to exclude gays and lesbians from the military a decade after "conservative" South Africa sought to conscript them. During the apartheid years the military made no distinction between heterosexual and homosexual conscripts. The minority regime required as many individuals as possible to shore up their military and ideological ambitions.

However, gays and lesbians (as elsewhere) served in the military structures on both sides of the armed struggle in South Africa. While the erstwhile South African Defence

---

[15]Letter addressed to the author, November 2, 1995.
[16]Media Statement by the national commissioner of the South African Police Service, Commissioner George Fivaz, Pretoria, November 15, 1995.

Force (SADF) made no exceptions to their conscription policy, Umkhonto weSizwe (the armed wing of the ANC) made conscious overtures, particularly to lesbians, for use in ordinance structures and cadres. The SADF's use of gay men was never openly acknowledged, however, and in 1993 when conscription was abandoned for a volunteer army, press statements made specific mention that gays and lesbians would not be welcome. That policy was bound to come under scrutiny after the interim constitution came into effect in April 1994.

The defense establishment has undergone a dramatic transformation since the advent of a democratically elected government. Defense structures have been subjected to civilian control by the establishment of the office of Defence Secretariat, the arms industry has been the subject of inquiry under the Cameron Commission, and the transformed South African National Defence Force (SANDF) has had to adapt to the integration of the SADF, the liberation armies and those of the previous homelands. The constitutional commitment to nondiscrimination against both women and homosexuals has created new pressures to reappraise past exclusionary policies. Accordingly, the Defence White Paper (Ministry of Defence, 1996) makes specific provision that "the SANDF shall not discriminate against any of its members on the grounds of sexual orientation" (par. 52). The paper provides further that "the Minister of Defence shall appoint a work group to facilitate and monitor the implementation of the policy regarding ... sexual orientation (par. 53).

These two provisions have been championed by the ANC within the parliamentary standing committee on defense. The debate has given a useful insight into the application of the interim constitution's guarantee of equality. The National Party has persistently attempted to open a broad debate along the line that allowing gays and lesbians into the armed services was allowing "sexual deviants in the barracks" that would "lead to indiscipline" and "undermine the military's effectiveness," according to National Party senator Mark Wiley ("Gays and Lesbians OK in Forces," 1995). By contrast, the ANC has been guided by the constitutional imperative of nondiscrimination. ANC parliamentarian Lindiwe Sisulu cast the debate uncompromisingly as a matter of principle when she noted: "It is a matter of principle. ... We are trying to get away from a situation in which we act in accordance with constitutional principles when it suits us, but we throw them away when it doesn't suit us" (*The Citizen*). Sponsor of the white paper proposal, Member of Parliament (MP) Thenjiwe Mtintso, told the parliamentary defense committee that the proposal was necessary because of the military's tendency in the past to overt discrimination against gays and lesbians: "They were referred to as sissies and moffies. While the Constitution does not allow discrimination on the basis of sexual orientation, this must also be articulated in the white paper" (*The Citizen*). Despite the National Party's protestations at the specific mention of sexual orientation ("Gay dienspligtiges nie aanvaarbaar nie–NP," 1996), the SANDF issued a press statement noting "the military respects their constitutional rights to be homosexual or lesbian as long as their activities do not interfere with military discipline, esprit de corps and morale" ("Gays Welcome in Defence Force," 1996).

Broadcasting and Access to Media

Censorship of information, including access to the public airwaves, has characterized South Africa's history. Central to the democratic process is the need to inform others, address prejudice, and enter dialogue (National Coalition for Gay and Lesbian Equality,

1995). The public broadcaster is an essential part of that process, and in 1993 the transitional arrangements leading to the adoption of the interim constitution provided for the establishment of an Independent Broadcasting Authority (IBA). The role of the IBA is to promote the provision of a diverse range of sound and television broadcasting services catering to a diverse range of communities [Independent Broadcasting Authority Act, ss. 2, 2(I)]. The interim constitution further provides that all media financed by or under the control of the state shall be regulated in a manner that ensures impartiality and the expression of a diversity of opinion [Republic of South Africa Constitution Act, 1993, s. 15(2)].

On June 8, 1995, in an address to the National Assembly on his budget vote, Dr. Pallo Jordan, then Minister for Posts, Telecommunications and Broadcasting noted that a public broadcasting service must "avoid characterisation of individuals and groups in its programming by means of unjustified racial, ethnic, gender, sexual orientation or other stereotypes." Since the advent of a democratic government, the public broadcaster has carried an unprecedented number of documentary programs on gay and lesbian issues.

Social Welfare

The South African social welfare system was one of the most discriminatory vehicles of social policy under apartheid. Under a new democratic government, social welfare policy and strategy are undergoing a radical reappraisal. This has positive implications for gays and lesbians. The government white paper specifically stipulates that social welfare services and programs should promote nondiscrimination, tolerance, mutual respect, diversity, and the inclusion of all groups in society. Women, the physically and mentally disabled, offenders, people with HIV/AIDS, the elderly, and people with homosexual or bisexual preferences may not be excluded (Republic of South Africa, 1996). The policy firmly encompasses extended families. These are defined as "individuals who either by contract or agreement choose to live together intimately and functionally as a unit in a social and economic system. The family presents itself in a variety of forms and structures, all of which are acknowledged" (p. ii). The implicit recognition of gay and lesbian families in this definition augurs well for the future development of family law and eventual legislative provisions for gay and lesbian partnerships.

Under even the present statutory regime, an unmarried or divorced person may adopt a child [Child Care Act, s. 17(b)]. A commissioner of child welfare may grant an adoption order if the applicant is possessed of adequate means [s. 18(4)(a)], is of good repute and is a fit and proper person to be entrusted with the custody of the child [s. 18(4)(b)], and if the proposed adoption will serve the interests and be conducive to the welfare of the child [s. 18(4)(c)]. The desirability of same-sex matching is also considered (*McCall v. McCall*, 1994). A difficulty for gay and lesbian couples is that the act makes provision only for an unmarried person to adopt a child. No provision is made for two unmarried persons jointly to adopt a child. Accordingly, the partner who is not granted custodial rights enjoys no security.

The first officially sanctioned lesbian adoption took place in August 1995, following the coming into force of the interim constitution, with the approval and support of the Johannesburg Child Welfare agency and the local child commissioner. Previously, gay couples had been allowed to foster only in limited circumstances. Despite the nondiscriminatory provisions of the Child Care Act, an administrative ban was enforced by the child welfare agencies who performed the initial screening of prospective adoptive parents.

Availability, sound health, energy, and commitment to care for the child are employed as screening criteria. Marionka Manias, a spokesperson for Johannesburg Child Welfare, stated in an interview with the *Mail & Guardian*: "We go along with the policy that anyone can apply to adopt a child…. We make sure that applicants really want children because they cannot conceive, and don't simply want children because they want to look like everybody else" ("Lesbian Couple," 1995). She further noted that a motivating factor for this official policy was the chronic oversupply of babies, many of whom are difficult to place because of birth defects or because they were born to parents with HIV. "Ideally we would want to place babies with families broadly representative of society. Gay men might find it harder to adopt a child than lesbian women. A man might not find it as easy to cope with a newborn child as a woman," she stated.

The first official adoption by a male gay couple has raised a more prejudiced view by the child commissioner. The couple from Pretoria, a traditionally conservative area, applied to adopt a baby boy who soon after birth tested positive to antibodies for HIV. The initial application for fostering rights was granted, and Child Commissioner Bischoff told the press, "I have nothing against them being homosexual and, according to the new constitution, we cannot be prejudiced, but I do not believe a homosexual couple provides the ideal environment for a child to grow up in." However, he found that there "were unfortunately no alternatives" and granted the fostering order. He observed that as the gay couple had a full-time nurse and the child was not going to live long anyhow, they should be allowed to take him. However, on application for the final adoption the child (as frequently happens with babies born to mothers with HIV) had tested negative for HIV. The couple was now told that they would not make suitable parents ("Gays May Lose," 1995). The decision was challenged, and in September 1996 the adoption was granted after the child commissioner had been replaced.

Decriminalization

The Department of Health's National AIDS Plan calls specifically for the decriminalization of all laws prohibiting sexual acts between males and for the enactment of equal ages of consent. The South African Law Commission, in a recent working paper on AIDS, was more conservative, claiming that "the existing criminalisation is not aimed at the prevention of HIV infection, but at the punishment of socially unacceptable behaviour" (South African Law Commission, 1996, p. 79). Rather than assist in combatting HIV infection by repealing discriminatory legislation, they recommended "a comprehensive, constructive and specific education programme to abandon high risk behaviour" (p. 81).

Numerous calls for the decriminalization of same-sex conduct have followed the adoption of the constitution (Gregan, 1994; Snyman, 1995; Submission, 1994; *S v. H*, 1993). Snyman has noted that the punishment of homosexual acts between consenting adults, including sodomy,[17] would seem to be incompatible with the interim constitution.

In 1994 a prisoner accused of sodomy approached the Supreme Court in Cape Town for a declaration that the offense of sodomy was inconsistent with the provisions of the interim constitution (*S v. Adendolf*, 1995). The ill-considered application was rejected by the court on the grounds that there was no consent between the parties. However, the

[17]In the Draft Criminal Code, which Snyman proposes, sodomy is defined in the following way: "(1) A male person commits sodomy if he unlawfully and intentionally is an active or passive party to anal intercourse with another male person, in circumstances in which the latter has not consented to the act. (2) The offence is complete upon penetration, whether or not there is an emission of seed" [Snyman (1995), p. 31].

judges did imply that had the case involved two consenting adults, the court would have entertained the argument. However, they were not inclined to do so in a purely theoretical and academic exercise without any factual basis.

That archaic provisions of the common law and statutory prohibitions against same-sex conduct dating from the apartheid era should still exist in South African law is a patent anachronism. This is an area that is likely to attract judicial or parliamentary scrutiny in the foreseeable future.

Education

The National Education Policy Act mandates the minister of national education to direct policy to protect every person against unfair discrimination on any ground whatsoever within or by an education department or education institution [s. 4(a)(i)]. The Gauteng Education Bill provides that admission requirements for public schools shall not unfairly discriminate on grounds of race, ethnic or social origin, color, sexual orientation, religion, conscience, belief, culture, and language [s. 9(2)]. The bill further makes provision for a number of directive principles and school education policies to be determined by the member of the executive council of the province responsible for education. These include provisions that no learner or educator shall be unfairly discriminated against by the department, a state-aided school, or a private school receiving a subsidy from the state [s. 4(c)]. There is a specific duty to foster the advancement of persons, groups, or categories of persons previously disadvantaged by unfair discrimination [s. 4(d)] and a duty to combat sexual harassment at schools and centers of learning [s. 4(e)]. The education process is mandated to promote a culture of tolerance [s. 4(f)] and the fostering of independent critical thought [s. 4(m)]. A court interpreting any provision of the bill may refer to these guiding principles in determining any dispute.

Access to Resources

A primary area of state control is the lack of adequate funding for gay and lesbian issues. Before 1994 no state funding for gay and lesbian infrastructure had been recorded. In 1994 the Transvaal Organisation for Gay Sport (TOGS) acquired a concessionary lease from the Johannesburg Metropolitan Council for a sports facility in Brixton. In 1995 a request for funding by the Gay and Lesbian Organisation of Pretoria (GLO-P) to fund a counseling service was rejected by the Pretoria Metropolitan Council. GLO-P appealed. In April 1996 the minister of arts and culture, Ben Ngubane, reported in the National Assembly that whereas 2.7 million Rand had been spent on minority Afrikaans cultural infrastructure such as the Voortrekker Museum and the War Museum of the Boer Republic, only a paltry 15,000 Rand had been spent on the 1995 Gay and Lesbian Film Festival ("Gay culture loses to 'Voortrekker' funding," 1996).

CONCLUSION

The period since 1991, when the first draft constitution of the ANC expressly disavowed discrimination on the ground of sexual orientation, has been exhilarating for gays and lesbians and those committed to equality for them. South Africans have since then, first in the interim constitution (1994–1996) and now, in the final constitution (1996), become the world's first nation whose constitution expressly proscribes anti-gay discrimination. This is no doubt the product of our peculiar history, where institutionalized discrimination against people on the ground of race was perfected through the legal system. The racial legacy has given the majority of South Africans a repugnance for the use of legal processes for irrational discrimination. Gays and lesbians have been among the direct beneficiaries. For all South Africans, however, the problem now is to reconcile constitutional promise with daily practice. For most, historical disparities are still reflected in desperately unequal living conditions, employment, and access to public services. For all, the promise of equality before the law and of protection from unfair discrimination must now be realized through legislative programs and in substantive changes in social conditions and attitudes. South Africa's gays and lesbians are no longer separate from, but are an integral part of, both the promise and the effort to put equality into practice.

CITED STATUTES

Child Care Act 74 (1983).
Criminal Amendment Act 16, Transvaal (1908).
Criminal Ordinance of Emperor Charles V (1544).
Criminal Procedure Act 51 (1977).
Gauteng Education Bill 1587-95 (1995).
Immorality Amendment Act 57 (1969).
Independent Broadcasting Authority Act 153 (1993).
Interception and Monitoring Prohibition Act 127 (1992).
Marriage Act 25 (1961).
Natal Criminal Act 22 (1898).
National Education Policy Act 27 (1996).
Obscene Photographic Matter Act 37 (1967).
Placaat of the States of Holland, 21 July (1730); Placaets of Holland, Vol. 6, folio 604.
Publications Act 42 (1974).
Publications and Entertainment Act 26 (1963).
Republic of South Africa Constitution Act 200 (1993).
Security Officers Act 92 (1987).
Sexual Offences Act 23 (1957).
Transkei Penal Code, Act 24 (1886).
Transvaal Immorality Ordinance 46 (1903).
Union of South Africa Act, 9 Edw VII c9 (1909).

CITED CASES

Baptie v The State, (1) PH H 96 (N) (1963).
Case and Another v The Minister of Safety and Security, judgment of the Constitutional Court (May 9, 1996).
Croft v Croft, PH B 34 (1923).
Cunningham v Cunningham, (1) SA 167 (1952).

McCall v McCall, (3) SA 201 (C) (1994).
McGill v McGill, NPD 398 (1926).
R v C, (2) SA 51 (1954).
R v C, (2) PH H 351 (C) (1959).
R v Curtis, CPD 386 (1926).
R v Gough & Narroway, CPD 159 (1926).
R v H, (1) SA 278 (SR) (1962).
R v Hardy, NLR 165 (1905).
R v K & F, EDL 71 (1932).
R v M, (2) PH H 338 (C) (1958).
R v M, (1) SA 328 (R) (1969).
R v Mateba, (2) PH H 130 (GW) (1950).
R v N, (3) SA 147 (T) (1961).
R v S, (2) SA 350 (SR) (1950).
R v S, (1) SA 649 (T) (1956).
R v Serei & Another, (1) PH H 15 (O) (1951).
R v Taleke, 5 EDC 180 (1886).
R v Taylor, CPD 16 (1927).
R v V, (3) SA 314 (AD) (1953).
R v Baxter & Another, AD430 (1928).
S v C, (2) SA 76 (W) (1987).
S v C, (2) SA 398 (ZHC) (1988).
S v E, (2) SACR 625 (A) (1992).
S v H, (2) SACR 545 (C) (1993).
S v K, (1) SA 87 (RAD) (1973).
S v M, (2) SA 357 (Tk) (1977).
S v M, (2) SA 167 (T) (1979a).
S v M, (2) SA 406 (RAD) (1979b).
S v M, (2) SACR 509 (E) (1990).
S v Matsemela & Another, (2) SA 254 (T) (1988).
S v R, (1) SACR 495 (ZH) (1992).
S v R, (1) SACR 209 (A) (1993).
S v S, (4) SA 405 (N) (1965).
S v V, (2) SA 17 (E) (1967).
Seedat's Executors v The Master Natal, AD 302 (1917).
State v Adendolf, unreported decision of the Cape Provincial Division of the Supreme Court, Case 170/94 (June 9, 1995).
van Rooyen v van Rooyen, (2) SA 325 (W) (1994).
W v W, (2) SA 308 (W) (1976).

References

Abel, R. L. (1995). *Politics by other means: Law in the struggle against apartheid, 1980–1994.* London: Routledge.
Adlam, R. C. A. (1981). The police personality. In D. W. Pope & N. L. Weiner (Eds.), *Modern policing* (p. 159). London: Croom Helm.

African National Congress. (1995). *Building a united nation: Policy proposals for the final constitution.* Cape Town, South Africa: Author.

Bleys, R. C. (1996). *The geography of perversion: Male-to-male sexual behaviour outside the West and the ethnographic imagination 1750–1918.* London: Cassell.

Boberg, P. Q. R. (1977). *The law of persons and the family.* Cape Town, South Africa: Juta.

Bonthuys, E. (1994). Awarding access and custody to homosexual parents of minor children: A discussion of van Rooyen v van Rooyen. *Stellenbosch Law Review, 3,* 298.

Boswell, J. (1980). *Christianity, social tolerance and homosexuality. Gay people in Western Europe from the beginning of the Christian era to the fourteenth century.* Chicago: University of Chicago Press.

Botha, K. (1995, October). *South Africa's chapter of fundamental rights: Establishing the foundation for an inclusive conception of nationhood.* Paper presented at the Southern African Colloquium on Gay and Lesbian Studies, University of Cape Town, South Africa.

Botha, K., & Cameron E. (1995). Sexual orientation. In R. Louw (Ed.), *South African human rights yearbook,* 1994 (5) (pp. 281–293). Durban, South Africa: Centre for Socio-Legal Studies.

Brits, J. J. (1994). *Toegang tot kinders, lesbianisme en die konstitusie.* (57) THRHR 710. Durban, South Africa: Butterworths.

Bunting, B. (1986). *The rise of the South African reich.* Shadowdean, London: International Defence and Aid Fund for Southern Africa.

Burchell, E. M., & Hunt, P. M. A. (1983). *South African Criminal Law and Procedure* (Vol. I) Cape Town, South Africa: Juta.

Burke, M. (1992). Cop culture and homosexuality. *Police Journal, 45,* 30.

Cameron, E., & Botha, K. (1993). Sexual privacy and the law. In N. B. Boister (Ed.), *South African Human Rights Yearbook, 1993 (4)* (pp. 219–227). Durban, South Africa: Centre for Socio-Legal Studies.

Cameron, E. (1993). Sexual orientation and the constitution: A test case for human rights. *South African Law Journal, 110,* 450–472.

Carpzovius, B. (1752). *Verhandeling der Lijfstraffelijke Misdaaden en haare berechtinge naar't voorschrift des gemeen rechts, getrokken uyt de schriften van den heer.* Rotterdam, The Netherlands: Hogewndorp.

Constitutional Assembly, Constitutional Committee. (1996). *Public Submissions, 19(1),* 72.

Constitutional Assembly, Theme Committee 4 (Fundamental Rights). (1995). *Public Submissions, Vol. 56(2616).*

Costa, A. (1994, December). Polygamy, other personal relationships and the Constitution. *De Rebus,* 914.

Council Debates. (1908). *Debates of the Legislative Council of the Transvaal,* Second Session of the First Parliament. Pretoria, South Africa: Transvaal Republic.

Court of Justice. (1652–1827). *Record and minutes of proceedings of the Court of Justice.* Cape Town, South Africa: State Archives.

Cronje, D. S. P. (Ed.). (1994). *The South African law of persons and family law* (3rd ed.). Durban, South Africa: Butterworths.

Cronje Commission. (1956). *Report of the Commission of Enquiry in regard to undesirable publications.* Pretoria, South Africa: Government Printer.

Damhouder, J. (1656). *Practijcke van Civil en Criminele Saecken.* Rotterdam, The Netherlands.

Davidson, G., & Neiro, R. (1994). Exit: Gay publishing in South Africa. In M. Gevisser & E. Cameron (Eds.), *Defiant Desire* (pp. 225–231). Johannesburg, South Africa: Raven Press.

De Klerk: Vrae Vreemd aan Kultuur. (1987; June/July). *Exit,* p. 2.

de Vos, P. (1994). The right of a lesbian mother to have access to her children: Some constitutional issues. *South African Law Journal, 12,* 687.

Debates of the House of Assembly. (1967). Republic of South Africa. Cape Town, South Africa: Creda.

Debates of the House of Assembly. (1969). Republic of South Africa. Cape Town, South Africa: Creda.

Debates of the Constitutional Assembly. (1995). Republic of South Africa. Cape Town, South Africa: Creda.

De Wet, J., & Swanepoel, H. L. (1975). *Die Suid-Afrikaanse Strafreg,* 3rd ed. Durban, South Africa: Butterworths.

Debates of the Legislative Assembly of the Transvaal, second session of the First Parliament, 7 August 1908 (1908). Pretoria, South Africa: Transvaal Republic.

Dynes, W. R. (Ed.). (1989). *An encyclopaedia of homosexuality.* New York: Garland.

Gardiner, F. G., & Lansdown, C. W. H. (1926). *South African criminal law and procedure* (Vol. 2). 2nd Ed. Cape Town, South Africa: Juta.

Gay culture loses to "Voortrekker" funding. (1996, April 10). *Business Day,* p. 1.

Gay dienspligtiges nie aanvaarbaar nie–NP. (1996, February 11) *Beeld* (Johannesburg), p. 7.

Gays and lesbians OK in forces — ANC. (1995, November 29). *The Citizen* (Johannesburg), p. 12.

Gays may lose baby boy — now that he's not dying. (1995, August 6). *Sunday Independent*, p. 6.

Gays not rejected. (1996, February). *Sunday Independent* (Johannesburg), p. 8.

Gays welcome in defence forces. (1996, February 9) *The Star* (Johannesburg), p. 5.

Gevisser, M. (1994). A different fight for freedom: A history of South African lesbian and gay organisation from the 1950's to 1990's. In M. Gevisser & E. Cameron (Eds.), *Defiant desire* (pp. 14–88). Johannesburg, South Africa: Raven Press.

Gevisser, M., & Cameron, E. (Eds.). (1994). *Defiant desire: Gay and lesbian lives in South Africa*. Johannesburg, South Africa: Raven Press.

Gregan, S. H. (1994). Enkele opmerkings oor die invloed van die Grondwet van die Republiek van Suid Afrika, 200 van 1993 op gemeenregtelike misdrywe in die strafreg. *Journal of Applied Law*, 50.

Groenewegen Van der Made, S. (1669). *Tractatus de legibus abrogatis et Institutatis in Hollandia Vicinisque Regionibus* (3rd ed.).

Helm, B. (1973). *Deviant or variant? Some sociological perspectives on homosexuality and its subculture* (Papers from the first Congress of ASSA). Durban, South Africa: Association of Sociologists of South Africa.

Hosten, W. J., Edwards, A. B., Nathan, C., & Bosman, F. (1983). *Introduction to South African law and legal theory* (2nd ed.). Durban, South Africa: Butterworths.

Hunt, P. M. A. (1982). *South African criminal law and procedure, vol. II: Common law crimes* (2nd ed.). Cape Town, South Africa: Juta.

Huussen, A. H. (1989). Sodomy in the Dutch Republic during the eighteenth century. In M. B. Duberman, M. Vicinus, & G. Chauncey (Eds.), *Hidden from history: Reclaiming the gay and lesbian past* (pp. 141–149). London: Penguin.

Isaacs, G., & McKendrik, B. (1992). *Male homosexuality in South Africa, identity formation, culture and crisis*. Oxford: Oxford University Press.

Joubert, W. A. (1981). *The law of South Africa* (Vol. 6). Durban, South Africa: Butterworths.

Justinian. *Institutions in the Corpus Juris Civilis*. Byzantine, 533 A.D.

Kersteman, F. L. (1768). *Hollandsen rechtsgeleert Woordenboek*. Amsterdam, The Netherlands.

Lesbian couple gets first official adoption. (1995, August 11–17). *Mail & Guardian*, p. 6.

Matthaeus, A. (1661). *De Criminibus ad lib XLVII et XLVIII Digestum Commentarius, adjecta est brevis, jurs municipalis interpretatio* (2nd ed.). *On Crimes, A commentary on books 47 and 48 of the Digest*. Amsterdam.

McLean, H., & Ngcobo, L. (1993). Abangibhamayo bathi ngimnandi (Those who fuck me say I'm tasty): Gay sexuality in reef townships. In M. Gevisser & E. Cameron (Eds.), *Defiant desire* (p. 158–185). Johannesburg, South Africa: Raven Press.

Menochius, J. (1583). *De Arbitrariis questionibus et causis libri duo*. Lyon, France.

Ministry of Defence, Republic of South Africa. (1996). *Defence in a democracy*. Self-published.

Mischke, C. (1995). Big law — little wrong: Discrimination on the basis of sexual orientation and the new South African constitutional order. *Codicillus*, 36(1), 33.

Mogoba, M. S. (1995). Letter to the Constitutional Assembly in support of sexual orientation, Theme Committee 4, *Constitutional Submissions*, 1995, 8 June.

Moodie, T. D. (1994). *Going for gold: Men, mines and migration*. Johannesburg, South Africa: Witwatersrand University Press.

Most parties state backing for gay rights. (1996, April 15). *The Star* (Johannesburg).

National Coalition for Gay and Lesbian Equality. (1995). *Submission to the Independent Broadcasting Authority inquiry into the viability and protection of public service broadcasting*, April 11, 1995 (unpublished).

Police Policy. (1995, September). *Gay and lesbian persons in the South African Police Service* (Principle of Policy, Change Management). Pretoria, South Africa: South African Police Service.

President's Council. (1985). *Report of the Ad hoc Committee of the President's Council on the Immorality Act* (PC 1-1985).

Republic of South Africa, Bureau of Statistics. (1962). *Special Report No. 272 on the statistics of offences and of penal institutions 1949–1962* (Report No. 272, No. 08-01-00). Author.

Republic of South Africa, Bureau of Statistics. (1964). *Report on the statistics of offences and of penal institutions 1963/64* (Report No. 08-01-01). Author.

Republic of South Africa, Bureau of Statistics. (1966). *Report on the statistics of offences and of penal institutions 1965/66* (Report No. 08-01-02). Author.

Republic of South Africa, Bureau of Statistics. (1967). *Report on the statistics of offences and of penal institutions 1966/67* (Report No. 08-01-03). Author.

Republic of South Africa, Bureau of Statistics. (1968). *Report on the statistics of offences and of penal institutions 1967/68* (Report No. 08-01-04). Author.

Republic of South Africa, Bureau of Statistics. (1969). *Report on the statistics of offences and of penal institutions 1968/69* (Report No. 08-01-05). Author.

Republic of South Africa, Bureau of Statistics. (1970). *Report on the statistics of offences and of penal institutions 1969/70* (Report No. 08-01-06). Author.

Republic of South Africa, Bureau of Statistics. (1979). *Report on the statistics of offences and of penal institutions 1968–1979* (Report No. 08-01-10). Author.

Republic of South Africa, Bureau of Statistics. (1980). *Report on the statistics of offences and of penal institutions 1979/80* (Report No. 08-01-11). Author.

Republic of South Africa, Bureau of Statistics. (1981). *Report on the statistics of offences and of penal institutions 1980/81* (Report No. 08-01-12). Author.

Republic of South Africa, Bureau of Statistics. (1982). *Report on the statistics of offences and of penal institutions 1981/82* (Report No. 08-01-13). Author.

Republic of South Africa, Bureau of Statistics. (1983). *Report on the statistics of offences and of penal institutions 1982/83* (Report No. 08-01-14). Author.

Republic of South Africa, Bureau of Statistics. (1985). *Report on the statistics of offences and of penal institutions 1984/85* (Report No. 08-01-16). Author.

Republic of South Africa, Bureau of Statistics. (1987). *Report on the statistics of offences and of penal institutions 1986/87* (Report No. 00-11-01). Author.

Republic of South Africa, Bureau of Statistics. (1988). *Report on the statistics of offences and of penal institutions 1987/88* (Report No. 00-11-01). Author.

Republic of South Africa, Bureau of Statistics. (1989). *Report on the statistics of offences and of penal institutions 1988/89* (Report No. 00-11-01). Author.

Republic of South Africa, Bureau of Statistics. (1990). *Report on the statistics of offences and of penal institutions 1989/90* (Report No. 00-11-01). Author.

Republic of South Africa, Bureau of Statistics. (1991). *Report on the statistics of offences and of penal institutions 1990/91* (Report No. 00-11-01). Author.

Republic of South Africa, Bureau of Statistics. (1992). *Report on the statistics of offences and of penal institutions 1991/92* (Report No. 00-11-01). Author.

Republic of South Africa, Bureau of Statistics. (1993). *Report on the statistics of offences and of penal institutions 1992/93* (Report No. 00-11-01). Author.

Republic of South Africa, Bureau of Statistics. (1994). *Report on the statistics of offences and of penal institutions 1993/94* (Report No. 00-11-01). Author.

Republic of South Africa. (1996). *White paper on social welfare policy and strategy for South Africa*. Pretoria, South Africa: Ministry of Social Welfare and Population Development.

Quistorp, J. C., von. (1970). *Grundzatze des teutschen*. Peinlichen Rechts (2 volumes).

Retief, G. (1993). *"Policing the perverts": An exploratory investigation of the nature and social impact of police action towards gay and bisexual men in South Africa*. Unpublished research report, Institute of Criminology, University of Cape Town, Cape Town, South Africa.

Select Committee, Republic of South Africa. (1968). *Report of the Parliamentary Select Committee into the Immorality Amendment Act* (Report 7-1968).

Singh, D. (1995). Discrimination against lesbians in family law. *South African Journal on Human Rights, 11*, 571–581.

Snyman, C. R. (1992). *Strafreg* (3rd ed.). Durban, South Africa: Butterworths.

Snyman, C. R. (1995). *A draft criminal code for South Africa*. Durban, South Africa: Butterworths.

South African Law Commission. (1996). *Aspects of the law relating to AIDS* (Working paper 58, project 85). Pretoria.

Submission to the National Minister of Safety and Security on behalf of gay and lesbian community organisations. (1994). *The role of the South African Police Service in furthering a national human rights ethos, addressing issues relevant to gay and lesbian police officers and the gay and lesbian community and dealing effectively with anti-gay hate crimes*. Johannesburg, South Africa: September 1994.

Swerling, J. B. A. (1978). *A study of police officers' values and the attitudes towards homosexual officers*. Doctoral dissertation, California School of Professional Psychology, Los Angeles, California.

Taberer, H. M. (1902–1934). *Archives of the Government Native Labour Bureau*, 229, 583/15/145, 16/2/16.

Theale, G. M. (1887). *History of the boers in South Africa, or The wanderings and wars of the emigrant farmers from their leaving the Cape Colony to the acknowledgement of their independence by Great Britain*. London.

Theale, G. M. (1905). Report of the Commissioners of Enquiry to Earl Bathurst upon criminal law and jurisprudence. In *Records of the Cape Colony from August to October 1827*, copied for the Cape Government from the manuscript documents in the public record office (Vol. XXXIII). London.

Toms, I. (1994). Ivan Toms is a fairy? The Defence Force, the End Conscription Campaign and me. In M. Gevisser & E. Cameron (Eds.), *Defiant desire* (pp. 258–263). Johannesburg, South Africa: Raven Press.

Transkei Report. (1883). *Cape of Good Hope, Report and proceedings with appendices of the government commission on Native Laws and Customs* (G4-1883).

Tutu, D. M. (1995). Letter to the Constitutional Assembly, June 2, 1995. Constitutional Assembly, Cape Town, South Africa.

Union of South Africa. (1923). *Statistics of crime, 1923* (Report No. 10). Author.

Union of South Africa, Office of Census and Statistics. (1927). *Report on the statistics of crime for the year 1927* (Report No. 4). Author.

Union of South Africa, Office of Census and Statistics. (1928). *Report on the statistics of crime for the year 1928* (Report No. 5). Author.

Union of South Africa, Office of Census and Statistics. (1929). *Report on the statistics of crime for the year 1929* (Report No. 6). Author.

Union of South Africa, Office of Census and Statistics. (1930). *Report on the statistics of crime for the year 1930* (Report No. 7). Author.

Union of South Africa, Office of Census and Statistics. (1931). *Report on the statistics of crime for the year 1931* (Report No. 8). Author.

Union of South Africa, Office of Census and Statistics. (1932). *Report on the statistics of crime for the year 1932* (Report No. 9). Author.

Union of South Africa, Office of Census and Statistics. (1933). *Report on the statistics of crime for the year 1933* (Report No. 10). Author.

Union of South Africa, Office of Census and Statistics. (1934). *Report on the statistics of crime for the year 1934* (Report No. 11). Author.

Union of South Africa, Office of Census and Statistics. (1935). *Report on the statistics of crime for the year 1935* (Report No. 12). Author.

Union of South Africa, Office of Census and Statistics. (1937). *Report on the statistics of crime for the year 1936–1937* (Report No. 13). Author.

Union of South Africa, Office of Census and Statistics. (1938). *Report on the statistics of crime for the year 1938* (Report No. 14). Author.

Union of South Africa, Office of Census and Statistics. (1940). *Special report on the statistics of crime for the year 1940 (abridged)* (Report No. 148). Author.

Union of South Africa, Office of Census and Statistics. (1947). *Special report no. 178 on the statistics of criminal and other offences and of penal institutions for the year ending 1947* (Report No. 178). Author.

van der Keesel, D. G. (1809). *Praelectiones in libros XLVII et XLVIII Digestorum*. Cape Town, South Africa: Juta.

van der Linden, J. (1806). *Regtgeleerd, practicaal, en Koopmans Handboek*. Amsterdam, The Netherlands.

van Leeuwen, S. (1662). *Censura Forensis theoretico-practica, id est totius Juris Civilis Romani usuque recepti et practici methodica collatio*. Leyden, The Netherlands.

van Niekerk, B. (1970). The "Third Sex" act. *South Africa Law Journal*, 87, p. 87.

Wasserfall, J., & Anderson, D. (1996). Interviews with the author, 2 February 1996. Cape Town, South Africa, 1996.

2

ZIMBABWE

OLIVER PHILLIPS

"VENUS MONSTROSA" AND "UNNATURAL OFFENCES"

> I find it extremely outrageous and repugnant to my human conscience that such immoral and repulsive organisations, like those of homosexuals who offend against the law of nature and the morals and religious beliefs espoused by our society, should have any advocates in our midst and elsewhere in the world.... I don't believe [homosexuals] have any rights at all. (President Robert Mugabe, opening the Zimbabwe International Bookfair on Human Rights and Justice, August 1, 1995)

> I would like to ask Mr. Chihuri the head of the police that police should be on the look-out and look for homosexuals and lesbians. They should take them and put them some-where they can never be seen because we cannot mix with such people. They will tarnish our image. We should look for ways of keeping these people separate from those who are normal. (Border Gezi, Member of Parliament (MP), during Zimbabwe Parliamentary Debate on "Homosexualism (sic) and Lesbianism," September 6, 1995)

The year 1995 was one of unprecedented political significance for homosexuality in Zimbabwe. This hitherto taboo subject was persistently raised by the president himself. Never before had such a sizable local gay and lesbian organization emerged that was prepared, not only to parry his attack, but to deliver a reposte as well. Demonstrations protesting his stance took place outside Zimbabwean embassies around the world and wherever else the president chose to travel.[1] Never before had Zimbabwean newspapers been obliged to typeset the word "homosexual" so many times. Never before had homosexuality merited a parliamentary debate in Zimbabwe. The focus of debate was not on the finer points of same-sex marriage or an equal age of consent, but on how to protect "the moral fibre of the nation," how to "chop off the festering finger,"[2] in the light of the seemingly preposterous claims that a homosexual orientation is a human right.

---

[1]Among others, protests occurred outside the Zimbabwean embassies in Washington, D.C. (August 17, 1995), and London (August 18, 1995), as well as upon the arrival of President Mugabe at Jan Smuts Airport in Johannesburg, South Africa (August 26, 1995); there were also two demonstrations (November 10 and 13, 1995) at the Commonwealth Heads of Government Meeting, which President Mugabe attended, in Auckland, New Zealand, as well as a demonstration on his visit to Maastricht for the World Bank-sponsored Global Coalition on Africa meeting (also in November 1995).

[2]"When your finger starts festering and becomes a danger to the body you cut it off. The purpose for cutting it off is to preserve the body. When your whole leg starts festering and refuses to be cured and you come to the conclusion that you cannot cure it, you cut it off in order to preserve the rest of the body.... The homosexuals are the festering finger endangering the body and we chop them off. The homosexuals are like a leg bitten by the black mamba or a viper and what the President is doing is to apply a tourniquet to reduce the danger from the invasion of the rest of the body by the poison from the black mamba, the black mamba being these vipers,

---

OLIVER PHILLIPS • Institute of Criminology, University of Cambridge, Cambridge CB3 9DT, England, United Kingdom.

Sociolegal Control of Homosexuality, edited by West and Green, Plenum Press, New York, 1997.

The history and mechanics of the laws around sodomy and "unnatural offences" provide a necessary backdrop for the current social context and inform the prevailing discourse in a number of ways. The very definition of what constitutes "homosexuality" is influenced by the perpetuation of a fundamental distinction between acts falling within or without the boundaries of "nature" — a division that has its roots in concepts of nature dating from an age and a place distant to Zimbabwe, that of Roman law. The 1979 Zimbabwe constitution provides that the common law is that in force in the colony of the Cape of Good Hope on July 10, 1891, as amended by subsequent legislation having effect in Zimbabwe.[3] Thus, the common law is Roman-Dutch law, obliging judges to follow the rules of precedent, referring frequently to South African cases, and binding lower courts to the decisions of the high courts and ultimately the Supreme Court.

> The Roman-Dutch writers lumped all unnatural offences together under the title *"sodomie," "onkuisheid tegen die natuur,"* or *"venus monstrosa."* Sodomy and bestiality as they are today understood were not separate crimes; they were simply means of conducting *venus monstrosa.* Broadly speaking, the crime was constituted by the "gratification of sexual lust in a manner contrary to the order of nature." But the writers, many of whom concern themselves more with punishment than the niceties of definition, are not always *ad idem* as to just what conduct falls within the description. (Hunt, 1982, p. 267)

It is clear that Zimbabwean law recognizes three classes of "unnatural offences":[4] sodomy, bestiality,[5] and what can be described as "a residual group of proscribed 'unnatural' sexual acts referred to generally as 'an unnatural offence'" (Hunt, 1982, p. 270). Any two men (both active and passive parties) who consent to engage in anally penetrative sex (sodomy) are guilty of an unlawful act.[6] The offenses of sodomy and bestiality carry specific requirements leading to precise definitions, but what is striking about the "residual group" is the very imprecision of their definition. For example, Hunt suggests that an "unnatural offence" is defined as "the unlawful and intentional commission of an unnatural sexual act by one person with another person or animal" (1982, p. 276). Such a tautologous definition implies that the limits of "natural" sex are defined by imagination alone,[7] and in this case it will be shown that the imagination of the Zimbabwean courts has been lamentably constrained. In effect, this vagueness enables any sexual act between men that falls short of the requirements for sodomy to be defined as an "unnatural offence."

It is clear that activities that constitute an "unnatural offence" when committed by a male with another male do not constitute an "unnatural offence" when committed by a

---

the homosexuals" (Anias Chigwedere, MP, Zimbabwe parliamentary debate on "Homosexualism and Lesbianism," September 28, 1995).

[3]Predominantly southern Rhodesian, federal, Rhodesian, Zimbabwe-Rhodesian, and Zimbabwean legislation.

[4]See S *v. C* (1976).

[5]The concern in this publication is to focus on homosexuality and the law; as such, attention will only be paid to bestiality where incidentally relevant.

[6]See Feltoe (1980). The only recognized defense for someone charged with sodomy is to show that he has been coerced into submission — the crime of rape requires penile–vaginal penetration [*King Kingsley Otis Ndebele* (1989); see also Feltoe (1980) and Hunt (1982) — so coercive anal penetration is classified as sodomy or indecent assault rather than rape.

[7]In Roman-Dutch times, sex between Jews and Christians and even self-masturbation were considered to be "unnatural acts" (Hunt, 1982).

heterosexual couple. The crime of heterosexual sodomy was said to be abrogated by disuse in 1968, a decision confirmed as settled law in 1979.[8] Oral, anal, masturbatory, or inter-femoral sex between a man and a woman is not considered to be an "unnatural offence" (Hunt, 1982, p. 277), but any such activity between men is considered to be such.[9] By neglecting to deliver a precise definition for this "residual category," the courts can use the rule of precedent to include any act previously mentioned in court as an offense, without being obliged to exclude any possibilities through defining the limits of an "unnatural act."

In *S v. Meager* (1977) the accused was convicted of seven separate charges of committing an "unnatural offence," and a brief glance at some of these charges indicates the importance of detailing each specific act in order to make clear their proscription. He was charged:

> Firstly,… with the crime of committing an unnatural offence, in that … being a male person, [he] did wrongfully, unlawfully and against the order of nature, *stroke the private parts of B … did suck his penis and go through the act of intercourse between his thighs*.
>
> Secondly, committing an unnatural offence, in that … the accused did wrongfully, unlawfully and against the order of nature, *masturbate the penis of C.*…
>
> Fifthly, committing an unnatural offence, in that … the accused, being a male person, did wrongfully, unlawfully and against the order of nature, *stroke the private parts of B aforesaid, over his trousers*, thereafter telling him to take off his clothes and did then *masturbate him, sucking his penis, and went through the motions of intercourse between his thighs, ejaculating between his legs*. (S v. Meager, 1977, p. 328, pars. C–H, emphasis mine)

The charges meticulously listed all the possible contraventions of "nature" to establish clearly the offensiveness of each particular action. From this case, oral and interfemoral sex, as well as mutual masturbation and any stroking of another man's penis (whether naked or clothed), can be construed as unnatural and unlawful. By leaving the definition of an "unnatural offence" so open, the court was able to use it as a kind of blank check to be filled in with the confessions of the parties involved in the offense. Their evidence lends an enveloping power to the legal scrutiny, enabling it to shift its focus and cover any new forms of activity that male sexual partners may think to explore. In this way, it is the imaginations of the offenders, rather than the judiciary or legislature, that map out the routes through which the courts traverse old conceptual boundaries and circumscribe new terrain.

S v. Meager (1977) illustrates this clearly. The appellant, "a married man aged 37 years" (p. 329, par. C), had been sentenced in the magistrates court to 2 years imprisonment with labor for committing these offenses with three "European male juveniles" (B., L., and C.) who were 15 or 16 at the time. All three consented to the act, and the court itself seemed ignorant as to "how the allegations came to light" (p. 330, par. F). It is not clear how the three juveniles became active "complainants," as at no stage did they "complain" about the appellant, but rather they openly expressed "love and affection" (p. 331, par. A) for him. While this may seem to mitigate the offense, the court, in confirming the sentence, took the opposite view in using this bond of affection to lend probative force to testimony that was otherwise problematically vague as to the precise times, dates, and locations of events:

---

[8] *R v. Masuku* (1968), S v. *Macheka* (1979); see also R v. *K & F* (1932) for a full consideration of the Roman-Dutch authorities.

[9] *S v. Meager* (1977).

> All three of the complainants were obviously most reluctant to be involved in the case, and there can be no suggestion that they were eager to give evidence against the appellant. L, in particular, was most anxious to exculpate the appellant, so that particular importance can be attached to his evidence where he inculpates the appellant.…
>
> It is clear that all the complainants were ashamed of what happened and that they were most embarrassed at having to testify and describe in court the depraved conduct in which they had become involved. (p. 331, pars. B–D)

It seems most probable that the shame of the "complainants" was not because of the sex per se, but was rather a reflection of their embarrassment at having to give a detailed confession to the court of their private sexual activities, particularly when this was done in the knowledge that they were likely to be branded as "depraved." The giving of testimony became a means of censure in itself. Those who testified, while not officially on trial, were made acutely aware at an intensely personal level that their behavior was "offensive" and "unnatural."

The law itself is thus only one technique used in the censuring of homosexuality. The mechanics of investigation, the extraction of confessions, the established rituals and due process of the trial — all provide immense opportunity for a greater diversity of targets and the simultaneous strengthening of effective censure.[10] The case of S v. Meager (1977) illustrates how the openness of the definition of an "unnatural act" not only allows the court to judge the "nature" of specific acts as they come to the attention of the court, but also facilitates the divulgence and exposure of intimate sexual details, thereby interweaving the process of categorization in law with a more direct form of censure within the mechanics of the trial itself.

There is no record of any case, in either South Africa or Zimbabwe, where two women have been prosecuted for committing an "unnatural offence." Both Hunt (1982) and Feltoe (1980) suggest that lesbian activity is probably not punishable, but leave the question fairly open. In view of the ruling that the "unnatural offence" of heterosexual anal penetration had been "abrogated by disuse" (R v. Masuku, 1968; S v. Macheka, 1979), it is submitted that sexual relations between women would also no longer be considered an "unnatural offence" and that it would be extremely difficult to bring a successful prosecution where there was no evidence of coercion, public indecency, or some other extraneous factor around which a charge could be based.

When these definitions are considered in conjunction with the fact that sexual activity with an animal that falls short of the legal requirements for bestiality (i.e., that of penetration) also falls into this "residual group of 'unnatural offences,' " a clearer pattern begins to emerge. This is that while an "unnatural offence" can be committed between a human and an animal, between two men, or just possibly between two women, it can never be committed between a man and a woman. This pattern is further elucidated by the fact that no other sexual offense that contains a heterosexual element is considered to be "unnatural": rape, indecent assault,[11] and incest are not considered to be outside the boundaries of

---

[10]The notion of censure used here is based on the theoretical development of a sociology of censure put forth by Sumner (1990).

[11]While consent is generally a valid defense to a charge of indecent assault, where the charge involves unlawful activity, such as sex between men, it has in the past been held that the defense of consent should be very restrictively viewed (S v. D, 1963); however, the more recent case of S v. Simon (1987) upheld a defense of consent to a charge of indecent assault, acquitting the accused in a case where he could have been successfully

nature. Thus, no heterosexual act is considered to be "unnatural," and any sexual act that is between two people of the same sex may be labelled as such.

The law is therefore operating within the narrow confines of a paradigm of heterosexuality not just as normative, but as exclusively "natural." Homosexuality is not defined through overt reference to either morality, or religion, or culture, but is rejected through the absolutist imputation that it lies outside the boundaries of "nature." While Hunt (1982) correctly recognizes that the definition of "unnatural" involves a value judgment, what demands further comment is the irony of attempting to disguise a value-laden judgment through resorting to the supposed value-free concept of "nature." The very fact that the courts are required to determine whether an act is "natural" or "unnatural" demonstrates that the concept of "nature" used is not one that arises out of an automatic and hylic unfolding of some biological or essential reality. Rather, the necessity for the court to delve into an analysis of intellectual and legal history in order to decide what constitutes "unnatural" sexual behavior shows that it is in fact very deliberately constituted discursively through social and intellectual construction. And while this particular concept of "unnatural" desire is, in this case, derived from Roman law (*contra naturam*),[12] contemporary courts are deeply implicated in this process of continually reconstructing their discursive ambit.

This classification of all sexual acts between males as "unnatural" regardless of consent has the further consequence of equating injurious sexual assaults with consensual sexual relations. Thus, an adult male who forcibly sodomizes a male child is charged with exactly the same offense as two adult men who engage consensually in an act of love that involves anal penetration. In each instance, the charge would be having "unlawfully and intentionally and against the order of nature had sexual intercourse *per anum* with another male" (*S v. Magwenzi*, 1994; *S v. Stanford*, 1992). This failure to discriminate between two very different situations has serious repercussions both practically and discursively. It necessarily carries the implication that male adult abusers of young boys, men who forcibly rape other men, and male homosexuals are all qualitatively the same — an assumption that runs counter to available evidence.[13] This approach focuses on the *a priori* "unnaturalness" of male–male sex, while the relationships of power and age existing between the two people involved are only taken into account as an aggravating or mitigating factor in sentencing (*S v. K*, 1972). It therefore suggests that where an assault (possibly violent) has taken place, it is of secondary importance to the fact that an "unnatural act" has occurred. This significantly undermines the existence of a victim in one case and the nonexistence of a victim in another. Issues of the possibility and intention of causing injury, or of the abuse of power and lack of consent, are far more material factors in the crime than whether

---

convicted of an "unnatural offence" (had such a charge been brought), as this pays no heed to the issue of consent.

[12]"The *lex Julia de alteriis* imposed the death penalty for unnatural practices between males, which were in addition expressly proscribed by Justinian in his novels" (Hunt, 1982, p. 267).

[13]There is a plethora of evidence to support this, but among others see D. J. West, *Homosexuality Reexamined* (1977, pp. 212–217) and *Homosexuality* (1967, pp. 118–119); "Comment, private consensual homosexual behavior: The crime and its enforcement," *Yale Law Journal*, vol. 70 (1961, pp. 623, 629); Institute for Sex Research, *Sex Offenders* (1965, p. 639); and M. Schofield, *Sociological Aspects of Homosexuality* (1965, pp. 147–155). Full citations of these are provided in Rivera (1991). The evidence suggests that most adults who abuse children tend to lead heterosexual lives, regardless of the biological sex of the children they abuse (see Schofield, 1965, and Institute for Sex Research, 1965; both in Rivera, 1991).

the survivor of the assault is male or female, yet they are dealt with simply as circumstances that might aggravate the main charge of same-sex activity.

It is in fact completely unnecessary to prosecute violent assaults or abusive relationships between males as "unnatural offences," as they could be dealt with under alternative charges.[14] The tendency of the prosecution and the courts to do so suggests that they do not fully appreciate the material distinction between sexual acts that are illegal because of their deviance and acts of abuse or assault that are injurious and produce traumatized victims. This seems to lead to considerable confusion in the lower courts, manifesting itself in two significant problems. First, the lower courts appear to be handing down far lighter sentences for the rape of young boys than those given for the rape of young girls, an apparent consequence of the fact that the former are charged as "unnatural offences," while the latter are charged as rape.[15] Second, the strong condemnatory language used by the higher courts in sentencing perpetrators of abuse and assault is translated into a similarly strong condemnation of consensual sexual acts between men in the handing down of sentences in the lower courts.[16] Analysis of high court decisions made on review or appeal show that the lower courts are regularly found to have punished consenting homosexual acts excessively and to have punished acts of abuse and assault between males leniently. But never have they been found to be too lenient on consenting adult partners (*Derks & Anor*, 1984; *Le Roux*, 1981; *R v. B*, 1969; *S v. C*, 1976; *S v. K*, 1972; *S v. Magwenzi*, 1994; *S v. Meager*, 1977; *S v. Roffey*, 1991; *S v. Stanford*, 1992). Such consistent harshness appears to derive from the lack of clarity in seeing that the really serious aspects of an "unnatural offence" are the aggravating factors rather than the offense itself.

The only way to prevent further miscarriages of justice regarding both consensual sexual acts and nonconsensual acts of abuse between males is to treat homosexual rape as the same as heterosexual rape, to charge an indecent assault as an indecent assault, to use the Criminal Law Amendment Act to protect both underage males and females from abuse (as is provided for), and to remove the muddling concept of an "unnatural act" from Zimbabwean law, thereby relying on present laws based around the notion of consent and the protection of bodily security. Such a transformation would require the support of the Supreme Court and Parliament, neither of which is likely to be forthcoming in view of a reluctance among the most senior members of the judiciary to countenance such a move[17] and recent government statements around the issue.

The Supreme Court will be obliged to at least discuss this possibility in the light of cases sure to arise in South Africa under the new constitution, which prohibits discrimination on the grounds of sexual orientation. While this constitutional provision is specific to South Africa, the fact that Zimbabwean courts make reference to South African precedent

[14]Either as indecent assault or, where applicable, under Section 12 of the Criminal Law Amendment Act (Chapter 58); see further the *obiter dictum* in *S v. Simon* (1987, p. 56, par. B).

[15]See *S v. Magwenzi* (1994), *S v. Beli Enock Dube* (1987); see also cases reported in "'Prophet' jailed for sodomy," *The Herald* (Harare, Zimbabwe), April 7, 1995; and the editorial, "Comment—Unacceptable sentence," ibid, p. 8.

[16]In *S v. Roffey* (1991), which concerned two consenting adults in a private home, the magistrate commented that "such unscrupulous acts do in my view stink in the nostrils of justice" (@50b) and handed down a sentence of 10 months imprisonment with labor, which on appeal was reduced to a small fine. Similarly, see *Derks and Anor* (1984).

[17]According to interviews with numerous judges of the High and Supreme Courts of Zimbabwe between January 22, 1993, and January 25, 1993.

will enable a defendant to ask the court to consider relevant South African cases that should soon find that sexual acts between men are no longer a crime.[18] But the Zimbabwean Supreme Court is in no way bound to follow this lead. Thus, while the most recent cases dealt with by the high courts in Zimbabwe suggest that consensual sexual behavior between adult men should no longer be punished with a custodial sentence (*Derks & Anor*, 1984; *S v. Roffey*, 1991), because of the tendency of magistrates' courts to punish such acts more severely, as was discussed earlier, those men whose sentences do not get reviewed or go on appeal are likely to continue serving harsh custodial sentences handed down by magistrates.

A RACIAL DIMENSION

The vast majority of the cases of "unnatural offences" that have gone on appeal or review to the high court or Supreme Court and are thus recorded in the law reports involve the participation of a white man.[19] In view of the fact that the white population of Zimbabwe amounts to less than 1 percent of the total population and that the same records for other sexual offenses show no such racial concentration, this is remarkable. A more detailed analysis of how this situation arises is given elsewhere (Phillips, 1997), but it is necessary to give a brief summary of some of the reasons here.

Economically, the white population in Zimbabwe is disproportionately powerful; this has two important consequences. First, the prosecution of a consensual act depends either on the testimony of a third party (a rare occurrence) or on the confession of one of the parties involved. Thus, the majority of cases that come before the courts tend to be the result of a dispute over payment or a refusal to succumb to blackmail.[20] Because of their economic power, white men are considerably more vulnerable to extortion than black men, with the result that they find themselves prosecuted more often for what were consensual acts. Second, they can more easily afford legal representation and so are more likely to appeal against a conviction or sentence, thus taking the case into the higher courts, the findings of which are recorded in the law reports. Further, a number of factors relating to social and kinship structures (including the overwhelming importance of marriage in Shona and Ndebele families) mean that in the past, white homosexual men have been

---

[18]At the time of this writing, the most recent South African case was that of *S v. H* (1993), in which the Cape Provincial Division, after a careful review of authorities in South Africa and elsewhere, held that a custodial sentence was not an appropriate sentence for consensual, adult private sodomy taking place under circumstances that pose no threat to any legitimate societal interest, the accused was discharged with a caution. The new constitutional "equality clause" should mean that a court will now find that sex between consenting men is no longer a crime.

[19]Cases dealt with in the magistrates' courts, and the archived proceedings of such cases, are not readily accessible to the public and are not reported in published law journals. They are, however, often commented on in the crime columns of local newspapers [e.g., in *The Herald* (Harare, Zimbabwe)].

[20]Interview with Director of Public Prosecutions Mr. Yunnus Omerjee, January 26, 1993; further, at the time of this writing (May 1996), the legal representative of Gays and Lesbians of Zimbabwe (GALZ) reported that during the first 5 months of 1996, he had been approached for assistance on five occasions by people threatened with blackmail because of homosexual activity. This only accounts for those people who have the confidence to approach GALZ; the most vulnerable to blackmail will be those who are not "out" and who are unlikely to approach GALZ—suggesting that most of the people being blackmailed are unable to effectively defend themselves.

more visible than their black Zimbabwean counterparts [see Phillips (1997) for more detail]. In addition to this, prior to Independence, where sex took place between two men of different races, the courts took a more serious view of the offense, ostensibly because of the fact that socioeconomic differences interfered with the possibilities of consent being freely given (see R v. B, 1969; S v. C, 1976; S v. K, 1972).

> The end result of this disparity in convictions is that it contributes to a discourse of discrimination which produces homosexuality as "a white man's disease." There is no doubt that some black Zimbabwean men do have sex with each other, and as with anyone else, this is carried out with varying degrees of furtiveness and openness by men occupying a wide variety of social positions. Yet the cases which go through the higher courts are predominantly those which involve the participation of a white man. This means that the cases passing before the senior judiciary, receiving publicity in the media, being recorded in public law reports, coming to the attention of government, and featuring in the market-place discussions of an insatiably curious populace are those which involve the participation of a white man. Public discussion of homosexuality becomes fueled with racial epithets and the primary definition of the issue includes the presence of a white man. (Phillips, 1997)

Hence, one can explain the claims by President Mugabe and other members of government that homosexuality is a white man's proclivity and is contrary to traditional culture.[21]

By claiming that homosexual activity was unimagined in Zimbabwe before the arrival of white settlers, Mugabe is suggesting that his ancestors were somehow deprived of an inventive capacity enjoyed by the rest of the continent. Professor Chavanduka [previously Chairman of the Zimbabwe Natural and Traditional Healers Association (ZINATHA)] stated in interview that traditionally homosexuality was thought to be normal in the lead up to and during puberty and that thereafter it was frowned upon.[22] Further, its existence across Africa is demonstrated by the fact that the Mandari (Buxton, 1973) and the Mbundu (Rachewiltz, 1964) severely punished homosexuality, whereas it was common practice for, among others, the Azande (whose warriors would have boy-wives) (Evans-Pritchard, 1970) and the Dahomey, Ila, Lango, Nama, Siwa, Thongo, and Wolof (Rachewiltz, 1964). Indeed, the Ekkpahians, the Abuan, and the western Ikwerri lavished great resources on constructing extravagant buildings specifically for homosexual sex, as it was considered to increase human and crop fertility by magical means (Talbot, 1967). Clearly, attitudes toward homosexuality varied according to social context, but to suggest that it did not exist is misleading.

Further, missionaries and other colonial agents of the "civilizing mission" successfully eliminated many practices from Shona and Ndebele circumcision and excision ceremonies because of their view that these practices were "lascivious," "indecent," and "obscene."[23] This not only suggests possible allusion to homoeroticism in traditional ceremo-

---

[21]Homosexuality "is mainly done by whites and is alien to the Zimbabwean society in general" (President Mugabe, quoted in GALZ 11, January 1994, p. 13).

[22]From a January 28, 1993, interview; Elizabeth Colson noted a similar attitude among the Tonga, neighbors to the Shona and populous in Zimbabwe, suggesting that this approach possibly has local resonance (see Colson, 1958).

[23]For example, see Bullock (1950) on the Ndebele ceremony of dunduzela and Gelfand's (1967) vague references to the "modified" nature of Mahungwe in Shona culture, where he is solicitous in his care to reassure us that this is a morally sanitized "training for marriage" (p. 63).

nies, but is also indicative of the extent to which settlers were effective in the reconstitution of "tradition." The pervasiveness of the notion of sin, the commercialization of both sex and the body in general, as well as later reproductive technologies of medical science, have all significantly altered constructions of sexual traditions. But to accuse the white settlers of unshackling "licentious" sexual practices is overly generous, as they are actually far more likely to be responsible for the introduction of a repressive concept of sexuality based on the binary division of heterosexual/homosexual in line with their concomitant Cartesian scissions of mind/body, culture/nature, civilisation/savagery, and discipline/lasciviousness.

The compulsory nature of heterosexual marriage in Shona and Ndebele societies would make it very unlikely that homosexuality was institutionalized to the point of veneration as in some other regions. Shona and Ndebele marriages were traditionally polygamous and based around reproduction and the creation of kinship links and social alliances rather than a notion of "romantic love."[24] Thus, while extramarital sex was not and is not presently condoned, it was not and is not uncommon. This suggests that any homosexual sex between adults that did occur in precolonial times would occur in a furtive manner, as it would necessarily be extramarital. The only difference in contemporary Zimbabwe is that while there are still many married men engaging furtively in homosexual sex, there are now also men and women resisting marriage on the openly avowed grounds of their sexuality.

OFFICIAL DISAPPROVAL

It is the open acceptance of an identity ("the homosexual/gay man/lesbian") with the late-twentieth-century implications of lifestyle, civil rights, and equality that is the source of political consternation in Zimbabwe, as frightened homophobes confuse a social identity that might not have a "traditional" precedent with an activity that certainly has. The common law on "unnatural offences" explicitly operates at the level of activity: "The offence in this case is not having a desire to commit an unnatural offence; men are not punished for their desires and their thoughts. The offence is yielding to that desire and giving way to it," (Beadle, C. J., in S v. K, 1972, p. 82, par. F).

But the law is not so innocent in this process as that statement would have us believe. Through its definition of the boundaries of "natural" sex and its perpetuation of a confusion between consensual homosexual sex and injurious sexual assault, the law serves not only to punish acts of sex between men, but also to facilitate a discourse of exclusion. "Men" are punished for their desires and their thoughts: The association Gays and Lesbians of Zimbabwe (GALZ) is refused access to public (even commercial) media, so it is unable to carry out educational work and advertise counseling services; nonerotic publications are continually confiscated by the authorities; and besides all the many other state interventions into "men's" desires and thoughts, the punishment of the fear that accompanies the realization that one is either gay or lesbian can sometimes be so great as to lead to death.[25]

While members of the Zimbabwean government have made statements derogating

[24]Romantic love was appeased through the not uncommon practice of elopement (kutiza/kutiziswa mukumbo) (see Bullock, 1950; Gelfand, 1975; Schmidt, 1990).

[25]Studies of suicide and attempted suicide show a strong link with the externally induced stress involved in the realization of a suicide's homosexuality (see Gonsiorek, 1991), though as of yet no such studies have been carried out in Zimbabwe.

the rights of same-sex lovers in the past, this has never been done so repeatedly, definitively, and publicly, as has happened since their attempts in August 1995 to exclude GALZ from the Zimbabwe International Book Fair (ZIBF), the theme of which was *Human Rights and Justice* (see Dunton & Palmberg, 1996). In both 1995 and again in 1996, Bornwell Chakaodza — the Director of Information in the Ministry of Home Affairs — attempted to expel GALZ from the bookfair. In 1995 this was done with the connivance of the ZIBF committee, and then in 1996, once the ZIBF committee had realized that their international credibility was more important than local government whim, through what the Supreme Court rejected as an "inappropriate" use of the Board of Censors. The effect of these repeated attacks has been to besmirch the government's international reputation with an open insistence on what became viewed as a fanatical bigotry, to draw attention to previously unnoticed infringements of human rights, and to make visible the insecurities of a government unable to conceive of relinquishing power but simultaneously unsure of its ability to sustain a democratic basis for that power.

At a local level, attacks by senior politicians set the terms of reference for public discussions of homosexuality, and the terms bandied about in parliamentary debate are shockingly abusive and far removed from a real engagement with the issues. Thus:

> [Homosexuality is] unnatural and there is no question ever of allowing these people to behave worse than dogs and pigs.... What we are being persuaded to accept is sub-animal behavior and we will never ever allow it here. If you see people in your areas parading themselves as Lesbians and Gays, arrest them and hand them over to the police. (President Mugabe to ZANU-PF Women's League, August 11, 1995)

The language of the president, Robert Mugabe, is restrained in comparison to that of his parliamentarians. Their position not only served to encourage homophobia but also actively paved the way for further violent assaults and blackmail. By suggesting that it is the duty of upstanding citizens to arrest anyone they suspect of being homosexual, he not only inspires people to take the law into their own hands, but also indirectly condones physical attacks on lesbians and gay men. This increases the vulnerability of homosexuals to the capricious opportunism of blackmailers not only by giving strength of purpose to what may have been simply a thought gestating in the mind of a blackmailer, but also by adding to the climate of fear in which isolated homosexuals live. In other words, the position of the government not only involves the denial of the right to be homosexual, but also implicitly promotes the right to attack homosexuals:

> Our Youth League must lead by example so that we can eradicate all the evil vices like homosexualism [sic] and lesbianism. We must remain steadfast and united as a people.... I challenge all those misguided foreign demonstrators to go and demonstrate in support of homosexualism and lesbianism kwaGutu, Muzarabani kanu kuTsholotsho [in Gutu, Muzarabani, and Tsholotsho — all small rural towns], and see whether they will come back alive. I can assure you they will be beaten and driven out of Zimbabwe by our heroic people. (MP Mudariki, adjourned debate on motion: "on the evil and iniquitous practice of Homosexualism and Lesbianism," Parliament, Harare, November 30, 1995)

Mr. Mudariki appears ignorant to the fact that there are Zimbabweans living in each of the towns mentioned who identify as gay and are members of GALZ. Indeed, through their homophobic invective at the time of the bookfair, the government managed inadvertently to increase considerably the size and strength of GALZ. While previously GALZ had found it difficult to negotiate many of the social, economic, and racial barriers that exist so endemically in Zimbabwe, homosexual men and women in Zimbabwe now found themselves asserting a common identity regardless of their backgrounds. Black men and women who identified themselves as gay or lesbian "came out" to insist that they did exist, making themselves publicly visible on an unprecedented scale. Many Zimbabwean same-sex lovers and transgendered people who had previously not heard of GALZ or had not considered membership now contacted and joined the organization. Members who had previously resisted using GALZ for anything other than social purposes now became politically motivated, leading to its rapid transformation into a much more politically directed organization. GALZ received a large number of new offers of support and alliance from many different nongovernmental and international organizations. In short, the remarks made by members of government merely emphasized the need for the organization of GALZ to exist, strengthened its ideological basis, and increased both the numbers and solidarity of its membership and supporters.

A POLITICAL DIMENSION

Without denying the genuineness of the homophobia displayed by members of government in public and parliamentary debate,[26] it is important to recognize that these attacks on same-sex lovers have been carried out in such a way as to assert a neotraditional rallying point around which to build a conservative and xenophobic national identity—a process similar to that used in attacks on other marginal groups (including students, squatters, and single women). For example, at Independence in 1980, the new government arrived in office with an open and official commitment to the emancipation and empowerment of women. The role of women in the liberation forces was recognized as a vital contribution to victory, and the promotion of sexual equality was seen as their due. Thus, in 1981 the government established a Ministry for Women's Affairs (now the Ministry of Constitutional Development and Women's Affairs) and in 1982 passed the Legal Age of Majority Act (LAMA).[27] The resistance of men (particularly the chiefs and elder men) to any such emancipation of women was vociferous and resentful and caused the government to backtrack on proposed changes to a dowry system (*lobola/roora*) that they had previously recognized as commodifying women through a financial transaction between men (Seidman, 1984). Instead, men's control over women was defended as "part of the national heritage" that should resist "western feminism,… a new form of cultural imperialism" (Seidman, 1984, p. 432). To this day, notions of "tradition" are regularly used as a means of controlling the behavior of women, censuring their independence (particularly sexual independence) and attempting to oblige them to seek the protection of a man.

In this case, members of government were able simultaneously to give vent to their

---

[26]MP Norbert Makoni has called for the whipping of gays and lesbians, and many MPs called for the "eradication" or "separation" of "evil" gays and lesbians from the Zimbabwean community of "normal" people in Zimbabwe parliamentary debates.

[27]Act 15 of 1982. Previous to this act, black women were perpetually minors with no legal status and were permanently under the authority of a male guardian, either their father, brother, husband, or uncle. The LAMA declared any person to be legally independent upon reaching the age of 18, thereby emancipating black women.

homophobia and, using notions of "tradition" mixed with conservative Christian doc-trine,[28] create a marshalling point for the frustrations and grievances of a despondent and anxious public. Curiosity and taboo are the primary ingredients of public discourse around sex in general in Zimbabwe, and self-identified "gay communities" have previously been small and relatively discrete or closeted. These dynamics mean that homosexuality is an "illicit" issue that excites the imagination of people around the country, displacing anxieties about other unfulfilled political expectations and manufacturing a source of "moral" consensus. At the same time, the government is able to propagate a concept of "national" identity by defining something as "outside" the boundaries of Zimbabwean culture. Through this process of creating others excluded from tradition, an attempt is made to construct a consensus around gender, nature, and national identity that excludes all those who identify themselves as homosexual.

This is in striking contrast with current trends in South Africa and emphasizes very different approaches to the issue of diversity within society. Apartheid was a system that relied on the manufacturing and perpetuation of differences in order to exclude people from political power and deny them access to concomitant economic and social benefits. Consequently, the new South Africa is being built through embracing difference, consider-ing alternatives, and acknowledging diversity as a positive source of power. There is an attempt to preempt conflict and encourage national strength and harmony through a conscious acknowledgment of difference and a recognition of diffuse possibilities. In Zimbabwe, public debate is markedly more restricted, difference is judged harshly as marginal groups are regularly attacked, alternative viewpoints are either denied access to the media or are ridiculed, and challenges to the hegemony of the ruling party are actively discouraged as detrimental to the national interest. Where Zimbabwe has spent the last 16 years papering over social divisions in its cautious refusal to transform political structures and genuinely engage in a process of reconciliation, the South African political system has undergone extensive and radical change in attempts to cement together a previously divided society by being open and forthright about the grievances that lie at the heart of those divisions.

While the homophobia of members of government is genuine, their attack on lesbians and gay men is symptomatic of more serious problems within the country — a lack of political dynamism; a conservatism borne of fear, inertia, and despondency; and an anxiety about the way the freedom being established in South Africa contrasts with the restrictive and fettered nation-building being undertaken in Zimbabwe. Such an approach, built as it is on exclusion and xenophobia, can only lead to a more isolated existence, interfering with Zimbabwe's ability to participate in increasingly interactive international development. Central to effective international interaction is an ability to understand the value of diversity and a refusal to see "difference" as a threat.

In its rejection of alternative viewpoints, the Zimbabwean government exercises short-term political expediency at the cost of social and cultural development, which is not only ultimately inevitable but also replete with potential benefits. Through its growing depen-

---

[28]Leviticus and other Old Testament references are frequently quoted in castigating homosexuality, often by ordained ministers of the numerous churches that have large congregations in Zimbabwe. With a few notable exceptions, the churches in Zimbabwe have supported and often promoted Mugabe's "anti-homosexual campaign" — the Zimbabwe Council of Churches being complicit in this.

dence on sustaining a highly conservative moral consensus, it not only causes much pain and division among its own citizens, but also stifles the ability of traditional local structures to negotiate their interaction with the wide variety of global influences that pour through all countries with increasing effect. This refusal to understand culture as dynamic leads to the government's failure to see the irony in this situation, in which the enforcement of their claims around African "tradition" relies on a law derived from Roman-Dutch law and imported by settlers imbued with Victorian sexual attitudes.

Cited Cases

Addison, AD-65-71 (1971).
Derks & Anor, HC-B-124-84 (1984).
Jordan, AD-7-75 (1975).
King Kingsley Otis Ndebele, SC-135-89 (1989).
Le Roux, S-172-81 (1981).
Mackie, HC-B-54-90 (1990).
Palmer, AD-112-73 (1973).
R v B, (2) RLR 212 (1969).
R v Bourne, 36 CR App Rep 125 (1952).
R v K & F, E.D.L. 71 (1932).
R v Masuku, (2) RLR 332 (1968).
S v Beli Enock Dube, HC-B-94-87 (1987).
S v C, (1) RLR 55 (1976).
S v D, (3) SA 263 (1963).
S v H, (3) SACR 545 (C) (1993).
S v K, (2) RLR 78 (1972).
S v Macheka, (1) RLR 49 (1979).
S v Magwenzi, HH-59-94 (1994).
S v Meager, (2) RLR 327 (1977).
S v Roffey, (2) ZLR 47 (1991).
S v Simon, (2) ZLR 53 (1987).
S v Stanford, (1) ZLR 190 (1992).

References

Bullock, C. (1950). *The Mashona and the Matabele*. Cape Town, South Africa: Juta.
Buxton, J. (1973). *Religion and healing in the Mandari*. Oxford: Clarendon Press.
Colson, E. (1958). *Marriage and the family among the Plateau tonga of northern Zambia*. Manchester, England: Manchester University Press.
Dunton, C., & Palmberg, M. (Eds.). (1996). Human rights and homosexuality in southern Africa. *Current African Issues, 19*.
Evans-Pritchard, E. E. (1970). Sexual inversion among the Azande. *American Anthropologist, 72*, 1428–1434.
Feltoe, G. (Ed.). (1980). A Guide to the criminal law. *Zimbabwe Law Journal, 20*.
Gelfand, M. (1967). The Shona attitude towards sex behaviour. *Native Affairs Department Annual (NADA), 4*(4), 61–65.

Gelfand, M. (1975). *Kutiza mukombo* and *kutiziswa mukombo*: Elopement in Shona law. *Native Affairs Department Annual* (NADA), 9(4), 443–448.

Gonsiorek, J. C. (1991). The empirical basis for the demise of the illness model of homosexuality. In J. C. Gonsiorek and J. D. Weinrich (Eds.), *Homosexuality: Research implications for public policy* (pp. 115–148). London: Sage.

Hunt, P. M. A. (1982). *South African criminal law and procedure* (2nd ed.). Cape Town, South Africa: Juta.

Phillips, O. C. (1997). Zimbabwean law and the production of a white man's disease. *Social and Legal Studies* (special edition) *Legal Perversions* (in press).

Rachewiltz, B. de. (1964). *Black eros: Sexual customs of Africa from prehistory to the present day*. Tr. Peter Whigman. New York: Lyle Stuart.

Rivera, R. R. (Eds.). (1991). Sexual orientation and the law. In J. C. Gonsiorek and J. D. Weinrich (Eds.), *Homosexuality: Research implications for public policy* (pp. 81–100). London: Sage.

Schmidt, E. (1990). Negotiated spaces and contested terrain: Men and women in colonial Zimbabwe, 1908–1939. *Journal of Southern African Studies*, 16(4), 623–647.

Seidman, G. (1984). Women in Zimbabwe: Post-independence struggles. *Feminist Studies*, 10(3), 419–440.

Sumner, C. (Ed.). (1990). *Censure, politics and criminal justice*. Buckingham, England: Open University Press.

Talbot, P. A. (1967). *Some Nigerian fertility cults*. London: Frank Cass and Co.

3

China

FANG-FU RUAN

Male Homosexuality

Ancient China

Probably the earliest record of male homosexuality dates from the Shang Dynasty (from approximately the sixteenth to eleventh centuries BC). Official Chinese historical records indicate that during the Spring-Autumn and Chin-Han eras (770 BC–24 AD), male homosexuality was considered neither a crime nor immoral behavior. For example, in the Western Han era (206 BC–8 AD), there were 11 emperors. Ten of the eleven had at least one homosexual lover or expressed some homosexual proclivities. During the Western and Eastern Chin and Southern and Northern dynasties (256 AD–581 AD), male homosexuality seemed acceptable in the broader upper-class society.

There are three famous historical episodes concerning Chinese male homosexuality. Each is the source of one of the widely used colloquial terms for homosexuality in the Chinese language. The first story was recorded in "The Difficulties of Persuasion" in *Han Fei Tzu*, the works of the famous philosopher Han Fei, who died in 233 BC. It concerns a king in the state of Wei named Ling (534–493 BC), who was in love with a very handsome man called Mi Tzu-hsia. According to the law of Wei, anyone who drove the king's carriage without permission would be punished by amputation of his legs. One day Mi Tzu-hsia learned that his mother had suddenly fallen seriously ill and used the king's carriage to rush to her side. Unfortunately, he had not had time to ask for the king's permission and was risking severe punishment. However, when the king learned what Mi had done, he not only did not punish him, but also praised his filial piety. Another incident showed the warmth of the affection between the king and his lover. While taking a walk in the king's garden, Mi picked an unusually sweet and delicious peach. Instead of eating the whole peach, Mi ate half and saved the remaining half for the king. King Ling was so touched by Mi's affection for him that he publicly acknowledged Mi's love. This story gave rise to the expression "sharing the remaining peach," or *yu-tao*, as a term for male homosexuality.

The second story, recorded in *History of the Former Han*, also involves royalty. Emperor Han Ai-ti (reigning 6 BC–1 AD) was once in love with the handsome young man Dong Xian and was so fascinated by Dong's beauty that he appointed him to a high position in the court. Dong accompanied the emperor in all his travels and always slept in the same bed. Once, when the two had been taking a nap, the Emperor awoke and saw that the long sleeve of his gown was trapped under the soundly sleeping Dong. He decided to have the sleeve cut off from the gown rather than disturb his lover's sleep. Thus, "the cut sleeve," or *tuan hsiu* became another literary expression for same-sex love (Hinsch, 1990).

FANG-FU RUAN • The Institute for Advanced Study of Human Sexuality, San Francisco, California 94109.

Sociolegal Control of Homosexuality, edited by West and Green, Plenum Press, New York, 1997.

The third episode was recorded in the "Book of Wei" in *Chan-Kuo-Tse* [*Intrigues of the Warring States*]. During the Warring States period of the Zhou Dynasty, a king in the state of Wei had a male companion, Lord Lung-yang. Lung-yang was the king's favorite lover and friend. Once on a fishing trip, after catching about a dozen fish, Lung-yang suddenly burst into tears. When the king asked the reason for this sudden sadness, Lung-yang replied that he was very happy when he caught the first fish, until he caught a larger fish. He was thinking of giving away the smaller fish when it struck him that he was in a similar situation. He knew there were persons more beautiful than himself in the world and feared the king might abandon him as he had been prepared to abandon the smaller fish. The king immediately reassured him that this would never happen and issued an order prohibiting the mention of anyone more beautiful than Lung-Yang. People who violated this order would be punished by having their entire families killed. Lung-yang's name thus passed into history as another synonym for male homosexuality.

In the Ming and Ching dynasties (1368 AD–1911 AD), several books about homosexuality were published, nonfiction and fiction. One noted collection of homosexual historical stories is *Tuan-hsiu-pien* [*Records of the Cut Sleeve*], edited by Wu Xia A Meng (an anonymous author's alias) about 190 years ago. This book sums up literary data on male homosexuality in 51 titles. Most of them came from Chinese classics, official histories, and unofficial histories; they are nonfiction. Some were taken from classical Chinese short fictions, including some mysterious, mythical, fox, and ghost stories. Three noted fictional tales of homosexuality are *Yi-Chun Xiang-Zhi* [*Pleasant Spring and Fragrant Character*], by Zuixifu Xinyuezhuren (pseudonym), published during 1627–1644 AD, 4 rolls of 20 chapters; *Bian Er Chai* [*Wearing a Cap but also Hairpins*], also by Xinyuezhuren and published during 1627–1644 AD, 4 rolls of 20 chapters; and *Ping-hua Bao-jan* [*A Mirror of Theatrical Life*] by Chen Sen; published in 1849 and commonly recognized as the best representative novel about homosexuality in China. The author, Chen Sen, eloquently praises the charms of catamites (young male homosexuals):

> Across tens of thousands of miles, through five thousand years of history, nothing and nobody is better than a catamite. Those who do not love a catamite should not be taken seriously.... They are like elegant flowers and not grass or trees; they are like beautiful women who do not need make-up; they are like a shining moon or tender cloud, yet they can be touched and played with; they are like rare books and grand paintings, and yet they can talk and converse; they are beautiful and playful and yet they also are full of change and surprise. (Ruan & Tsai, 1987)

Despite these glorifications, homosexuality in China after the Song Dynasty (960–1279 AD), while not extensively and severely punished, received its share of condemnation. In other words, homosexuality was considered deviant behavior. During the Ming Dynasty, Zhang Jun-ying wrote a book entitled *Ren Jing Jing* [*The Canon of Using Human Beings as a Mirror*], published in 1641. In it he explicitly portrayed homosexual behavior. However, he quickly added in his book that a mirror (the key word of the title) reflects both virtue and evil, and homosexuality was the evil his "mirror" wished to reflect. Even fiction with the most explicit and detailed description of homosexuality, *Yi-Chun Xiang-Zhi* [*Pleasant Spring and Fragrant Character*], found it necessary to denounce its homosexual characters and have them cruelly punished. In Book Two of this work, the main homosexual character is portrayed as very beautiful and is sought by many men, many of whom lose their fortunes and remain unmarried to earn his love. Yet his death is especially cruel: An object like a fishhook is forced into his anus and used to pull out pieces of his intestines slowly and repeatedly until he dies. Perhaps this was the author's way of escaping punishment for his detailed description of homosexual behaviors. It also reflects society's reaction toward homosexuality for the last 1000 years. These stories from ancient China were certainly the opposite of a glorification of homosexuality.

Modern China

Considering the many and varied records of homosexuality in ancient China (Ruan & Tsai, 1987), one would expect to find evidence of it in modern China. However, literature regarding contemporary homosexuality is scarce at best. In Weinberg and Bell's (1972) 550-page book *Homosexuality: An Annotated Bibliography*, for example, not a single study or recording of Chinese homosexual life is listed. In Parker's (1971, 1977, and 1985) three-volume edition, *Bibliography on Homosexuality*, in which 9924 items were included, only two articles (from gay publications) on Chinese homosexuality were listed. This scarcity of literature on Chinese homosexuality is at least partially due to the prohibitions against it, which are especially strong in contemporary China. Thus it was a real breakthrough when, through an unusual and unexpected set of events, the present author published in 1985, under the pseudonym Jin-ma Hua, an article entitled "Homosexuality: An Unsolved Puzzle," in a widely circulated health magazine, *To Your Good Health* (Ruan, 1985a). The article pointed out that homosexuality has occurred in all nations, in all social strata, and in all eras in human history. It acknowledged that in some countries, in some historical periods, homosexuals were severely punished and sometimes even received the death penalty, adding that such persecution was perhaps an example of how majorities subjugate minorities in human societies. The article went on to assert that homosexuals should not be persecuted for failing to reproduce, that the number of homosexuals in any society is substantial and greater than laypeople realize, that homosexuals' problems should not be ignored, that they deserve a reasonable social status, and that homosexuals do not differ from heterosexuals in such qualities as intelligence, physical strength, creativity, or the ability to maintain stable relationships.

The publication of this article attracted considerable attention. Some readers of *To Your Good Health*, most of them gay, wrote to the magazine's editor in response to the article. Then, 5 months after its first publication, the bulk of the article was reprinted in the most popular and widely read magazine in China, *The (Chinese) Reader's Digest*. Letters received by the editor of *To Your Good Health* were forwarded to this writer. A striking aspect of the letters from gay men is their immense relief at having an opportunity to express their feelings:

> Hua's article on homosexuality provides me with a soothing sense of relief never before experienced in my life. It also gives me hope about my life and my future. (letter #11)
> I am extremely grateful for Hua's objective, humane, scientific and fair critique on homosexuality. (#24)
> The publication of this article is a great event in the medical field. It is a salvation of thought, a fruit of progressive advancement. To homosexuals, it is true "good news." We admire your courage and scientific attitude toward this matter. (#25)

This article is truly great. It gives us, a small number of homosexuals, a spiritual uplift. It gives me the second life and takes me to the spring of my life. (#28, written by a college student who had attempted suicide)

Of the two letters expressing disapproval of homosexuality, one (#57) came from a medical college in the northwest region of China, and the other (#58) came from a teacher in a factory training center in the northeastern region of China:

Hua's article is attempting to legitimize homosexual life and is not an objective treatment of the subject matter. (#57 and #58)

Homosexuality is an evil product of capitalistic society. Homosexuality brings with it bad influence on our socialist society. It is our obligation to point out our view in stopping this product of spiritual pollution. (#57)

In a tone reminiscent of the Cultural Revolution, the writer of letter #58 added:

We should absolutely prohibit homosexuality.... Widespread homosexuality will lead to epidemic deterioration of our racial spirit and destroy our society.... The reason that people despise, prohibit, punish and persecute homosexuals is precisely that the behavior is evil, ugly, opposed to human morality, and an insult to human dignity, promotes crime among youth, ruins their mental and physical health, leads to the destruction of our race and civilization.... It is imperative that we expose homosexuality lest it create a flood that sweeps away our marital, moral, legal and customary dam and destroys our socialist civilization. (#58)

Many letters expressed their writers' pain and conflicting desires for confidentiality and a chance to overcome their isolation.

I am a 29 year old young man.... I am not interested in the female sex at all. I do not even want to have any physical contact with them. However, among the men that I have encountered, some would occupy my body and soul.... I am particularly interested in one man and my love for him is beyond description. He is a little smaller than I am, but I fall for him in every respect I can think of. This feeling deepens every day. It has been ten years but my feeling for him has not been changed.... Frequently when I thought of him I would masturbate to fulfill my sexual desire.... During the last 10 years or so, my life had an interesting twist. When I was 25 years old, a woman fell deeply in love with me. I could not tell her about my true feelings. She insisted on marrying me no matter what. I could not do anything to discourage her. Finally I gave in and married her. I was living in a completely different world. I seldom had sexual relations with her. But on one of those very rare occasions I impregnated her. She knows nothing about my deep secret. This relationship has created pain in my heart and my life. I have been in love and devoted my love to him all this time. I think my love for him will never change for the rest of my life. However, the love is a deep secret. He would not understand nor would he be aware of this. My heart is full of contradiction and pain. (#1)

The pain that homosexuals suffer most lies not in homosexuality per se, but in the men's inability to find suitable lovers for fear of being discovered.

I am longing to love others [homosexuals] and to be loved. I have met some other homosexuals but I have doubts about this type of love. With all the pressure I was afraid to reveal myself and ruined everything. As a result, we departed without showing each other homosexual love. As I am growing older my homosexual desire increases. This is too troublesome and too depressing for anyone. I thought about death many times. When you are young you cannot fall in love and when you are old you will be alone. Thinking of this makes the future absolutely hopeless. (#8)

The pain and sometimes unbearable anxiety experienced by China's gay men derives chiefly from the fear of societal punishment, including arrest and possible sentence to labor reform camps or prisons. Those who were serving prison terms for their homosexuality at the time Hua's article appeared could not possibly have read it, much less responded to it. However, letter #22 described the testimony of one man who had been imprisoned. He was a physics teacher and had been director of academic affairs in a high school. His homosexual relationships had been consensual and initiated by others. He was arrested in September 1983 and sentenced to a 5-year prison term for his homosexual acts. Since the publication of Hua's article, this man's colleagues, friends, and relatives were reported to have changed their negative attitudes toward him. His superior had visited him in prison. His sentence, however, remained unaltered.

The social pressure, pain, and inner conflict homosexuals suffer can be so intense that they come to consider or attempt suicide. Of the 56 who responded to Hua's article, 15 mentioned suicide attempts.

Of the hopes and dreams expressed in these letters, three types of aspirations were outstanding. The first concerned human rights — the belief that society should accept homosexuals and their right to express their sexuality without social or legal condemnation. The second concerned the issue of freedom to interact with other homosexuals — the wish that society would provide them with means to make contacts and form relationships, just as it does for heterosexuals. The third concerned the issue of knowledge — the wish that objective and scientific studies would be conducted and publicized in order to improve societal understanding.

FEMALE HOMOSEXUALITY

Ancient China

In ancient times, Chinese culture was characterized by a very tolerant attitude toward lesbianism. One important reason was that women's supply of yin (the substance and/or energy which is essential for the body) was believed to be unlimited in quantity; from this point of view, female masturbation would be harmless. It was also recognized that when a number of women are obliged to live in continuous and close proximity, as did many women living in polygamous households, there are many opportunities for lesbian relationships to develop. Many considered such relationships inevitable, certainly to be tolerated, and, according to some, even encouraged.

The Chinese use the picturesque term *mojingzi* (rubbing mirrors, or mirror grinding) to describe lesbian sexual behavior. The image of two flat, mirrorlike surfaces in contact, without any intervening stemlike projection (such as the penis), effectively conveys the idea of genital contact between two women. People use the related term *mojingzhe* (mirror rubbers) to mean lesbians, offering the following definition: "Two women who are aroused by sexual desires, and having no help, rub their mons pubis for each other" (Yao, 1941).

Modern China

In modern times, lesbians in China are even more closeted than gay males. When this writer received letters from homosexuals all over China in 1985 and 1986, not one was from a woman. Some women who have been willing to discuss their homosexuality have already been imprisoned and have little to lose. The writer was the main speaker at the first national workshop on sex education held in Shanghai in August, 1985. Afterward, he received an invitation from the Shanghai Public Security Bureau to visit the Shanghai Women Delinquents Correction Institution. As the correction officer's counselor, he was asked to interview three women. One, Ms. Za, was a "sex criminal":

> Ms Za was 26 years old, born into an intellectual's family. Her first sexual encounter, with a male classmate, occurred while she was still in high school. She enjoyed sex very much, and had sex with about 30 different men altogether, never taking any money. Because of her sexual "delinquency," she was jailed many times. During one jail term, Ms Za shared a room with Ms X, who had been arrested and jailed for lesbian behavior. Ms Za had never even heard of homosexuality before she met Ms. X. In jail, Ms X treated Ms Za like a lover, touching her, petting her, and telling her that even without a man two women can have very good sex. After her initial surprise, Ms Za greatly enjoyed receiving manual and oral sexual caresses from Ms X. Later, Ms Za actively seduced other women. She felt that orgasms resulting from homosexual sex were as strong as those from heterosexual sex, though she preferred male partners. Now, Ms Za began receiving jail sentences for homosexual "sex crimes," as well as heterosexual promiscuity. (Ruan, 1991, p. 141)

Another, Ms. Jia, was reported by attorney Dun Li.

> Ms Jia, who had been deeply in love with another young woman, Ms Yi. They were constant companions, fond of calling each other "sister," and shared a bed all night as often as they could manage. Yi had been married 6 months, reluctantly having intercourse with her husband. She only wanted to have sex with Miss Yi. Later, Miss Yi became engaged, but before the wedding, Jia killed her. In court, Jia confessed that she loved Yi so intensely that she wanted to divorce her husband and live with Yi forever. When Yi disagreed, Jia decided that it was better to die herself after killing her lover. (Ruan, 1985b, p. 187)

An exception to the usual difficulty in locating lesbians is the experience of Chinese journalists He and Fang (1989), who were actually more successful in contacting lesbians than gay males in their 1989 survey of homosexuality in China. They wrote six stories about lesbians compared to one about a gay male. Three of these stories are summarized below:

> In the autumn of 1988, in a factory in "C" city, Miss Wang, an engineer, used strong acid to burn her colleague and homosexual partner Miss Li, both to prevent and to take revenge for Li's plans to marry a man.
>   Mr. Wu was a worker who was still single at 30; he had trouble finding a wife because he was so short, but finally he was introduced to Miss Xia. On their wedding night, another woman, Miss Jiang, roughly knocked on the door of the new couple's bedroom. Jiang was Xia's lover, and refused to accept the marriage unless Mr. Wu would agree to take both of them as wives, so the lesbian relationship could be maintained. Jiang forced Mr. Wu to have intercourse with her first, with his new wife Xia second, and then to join them in a menage a trois. Xia was displeased by the good sexual relationship

that formed between Wu and Jiang, and reported it to the authorities. Wu was arrested, and Xia and Jiang were forced to separate.

In "Y" county, in the Moon Buddhist Nunnery, there were more than 30 nuns. One day, a very beautiful girl, Miss Wang, insisted on becoming a nun and cutting her long hair. She took the Buddhist name Huimei, and became the lover of another nun, Huiming. Huiming's former lesbian lover, another nun named Huiyuan, was jealous and broke in on Huiming and Huimei while they were making love. When she broke the door down, their secret came out. Huiming and Huimei had to leave the nunnery and were no longer allowed to be nuns. Huiming said that it was other, older nuns who had originally seduced her. (He & Fang, 1989)

Among people who had every reason to fear discovery, He and Hang encountered the usual reluctance to be interviewed. They, too, had to rely on interviews with women who were jailed for "sex crimes," or crimes of violence inspired by sexual jealousy. Because so many investigations of female homosexuality are based on interviews with prisoners, it has been all too easy for Chinese people to develop a stereotype of lesbians as immoral, frustrated people. Thus Shui (1989), in an article in which it is impossible to separate fact from fiction, describes a secret "Lesbians' Company," a band of women who engage in murder and other crimes because they have been hurt and rejected by men. This story, one of the few publications in which homosexuality in mainland China has been discussed, is probably representative of common negative attitudes toward lesbianism.

It is clear that many lesbians do live difficult lives marred by fear and jealousy. But it is impossible to develop a complete and balanced picture of their lives under current conditions. Even anecdotal evidence must be distorted when the majority of those who supply it do so only because they are coerced by legal authorities. Given the general lack of sex information in China and the repressive attitudes of the leadership, it will be a long time before Chinese homosexuals can hope to live normal and happy lives.

The Current Situation of Homosexuals in China

Regarding the legal situation of homosexuals in mainland China now, although there is no specific statement concerning the status of homosexuals, in the current *Criminal Law of the People's Republic of China* Article 106 says: "All hooliganism should be subjected to arrest and sentence." In practice, homosexual activity has been included as hooliganism. As noted earlier, even the small sample of letters Ruan received contained a report of a man given a 5-year jail term for homosexuality, and additional examples will be cited later in this chapter.

Silence, especially a silence based on repression and enforced ignorance, must not be mistaken for approval or tolerance. When public figures do speak out on homosexuality, it is usually to condemn it. For example, a famous attorney in China today, Mr. Dun Li, when asked to express his opinion concerning homosexuality, said: "Homosexuality, though it exists in different societies and cultures, with some minor exceptions is considered abnormal and disdained. It disrupts social order, invades personal privacy and rights and leads to criminal behavior. As a result, homosexuals are more likely to be penalized administratively and criminally" (Ruan, 1985b, p. 186).

In 1987, a leading forensic psychiatrist, Dr. Zheng, Zhanbei, expressed himself in similar terms, asserting that homosexuality is against social morality, interferes with social security, damages the physical and mental health of adolescents, and ought to be a crime (Wan, 1988).

Another common reaction to the question of homosexuality in China is denial. For example, Mr. Z. Liu, a well-known newspaper reporter and editor of a famous magazine, after 2 years of study in Chicago, described his American experience in *Two Years in the Melting Pot* (1984):

> One group on campus, calling itself the gay and lesbian Illini, met every week.... One of my friends argued that love between those of the same sex is natural and has existed throughout history—during the Roman Empire, it was even made legal, he said. I disagreed, saying that it wouldn't be good for society to open up this issue. In old China, homosexuality was practiced by a few rich people, but the general public didn't approve. (Ruan, 1991, p. 131)

Evidence of the official denial of homosexuality was provided by Richard Green, series editor of *Perceptives in Sexuality: Behavior, Research, and Therapy* (which includes this volume). In his "Series Editor's Comment" for my *Sex in China: Studies in Sexology in Chinese Culture* (Ruan, 1991), he wrote: "Less than a year before the 1989 massacre in Tiananmen square, I lectured on human sexuality at Peking Union Medical College. I described my research on the nonsexual behaviors of young boys that predicted later homosexuality. I asked the physicians in the audience whether comparable childhood behaviors were found among Chinese boys. I was told that there were no homosexuals in China" (p. v).

This official attitude of denying homosexuality in China can no longer be justified. Recently officials in Shanghai, the largest city in China, recognized that there are about 10,000 homosexuals in the city. Actually, the number could be over 200,000.

Changzheng Hospital in Tianjin, the third-largest city in China, reported in a medical paper that in the past 4 years, out of 366 cases of sexually transmitted diseases (STDs), at least 61 cases of syphilis resulted from male homosexual behavior, 80% of the cases involved anal sex, 10% oral sex, and the other 10% both anal and oral sex. Most of the cases (80%) had participated in sexual activity in public toilets. Most of their homosexual partners (more than 80%) were anonymous. Their age ranged from 16 to 60, with two-thirds of the group falling between the ages of 20 and 30. Most of them were workers, some were officials, teachers, and members of other professions.

Yet another reaction is to admit that perhaps homosexuality does exist in China, but to insist that when it occurs it is the result of Western influence. This was what was meant when, in rigid ideological fashion, letter #57 referred to "spiritual pollution." A formal expression of this view appeared in an official newspaper, the *Beijing Daily News*, which identified homosexuality as one of the "Western social diseases," originating in "Western ideology and thoughts" (United Press International, February 4, 1987).

Finally, there are those who, when faced with undeniable evidence of homosexuality, respond by seeking to eliminate it. Thus Wan Ruixiong, a writer who, after spending considerable time conducting interviews, wrote a lengthy report on homosexuality in China, concluded that homosexuality is a crime, and expressed the hope that it will some day be abolished (Wan, 1988).

Many physicians do not consider homosexuality an acceptable sexual orientation. In Harbin, one of the largest cities in northeastern China, physicians attempt to change homosexuality with aversive techniques. According to one report:

When homosexuals are treated for what most Chinese doctors regard as their mental illness, they are sometimes given painful electric shocks to discourage erotic thoughts. An alterative approach is to offer herbal medicines that induce vomiting. In either case, the idea is to stimulate an extremely unpleasant reaction that will be associated thereafter with erotic thoughts and thus reduce the patients' ardor. Both approaches … are hailed by doctors in China as remarkably successful in "curing" homosexuality. (Kristof, 1990)

The people who experienced this treatment had not had any criminal charges brought against them, but were sent by family members who were upset by their homosexuality.

These attitudes contribute to a number of problems. Today in mainland China there is an acute housing shortage. Since there are virtually no private rooms for anyone in the family home, many homosexuals are forced to meet elsewhere. Public toilets are one of the few available locations for social and sexual liaisons. In these unsanitary conditions, gay men are forced to increase their risk of contracting and spreading contagious diseases, including AIDS and other STDs. It is past the time for the Chinese government to change its policies. Not only must it recognize the rights of gay people and develop educational programs promoting public acceptance of their lifestyle, but it must also begin promoting safe sex practices, ultimately preventing the premature deaths of perhaps millions of innocent people (Ruan & Chong, 1987).

Changes are coming, however. For instance, it was reported that two young lesbians in Wuwei County, Anhui Province, were deeply in love, but their parents opposed this homosexual relationship very much. At last, the angry parents reported the affair to the local police department. After several months of investigation, the police department of Wuwei County arrested these two female lovers and restrained them 15 days on charges of misconduct. The Wuwei County police department referred the case to higher institutions until the Public Security Department of Central Government in Beijing heard the case. The Public Security Department replied and instructed the county police that since under current laws there is no article that specifies punishment for such behavior and relationship, it could not treated as misconduct. Therefore, the Wuwei Police Department released the two women, and let them live together as "husband" and "wife." Usually the elder one takes the role of husband and wears male clothing, while the younger one takes the role of wife and prefers to stay in the home (reported in *Guizhou Ribao*, the official daily news of Guizhou Province). Also, on January 16, 1989, at Diyuan Village in Fujian Province, a 26-year-old man, a veteran, as the bride, married a 30-year-old man, a peasant, as the groom in a formal ritual. About 100 relatives and friends attended their wedding (reported in the *Centre Daily News*, February 27, 1989). If these reports are true, they reveal that some police officers and local officials, especially among the higher ranks, have started to change their attitude toward homosexuality.

The past decade of economic and social reform spawned a new permissiveness. For the first time, Chinese sociologists and sexologists have conducted extensive surveys to document the sexuality of the world's most populous nation (Liu, 1992; Li, 1991; Li & Wang, 1992; Peng, 1993). One main conclusion is that like most other populations, at least 1% to 5% of the Chinese are homosexuals (Chen, 1995).

In the noted sexual social survey, *Sexual Behavior in Modern China — A report of the Nationwide "Sex Civilization" Survey on 20,000 Subjects in China*, by Liu, Dalin (1992), a professor at Shanghai University and the head of the Shanghai Sociology of Sex Research Center, it was found in China that 0.5% of urban married people, 2.3% of rural married people, and 7.5% of college and university students have engaged in homosexual behavior.

Several academic books on homosexuality have been published. A sociological survey and studies book, *Their World — Perspectives of Male Homosexual Groups in Mainland China*, by Li, Yinghe and Wang, Xiaopo, was published in 1992 by Shanxi People's Publication House in Taiyuan, Shanxi Province. It is the first monograph (273 pages) on male homosexuality in China. An academic book of 675 pages (over 50,000 Chinese characters), *Same Sex Love* by Dr. Zhang, Beichuan, a dermatologist, was published in 1994 by Shantong Science & Technology Press. It was the first comprehensive academic book on homosexuality in mainland China, and the first time a book carried this type of nonjudgmental title. The authors Li, Wang, and Zhang are all heterosexual scholars. Their support for the normality of homosexual orientation and lifestyle may prompt progress in the acquisition of human rights for homosexuals in mainland China.

References

Chen, Zishan. (1995, September). A new look into the banned area of the studies of homosexuality in mainland China. *Ming Bao Monthly*, 116 [in Chinese].
The edition used for this chapter is an undated Ching Dynasty edition at the Beijing Library. There are a total of 20 volumes.
He, Cheng & Fang, Qian. (1989, April). The sex-love of Yin-Yang inversion: An inquiry into homosexuality in China. *Qinghai Quncong Yishu*, 103, 2–23 [in Chinese].
Hinsch, B. (1990). *Passions of the cut sleeve: The homosexual tradition in China*. Berkeley: University of California Press.
Kristof, N. D. (1990). "Curing" homosexuals in China. *San Francisco Chronicle*, January 31.
Li, Yinghe. (1991). *Love and marriage of the Chinese*. Zhengzhou, China: Henan People's Publication House [in Chinese].
Li, Yinghe, & Wang, Xiaopo. (1992). *Their world — perspectives of male homosexual groups in mainland China*. Taiyuan, China: Shanxi People's Publication House [in Chinese].
Liu, Dalin. (1992). *Sexual behavior in modern China — A report of the nationwide "Sex Civilization" survey on 20,000 subjects in China*. Shanghai, China: Shanlian Shudian [in Chinese].
Liu, Z. (1984). *Two years in the melting pot*. San Francisco: China Books & Periodicals.
Parker, W. (1971). *Homosexuality: A selective bibliography of 3,000 items*. Metuchen, NJ: The Scarecrow Press.
Parker, W. (1977). *Homosexuality bibliography: Supplement, 1970–1975*. Metuchen, NJ: The Scarecrow Press.
Parker, W. (1985). *Homosexuality bibliography: Second supplement, 1976–1982*. Metuchen, NJ: The Scarecrow Press.
Peng, Xinhua. (1993). *Sexual deviances and crimes*. Beijing: Police Officers Education Press [in Chinese].
Ruan, Fang-Fu (under pseudonym Hua, J. M.). (1985a). Homosexuality: An unsolved puzzle. *Zhu Nin Jiankang* [To Your Good Health], 3, 14–15 [in Chinese].
Ruan, Fang-Fu. (1991). *Sex in China: Studies in sexology in Chinese culture*. New York: Plenum Press.
Ruan, F. F., & Chong, K. R. (1987, April 14). Gay life in China. *The Advocate*, 470, 28–31.
Ruan, F. F., & Tsai, Y. M. (1987). Male homosexuality in the traditional Chinese literature. *Journal of Homosexuality*, 14, 21–33.
Shui, Shui. (1989). Nu Tongxinglian Gongsi [Lesbians' company]. In *Junlu Yanqing* [The Love Stories in the Military Tour], Shengyang: Liaonining Mingzu Press, pp. 66–95.
Wan, Ruixiong. (1988). The bigger variations of sex and love — about the problems of homosexuality in China. In Wen Bo (Ed.), *Nu Shi Ren Tan* [The ten women's tales] (pp. 78–109). Beijing: China Social Sciences Press.
Weinberg, M. S., and Bell, A. P. (1972). *Homosexuality: An annotated bibliography*. New York: Harper & Row.
Yao, L. X. (1941). *Siwuxic shaozi* [Yan Hai, The Sea of Words], Tianjin: Tianjin Books [in Chinese].
Zhang, Beichuan. (1994). *Same sex love*. Jinan, China: Shantong Science & Technology Press [in Chinese].

4

Japan

STEVEN D. PINKERTON AND PAUL R. ABRAMSON

Introduction

Ostensibly, this chapter concerns the legal regulation of homosexuality in Japan. If this description were taken literally, however, this chapter would be exceedingly brief and unduly deceptive. There are, in fact, no legal proscriptions of homosexuality in Japan, nor any laws concerning the practice of sodomy. When viewed from a Western perspective, this situation is both curious and instructive. Historically, homosexual behaviors among Japanese men are very well documented, especially among the samurai and certain sects of Buddhist monks. Homosexuality is also implicated in the historical development of the Japanese arts, including *kabuki, noh,* and other dramatic forms (Bowers, 1974); woodblock prints (*ukiyoe*); watercolors; and Japanese literature. The influence of an established homosexual tradition is also evident in modern Japanese fiction [e.g., Yukio Mishima's *Forbidden Colors* (1968) and Yasunari Kawabata's *Beauty and Sadness* (1964)]. Gay and lesbian organizations also exist, as do businesses catering to a gay and lesbian clientele. Thus, Japan has homosexuality (and homosexual behavior), but no specific legal provisions against it.

This, of course, does not mean that homosexuality and homosexual behaviors in Japan are void of statutory regulation. Laws relating to obscenity, prostitution, freedom of expression, or the family may suffice to exert constraints. Additionally, the absence of legal codes forbidding homosexuality is somewhat illusory, because societal rather than statutory regulations are preeminent in Japan. These societal restraints are organized along the principal dimensions of duty, honor, and responsibility to the family. In Japan, public welfare is a more compelling leitmotif than individual rights.

Social regulation of behavior is also facilitated by the homogeneity, both racial and cultural, of Japanese society (although, like many other aspects of Japan, this too is undergoing rapid change). Traditionally, conformity rather than individuality has been the chief virtue of this social system (Benedict, 1946). Sociocultural norms, in general, are therefore well respected. Chief among them are obedience to the intricate system of obligations (*giri*) and duties that govern interpersonal relationships [including specific obligation to one's name/family and other relevant incurred obligations (*on*)], as well as behaving in accord with one's place in the many hierarchies (including social, familial, and work-related) that constitute the backbone of Japanese society. As a corollary, the Japanese are usually quite respectful (even deferential) to authority, which derives legitimacy from the same forces of conformity and duty that govern Japanese society as a whole. Personal

STEVEN D. PINKERTON • Department of Psychiatry and Behavioral Medicine, Center for AIDS Intervention Research, Medical College of Wisconsin, Milwaukee, Wisconsin 53226.   PAUL R. ABRAMSON • Department of Psychology, University of California–Los Angeles, Los Angeles, California, 90024.

Sociolegal Control of Homosexuality, edited by West and Green, Plenum Press, New York, 1997.

disagreements and social disruptions are more often settled by compromise than by confrontation, with significant consequences for the Japanese legal system. In Japan, the governance of behavior is socially rather than legally enacted, in obvious contrast to most Western cultures. This is reflected in the legal and social status of homosexuality in Japan, which is the topic of this chapter.

Perhaps the best way to understand how homosexuality is regulated and shaped by Japanese society, as well as how homosexuality itself molds aspects of Japanese culture, is to examine it in both historical and contemporary perspectives. This stratagem is pursued in the sections that follow, which examine, in order (1) the historical expression of homosexuality in Japan, (2) Japanese constitutional issues relating to the regulation of homosexuality, and (3) the implications of the global AIDS crisis on Japanese homosexual and bisexual men (and other men who have sex with men, though they may not self-identify as gay, homosexual, or bisexual). A brief conclusion summarizes, integrates, and extends the arguments advanced in the preceding sections.

Homosexuality in Japan: A Brief Historical Overview

In Japanese folklore it has long been claimed that male homosexuality, or *nanshoku*, was imported from China along with other cultural practices in early historical times. According to one legend, homosexuality was introduced into Japan in the ninth century by the Shingon Buddhist monk Kukai (also known as Kobo Daishi, 774–835). Although homosexual behavior most certainly existed in Japan prior to the return of Kukai from his travels in China, just as it exists in essentially all known cultures, there are nevertheless few records of such activity predating the tenth century (Leupp, 1995). Moreover, it is likely that Japanese imitation of elements of Chinese culture is responsible for the development of male–male sexual behaviors into an aesthetic, or "way" (*shudo*, the way of youths). (Little is known of the history of lesbianism in pre-modern Japan, due, in part, to the lesser status accorded women in traditional Japanese society.) In early Japan, like China, a courtly tradition of homosexuality was also established within the walls of the imperial palace during the Heian period (794–1185). [The eleventh century masterwork, *The Tale of Genji*, contains one of the best-known allusions to courtly homosexuality in pre-modern Japan. In the passage in question, young Prince Genji beds the brother of a lady who has refused his advances, finding the youth "more attractive than his chilly sister" (Seidensticker, 1976, p. 48).]

That a Buddhist monk, Kukai, is credited with introducing *nanshoku* into Japan is really not surprising in view of the well-established homosexual tradition in Japanese Buddhist monasteries from the thirteenth century. Although technically a violation of scriptural injunctions against involvement in sexual activity of any kind, many Buddhist monks viewed partaking in homosexual pleasures as a lesser offense than heterosexual intercourse (Leupp, 1995). Women, it was thought, were intrinsically polluting, and according to Confucian yin–yang principles, too much sexual contact with women could be spiritually enervating and was therefore to be avoided. In contrast, homosexual intercourse entailed no loss of the vital masculine yang essence. Because intercourse with women was strictly forbidden, and since neither Confucianism, another Chinese import, nor the native Shinto belief system condemned or otherwise discouraged homosexual behavior, the uniquely Japanese adaptation of Buddhism easily accommodated such practices, which were viewed as providing a "tolerable outlet for the monks' feelings" (Leupp, 1995, p. 38). (*Nanshoku* remained forbidden in some Buddhist sects, however.)

In the Buddhist monasteries of Japan, homosexual relationships incorporated a pedagogical aspect in addition to the overt sexuality (Conner & Donaldson, 1990). In a typical relationship, an older monk would assume responsibility for a young acolyte's religious education and general well-being, in exchange for emotional and sexual closeness. Anal intercourse was the preferred sexual practice, with the older monk enjoying the insertive role and his younger partner the receptive. Acolytes were often dressed in imitation of women, with makeup, perfume, and appropriate coiffures. Thus, it appears that monastic *nanshoku* was motivated, at least in part, by the monks' limited access to women.

Similarly, by the fourteenth century a distinct tradition of *nanshoku* had arisen among the samurai warrior class (Leupp, 1995). In the palaces of the shogun, sexual relationships were common among military leaders and their sexual favorites. The samurai kept their young male lovers (often attendants or menials) close during military campaigns in the field as well (DeVos, 1973; Schalow, 1990b). As with monastic homosexuality, samurai *nanshoku* was rigidly age structured, with the older (samurai) partner assuming the insertive role in anal intercourse.

Thus, the available evidence suggests that *nanshoku* was widespread among the monastic, aristocratic, and samurai classes in the long medieval epoch (1185–1868) that preceded the influx of Western influences during the Meiji period (1868–1912). Indeed, in the Tokugawa (or Edo) period (1603–1868), homosexual behavior was socially normative among the upper classes of Japanese society, at least in the cities. As succinctly summarized by the Japanese social historian Gary Leupp (1995), "Although we know next to nothing about the popular view of *nanshoku*, the historical record left by the literate strata of society suggests that most people would have inquired not why a given man *had* taken male lovers but rather why he had *not* done so" (p. 55, emphasis in original).

The reunification of Japan in the late sixteenth century and the establishment of the Tokugawa shogunate was accompanied by an explosion in the populations of Japan's larger cities and a rapid expansion of the bourgeoisie. With the rise of the middle and merchant classes emerged a new *nanshoku* tradition, one based on the commercial prospects of male homosexuality (Leupp, 1995). During this period thousands of Japanese migrated from small villages to large castle-towns where they were exposed, perhaps for the first time, to the socially accepted forms of male–male sexuality practiced by the ruling classes. The upper crust of Japanese society thus provided a model for the burgeoning bourgeoisie to emulate. Moreover, the available heterosexual outlets were severely limited by the very high male-to-female ratios evident in the rapidly growing cities and castle-towns (Leupp, 1995). The result of this rather unique set of circumstances was the development of a vast sexual marketplace trading in male as well as female prostitution.

In this newly established commercial world, sex was divorced from the commitment inherent in the stylized homosexual relationships of monk and acolyte or samurai and retainer. Men from all walks of life could partake of the entertainments, both heterosexual and homosexual, of the extensive pleasure districts in Edo (Tokyo) and other large cities. During this period, male bisexuality and numerous extramarital involvements became the accepted norm in Japanese society (Leupp, 1995). One's sexual and family lives were largely kept separate, with the wife (typically the product of an arranged marriage) fulfilling maternal and domestic duties, and male and female lovers (especially prostitutes) offering various sexual possibilities.

In keeping with Confucian principles, sexual dalliances with either sex were unproblematic, provided that they did not interfere with familial commitments. Neither Confucianism nor the native Shinto religion forbid extramarital or same-sex affairs (indeed, Shinto celebrates the sexual as an expression of nature), and Buddhist restrictions on sexual activity apply primarily to the clergy rather than the laity. Sex, whether with a man or woman, was not conceived of as sinful in any influential native or imported belief system until the influx of Western ideals during the Meiji period (1868–1912), when homosexuality was briefly and unsuccessfully outlawed (Schalow, 1990b). In the latter half of the nineteenth century, the rulers of Japan, newly opened to foreign trade, hoped to convince Westerners of Japan's advanced civilization, and it was rightfully believed that the widespread acceptance of homosexuality would be an abomination in Western eyes. Homosexuality, however, persisted despite the Meiji repression, although somewhat more clandestinely than before.

And so, Japanese homosexuality — or more often, bisexuality — persists into present times with only relatively minor alterations in basic patterns. Homosexual behaviors are neither forbidden nor heavily stigmatized in modern Japan, provided they respect the prevailing framework of social and familial responsibilities. According to Confucian principles, one's primary responsibility is to one's family, including both future and past generations. The socially inescapable duty of every Japanese person is to marry and reproduce, in order to perpetuate the family lineage, and in so doing, to respectfully pay homage to past generations. Any activity that interferes with this goal, whether it be drinking sake to excess or visiting prostitutes too frequently, must be curtailed so that the most important function of life, procreation, can be pursued. In Japan, a person is not fully recognized as a social adult until he or she is married, an occasion that is often marked with a substantial raise and promotion at work, in anticipation of the added expense of raising a family.

Thus, until very recent times, homosexuality has expressed itself within a sometimes artificial context of bisexuality, in which a gay man or woman is expected to marry and have children and, having fulfilled this familial responsibility, is free to follow his or her true inclinations with members of the same sex, provided that a modicum of discretion is exercised. However, there remains no place in Japanese society for the exclusively gay or lesbian individual who is unwilling or unable to sublimate his or her sexual identity and pursue the charade of marriage.

Only recently has the notion of homosexuality as an orientation, rather than simply a behavioral option, emerged as a theoretical construct (Miller, 1992). It is unclear what the ultimate impact of this challenge to traditional Japanese family and social structure will be. As discussed further in the following section, with the brief exception of Meiji legislation in the 1870s, homosexual behaviors have never been outlawed in Japan. But, homosexual behaviors, per se, do not endanger the social fabric, whereas it might appear that *homosexuality* (as an exclusive sexual preference) has power to do so. As argued in the following section, although this power is illusory, reactionary responses to the threat it engenders are not.

GENERAL MACARTHUR AND THE LAW OF JAPAN

Any discussion of contemporary Japanese law must consider the circumstances under-lying the current Japanese Constitution. Recognized in Japan as the *Nihonkoku kenpo* [*Constitution of the Japanese Nation*], it is known throughout the rest of the world as the MacArthur Constitution. The attachment of General MacArthur's name to the Japanese constitution provides explicit recognition of the fact that the constitution was developed in conjunction with — though some have argued it was imposed by — American occupation forces residing in Japan following the end of World War II (General MacArthur was the Supreme Commander of the Allied Powers, hence the nomenclature).

The Japanese constitution represents the melding of two disparate cultures and legal perspectives. Although it may seem somewhat unusual that the future of Japanese law should have been predicated upon an uneasy union of the victors and the vanquished, the imposition of the victor's will upon the legal landscape of the conquered nation is common in the aftermath of war or colonial occupation; the post-World War II German constitution and the 1935 Philippine constitution are other obvious examples. International legitimacy for imposing a foreign constitution is derived from Article 43 of the 1906 Hague Convention, which states: "the authority of the legitimate power having in fact passed into the hands of the occupant, the latter shall take all the measures in his power to restore, and ensure, as far as possible, public order and safety, while respecting, unless absolutely prevented, the laws in force in the country."

Did the American occupation forces, in keeping with the Hague Convention, "re-spect" Japanese law, or did they substantially alter the Japanese constitution during the postwar period? Many Japanese politicians (and their constituents) believed the latter to be the case and came easily to resent the constitution of 1946. In fact, 10 years after its adoption, the National Diet passed a statute to create a Constitution Investigation Commit-tee to "undertake an examination of the Constitution of Japan, to investigate and deliberate on the various problems related thereto and to report the results to the Cabinet and through the Cabinet to the National Diet" (Takayanagi, 1967, p. 2). The final report of this committee was submitted to the Cabinet on July 3, 1964. Surprisingly, the committee did not recommend any revisions. The chairman of the committee, Kenzo Takayanagi, summarized the rationale for retaining the constitution: "when I participated, as a member of the House of Peers, in the enactment of the new Constitution, my first impression was that it was not revolutionary in content, but that it constituted a moderate and impartial reform following the lines of democratic tendencies of the Meiji Constitution [promul-gated in 1889] and that, in general, it was a Constitution that would serve the future of Japan" (Takayanagi, 1967, p. 4).

As Takayanagi noted, the 1946 constitution advanced the democratization of Japan. Unlike its predecessor, the Meiji Constitution, which was primarily a set of guiding principles for the rulers of Japan, with no legal consequences for unconstitutional acts, the 1946 constitution allows questions regarding the constitutionality of actions by the National Diet or the executive branch to be adjudicated by the courts; if deemed unconstitutional under the new constitution, such actions become legally null and void. This obviously significant difference between the two constitutions has considerable relevance to the enactment of laws today. However, in contemporary Japan, the actual process of judicial review is largely constrained by internal factors. Supreme Court and district court justices tend to be very conservative, similarly disposed, and few in number. Furthermore, their tenure is short, and they are burdened with considerable administrative responsibilities. Moreover, judicial review itself is limited by parliamentary supremacy (Bolz, 1980).

Unfortunately, the democratic principles evident throughout the 1946 constitution are threatened by the decidedly undemocratic "public welfare standard," codified as Articles 12, 13, 22, and 29. Under the constitution, the Japanese Supreme Court has often upheld the constitutionality of laws limiting free expression by appealing to concerns about the public welfare (or questions of political doctrine) (Kamiya, 1987; Masami, 1963). Thus, although the Japanese constitution emphasizes freedoms of speech and press (Article 21) and academic freedom (Article 23), Japanese law construes these constitutional guarantees very narrowly and burdens the individual with the responsibility of demonstrating that public welfare is concomitant with personal liberty (Brown, 1979). Moreover, sexual morality is often included within the purview of public welfare. In 1957 the Japanese Supreme Court proclaimed that "there can be no doubt that the protection of the sexual order and the maintenance of a minimum degree of sexual morality constitute the contents of public welfare" (Hoshii, 1987, p. 243).

Finally, Japanese law cannot be separated from attitudes about litigation, which are subsumed more generally within Japanese concepts of obligation. Japanese personal and social structures are based upon a series of obligations that effectively ensure the integrity of the family, the neighborhood, the workplace, and the nation (Benedict, 1946). Thus, the initiation of a civil lawsuit (or the continuation of an appellate process to challenge the constitutionality of a law) is often perceived as being inconsistent with the interdependency that characterizes Japanese social structures (Hendry, 1987). Although Japanese attitudes about civil lawsuits may have a long and humorous history (Ramseyer, 1995), it nevertheless remains true that the development of Japanese law is limited, to some extent, by the paucity of challenges it faces.

Similar attitudes are manifested toward criminal proceedings. The keys to Japanese criminal law are repentance and rehabilitation, rather than punishment or retribution (Haley, 1984). As such, the courts are receptive to expressions of guilt and remorse, as well as offers of compensation to victims (or other means of rectifying actual or perceived wrongs). The primary goal of the criminal justice system is the successful reintegration of the offender into the social fabric of Japanese life, where the elaborate network of obligations and responsibilities, and the individual's own sense of shame (*haji*), can once again be used to exercise social control over the offender. Thus, "at every stage, from initial police investigation through formal proceedings, an individual suspected of criminal conduct gains by confessing, apologizing, and throwing himself upon the mercy of authorities" (Haley, 1982, p. 229; quoted in Haley, 1984, p. 2). Of course, it is only through the uniformity and social cohesion of Japanese society that this approach to criminal justice succeeds.

REGULATING SEX

Although Japan, like all civilized nations, maintains criminal codes against sexual crimes (including rape), institutional forms of sexual regulation typically fall within the sphere of family law (as it relates to marriage and descendants) or the freedom of expression.

This is especially true in regard to the regulation of homosexuality, because in Japan there are no criminal codes specific to either homosexuality or sodomy. Homosexual behavior (and sexual choice in general) is constrained not by criminal law, but by social sanctions and expectations.

Because homosexual relationships — as opposed to homosexual acts or behaviors — are not deemed familial (being void of possible reproductive consequences), family law is potentially an avenue for discriminating against homosexuals. In Japan, however, this is not the case, perhaps because homosexuality itself has never been perceived as precluding either marriage or raising a family. As noted earlier, this was true of the samurai, who maintained both families and same-sex lovers, and was (apparently) also true of one of Japan's most famous contemporary artists, the playwright and novelist Yukio Mishima, who was married and had children, despite achieving notoriety for the homoerotic elements in both his artistic work and his life.

Japanese tolerance of nonexclusive homosexual behavior raises fundamental questions about the conceptual generalizability of homosexuality and about the proper scope of Japanese family law. The later issue will be considered first. The Potsdam Declaration (which governed Japan's surrender following World War II) required the Japanese government to "remove all obstacles to the revival and strengthening of democratic tendencies … [and to establish] freedom(s) of speech, of religion, and of thought as well as respect for the fundamental human rights" (Oppler, 1949, p. 293). The 1946 constitution, as discussed earlier, was adopted to implement this policy. Marriage was a specific focus of the new constitution, and Article 24 in particular. This article declares that "marriage shall be based only on mutual consent of both sexes and shall be maintained through mutual cooperation with the equal rights of husband and wife as a basis." It also states that "with regard to choice of spouse, property rights, inheritance, choice of domicile, divorce and other matters pertaining to marriage and the family, laws shall be enacted from the standpoint of individual dignity and the essential equality of the sexes" (Kawashima, 1983, p. 54).

As Kawashima (1983) notes, in order to fulfill these new objectives, the Meiji Civil Code on family law had to be drastically revised. Under Meiji law, the family was organized into a system called the House. Family rights resided in the head of the House, and inheritance was determined by headship. Marriage could not be entered into without the consent of parents and the House head. Wives had diminished legal rights (limiting alimony and inheritance), and parental authority resided exclusively in the father. Moreover, adultery was a crime, but only for wives.

In contrast, under the civil codes adopted after 1946, marriage was recognized as a union of two individuals based exclusively on their free agreement. All limitations on the legal capacity of a married woman were eliminated. The new code also guaranteed individual ownership of property and provided an intestate share for the surviving spouse even when there were surviving descendants. Similarly, it abolished the various rules giving the eldest son a predominant position as heir to the House and made all children equal successors. Finally, parental authority was transformed into a guardianship to be exercised jointly by both parents in the best interests of the child (Kawashima, 1983).

Although the Meiji and modern family civil codes differ in substantial ways, both are premised upon fundamental beliefs about descent and descendants. The purpose (and presumably *savoir vivre*) of marriage is to produce exemplary offspring, hence an exemplary spouse must be procured. Even today, an extensive system of private detectives exists solely to obtain "objective" (or at least surreptitious) information on prospective spouses and in-laws. Invasive screening procedures are deemed necessary to ensure the stability and salience of the family lineage. Assurances that a prospective mate is responsible, financially secure, and socially adequate are required because the future of the family depends upon it.

Japanese attitudes toward adoption provide compelling evidence of the cultural emphasis on descendants. In Western countries, the primary objective of adoption law is to protect children, particularly children born out of wedlock. Although the practice (and cultural perceptions) of having children outside the confines of marriage has drastically changed in the West, the relevant adoption law remains unaltered. In contrast to the Western view of adoption as an institution that benefits children primarily, and adults only secondarily, in Japan adoption is designed to foster *both* parental and child interests. As a consequence, a wide variety of different adoption arrangements exist. For example, Japanese family law permits adoption of: (1) an adult; (2) a child, with parents, who does not necessarily need any protection or care; (3) a parentless child who needs care; (4) a stepchild; or (5) one's own "illegitimate" child (Kawashima, 1983). The most unusual aspect of this law, at least from a Western perspective, is the permissible adoption of an adult. Yet, if adoption is conceptualized more broadly (as it is in Japan) as serving the interests of the family (or House), there are obviously many compelling reasons for legally adopting an adult. For example, a son-less couple might adopt a son-in-law (*muko yoshi*), who thereafter assumes the family surname and whose future children continue the line of descendence unbroken.

Also relevant are Japanese patricide laws. The Japanese penal code provides stiffer penalties for killing an ascendant than for killing any other person. Obviously, killing an ascendant bears directly on descent and familial continuation. Consequently, it is punished more severely in Japan, where descent (and descendants) reign supreme within the culturally predominant concept of family and familial obligation. In Japan, patricide is viewed as an act of treason against the family, and is punished accordingly.

This material has been introduced herein because it has relevance to both the legal and social regulation of homosexuality in Japan. Japan is a culture with an extraordinary investment in family and descent. Thus, activities or circumstances that interrupt or interfere with either are heavily scrutinized and legally regulated. Now, from a Western perspective, the focus of such regulation would undoubtedly include homosexuality, or sodomy at the very least (since oral and anal sex are nonreproductive). However, this unnecessarily presumes that homosexuality (or engaging in homosexual behaviors) precludes heterosexuality and the conception of children. Obviously where sodomy is concerned, heterosexual couples can occasionally engage in oral or anal intercourse without adversely affecting their reproductive prospects. Thus, within the Japanese cultural system, heterosexual sodomy is a tolerated diversion because it does not necessarily disrupt family and descent. Furthermore, sodomy, like sex in general, is presumed to be regulated internally — and subordinately — within the hierarchy of Japanese familial and social obligations (Abramson, 1986; Benedict, 1946).

"Homosexuality" is similarly conceived within Japanese social systems, where, traditionally, sexual behavior has not been conceptualized among an identity dichotomy of homosexual and heterosexual, or gay and straight. Although the notion that one *is* either heterosexual, homosexual, or bisexual has become more influential in recent years, in the past a person was not necessarily categorized by his or her sexual preferences. Having male lovers did not make a man a homosexual any more than having a wife made him a heterosexual. Such distinctions were essentially irrelevant; homosexual and heterosexual behaviors were simply two sides of the same sexual coin. Homosexuality was tolerated (and, at times, even encouraged) in Japan because homosexual relations typically coexisted with heterosexuality, family, and reproduction. Thus, a Japanese man (or woman for that matter) can fulfill his or her familial obligations — in both the literal (offspring) and figurative (*giri*) sense — without renouncing or avoiding a reproductively "irrelevant" diversion, such as engaging in homosexual behaviors. Homosexual relations were (and largely remain) irrelevant in Japan, because they did not disrupt family and descent.

Is the cultural attitude toward homosexual behaviors displayed by the Japanese unusual? Only within a strict Western (or Judeo-Christian) tradition. As demonstrated in our book *With Pleasure* (Abramson & Pinkerton, 1995), it is more accurate to speak of "homosexualities," rather than "homosexuality," because same-sex sexual relations exhibit extraordinary cultural and interpersonal variability. Clearly, the manner in which people express their sexuality is not necessarily monolithic, but is instead embedded in a larger network of cultural meanings. In some cultures, homosexuality is ritualized, age structured, and transient for all males (e.g., the Sambia of Papua New Guinea), whereas in other cultures (e.g., North American Indian) it is role specialized. Similarly, in some cultures (e.g., in Latin America, the Middle East, and among street "punks" in the United States) the designation of "homosexual" is reserved for the passive or receptive partner in male–male sexual relations. Japanese attitudes represent another variant within this continuum, in which homosexuality is tacitly accepted (and therefore not explicitly legally regulated) because it need not usurp marriage and family. Thus, although family law specifies the necessity of opposite-sex marriages, it does not go on to further admonish homosexuality or sodomy because both are deemed irrelevant to the main function of marriage.

FREEDOM OF EXPRESSION

In many societies, obscenity law is another vehicle for punishing or pathologizing homosexuality. In the United States, for example, prosecutors often utilize gay pornography as a ploy to facilitate obscenity convictions, acknowledging that it is easier to convince juries that explicit portrayals of male homosexuality (as opposed to heterosexuality) are either prurient, lack value, or violate community standards (Abramson & Pinkerton, 1995). However, in Japan, this strategy is conspicuously missing, suggesting once again that homosexuality is a diversion, neither publicly admitted nor vilified, because it is tangential to marriage and family.

The 1946 constitution formally provides for free expression in Article 21, where it states, "Freedom of assembly and association as well as speech, press and all other forms of expression are guaranteed.... No censorship shall be maintained, nor shall the secrecy of any means of communication be violated." This proviso notwithstanding, speech and press are routinely censored under the guise of public morals or shameful reactions. Yet, images of homosexuality, per se, have not been the focus of inordinate censorship in Japan, unlike the United States and Great Britain, which have a long-standing, shared tradition of condemning homosexual expression in novels, films, and the arts.

The term *waisetsu* (obscenity), and punishment for the public display or sale of obscene materials, first appeared in Japan in Article 259 of the Criminal Code of 1880. Article 175 of the 1907 revised Criminal Code is currently the primary legal provision concerning obscenity. The other major pre-World War II enactment still in force is the Customs Standards Law of 1910, under which the Customs Bureau can scrutinize and censor imported material. Additionally, obscene materials can be regulated under the Entertainment Facilities Law, the Law Regulating Businesses Affecting Public Morals, the Radio Law, the Broadcast Law, the Prison Law, and 39 local youth protection ordinances. These laws, in turn, are supplemented by self-regulatory codes administered by various industry ethics committees (e.g., booksellers, the film industry, etc.) (Beer, 1984).

In 1957, the Japanese Supreme Court defined obscenity as follows: "In order for a writing to be obscene, it is required that it wantonly arouse and stimulate sexual desire, offend the normal sense of shame, and run counter to proper concepts of sexual morality" (Beer, 1984, p. 348). This definition was offered in an appellate consideration of D. H. Lawrence's novel *Lady Chatterly's Lover*, which was deemed obscene under this definition. Similarly, in 1969, the Marquis de Sade's writings (e.g., *Julliette*) were held to be obscene by the Japanese Supreme Court, which further concluded that the inclusion of one or more obscene passages was sufficient to render an entire work of artistic or intellectual merit obscene.

In 1980, the Supreme Court Petty Bench clarified the definition of obscenity in ruling on the appeal of the editor of the magazine *Yojohan*, who had been convicted of publishing an obscene story dating from the Meiji era, "The Underlay of the Sliding Door of the Four-and-a-Half Mat Room" (Hoshii, 1987). Under the revised definition, whether a particular work is obscene depends on (1) the relative boldness, detail, and general style of its depiction of sexual behavior; (2) the proportion of the work taken up with sexual description; (3) the relationship in a literary work between such descriptions and the intellectual content of the story; (4) the degree to which artistry and thought content mitigate the sexual excitement induced by the writing; and (5) the relationship of sexual portrayals to the structure and unfolding of the story (Beer, 1984). However, a work could no longer be judged obscene on the basis of isolated sexual content; instead, the work, when taken as a whole, must be lewd and lascivious and appeal to the reader's prurient interests (Hoshii, 1987).

Clearly, if the Japanese Supreme Court deemed *Lady Chatterly's Lover* and *Julliette* obscene — and prosecutors later (in 1979) claimed that the popular Japanese movie, *The Realm of the Senses*, was also obscene — it would not be surprising if homosexual literature and films were similarly condemned, especially given the legal definition of obscenity, which includes language about offending the normal senses of shame and running counter to proper concepts of sexual morality. If ever there were a justification for penalizing the distribution of homosexually relevant material, this language would seem to suffice. However, homosexuality has *not* been a target of anti-obscenity zealots in Japan, and thus has not been rigorously prosecuted or demonized for political purposes.

Instead, in contemporary Japan the battle over obscenity is primarily fought on the battlefield of genitals and pubic hair, with depictions of either a possible violation of existing statutes, at least until recently. Presumably, the official abhorrence of genitals and pubic hair in sexually explicit material (whether heterosexual or homosexual) derives, in part, from Japanese concessions to the United States following World War II (Abramson & Hayashi, 1984). American regulations in the postwar period prohibited the visual depiction of genitals and pubic hair, and the Japanese readily endorsed these restrictions. However, despite a subsequent relaxation of such prohibitions in the United States, the Japanese persisted with this restriction until 1991, at which time depictions of pubic hair (*hea-nu-do*, "nude with exposed pubic hair") became permissible.

This raises a question: Why should a country with a sizable sex industry (ranging from hostess clubs, illegal prostitution, pornography vending machines, explicitly sadomasochistic sexual comics, sex junkets, dial-a-porn, etc.) actively prohibit the depiction of the genitals and pubic hair, but permit portrayals of enemas, anal eroticism, feigned (hence shaved) prepubertal females, sadomasochism, misogynistic violence, and so forth (on the vast Japanese sex industry, see Baruma, 1984; Bornoff, 1991; or simply surf the World Wide Web). Allison (1996) suggests that this particular prohibition is ultimately designed (at least symbolically) to protect the sanctity of family, home, and motherhood by prohibiting genital realism.

Because the genitals are necessary for reproduction, hence the continuation of family, Japanese law endows them with substantial ideological significance. [The social significance of the sex organs is readily apparent in the exaggerated focus and depiction of both female and male genitalia in pre-modern Japanese art (*Shunga*) and in the phallicism of the autochthonous Shinto religion.] By excising genitals from the public ideography, the lofty status of reproduction and the family is protected from being cheapened. However, sexual activities that do not overtly prevent reproduction — implied homosexuality among them — are not actively criminalized within obscenity law. Thus, homosexuality escapes the scrutiny and stigma of obscenity because it does not explicitly challenge reproduction and the family (at least according to Japanese customs and perspectives).

THE RIGHT TO PRIVACY

Restrictions of the right to privacy provide another judiciolegal mechanism whereby homosexuality can be punished or pathologized. This is certainly true in the United States, where specific forms of sexual expression among consenting adults, such as sodomy, remain outside the right to privacy (e.g., in Georgia). However, this strategy has apparently not been pursued in Japan. Though sexual issues have often arisen within the context of the right to privacy (particularly with regard to voyeurism and the media's intrusions into the sex lives of the famous), the statutory basis for privacy protection, and other legal provisions for privacy, have never been challenged for the purpose of trying to prohibit a particular lifestyle (e.g., homosexuality) or a particular behavior among consenting adults (e.g., oral or anal sex).

HOMOSEXUALITY AND THE AIDS EPIDEMIC IN JAPAN

It is nearly impossible to discuss the legal regulation and social control of homosexual behavior in Japan without addressing an issue of supreme importance to gay men everywhere (including Japan), namely, the acquired immunodeficiency syndrome (AIDS).

Harking back to the Meiji period in the latter half of the nineteenth century, the Japanese homosexual — or more precisely, the Japanese man with male lovers (lesbians are little affected) — is once again threatened from without, but the present crisis derives not from Westerners themselves, but from a particular virus now epidemic in most Western and many non-Western nations, namely the human immunodeficiency virus (HIV) — the reputed cause of AIDS — and from reactionary societal and governmental responses to the epidemic as well.

A surveillance system for the detection of AIDS was established by the Japanese Ministry of Health and Welfare in 1984, and in 1985 the first AIDS case in Japan was reported in a homosexual man who had traveled abroad (Miyazaki & Naemura, 1994). Although the Japanese AIDS epidemic has thus far remained relatively small, it has continued its inexorable growth little affected — or perhaps, negatively affected — by governmental AIDS policies. As of August 1994, a total of 713 people had been diagnosed as having AIDS, and 3022 had tested HIV-positive (Hoshino, 1995). However, the true extent of the HIV/AIDS epidemic in Japan is likely to be much greater than suggested by these numbers. Conceding the inaccuracy of governmental HIV prevalence figures, one Ministry of Health and Welfare official estimated that between 15,000 and 20,000 people were already infected by 1994 (Sesser, 1994). Moreover, in the same year, the Ministry of Health and Welfare's AIDS Surveillance Committee officially estimated that by 1997 there would be 26,000 HIV-infected people in Japan (Audet, 1994).

Another reason to suppose that the extent of the epidemic is vastly underestimated is the evidently widespread reluctance among sexually active Japanese men and women to be tested for HIV (this is discussed further, later in this chapter). Indeed, only 11% of nonhemophilic people diagnosed with AIDS as of April 1993 had previously been tested for HIV (Kitamura, 1994). [Many hemophiliacs also remain ignorant of their serostatus despite having been tested, due to the reticence of some Japanese physicians to inform patients of possibly life threatening conditions, including cancer, as well as HIV disease (e.g., see Feldman & Yonemoto, 1992).] Thus, there is likely to be a substantial pool of HIV-infected people who are not included in official surveillance estimates.

Fifty-nine percent of those infected with HIV through August 1994 were the unfortunate victims of a Japanese government that permitted the use of untested, non-heat-treated blood and blood products imported from the United States through 1986, nearly 2 years after the attendant risks became known (Hoshino, 1995; Ross, 1995). The Japanese government and several pharmaceutical companies were subsequently sued for negligence in 1989 by multiple groups of hemophiliacs, their families, and survivors. Although the case remains unresolved, in October 1995 the Tokyo and Osaka district courts recommended compensation in the amount of 45 million yen per patient, with the Japanese government responsible for 40 percent of the settlement and the pharmaceutical manufacturers the remainder (Guest, 1995; Ross, 1995). Unfortunately, by the time mandatory HIV screening and heat treatment of blood products had been instituted in 1985–1986, at least 37 percent of Japan's 4171 hemophiliacs had been infected with HIV, 324 of whom had developed AIDS by December 1991 (Miyazaki, O'Brien, & Naemura, 1995; Yamada, 1992). Since 1986 there have been no reported cases of new HIV infections attributed to clotting-factor or transfused blood (Hoshino, 1995; Miyazaki & Naemura, 1994). The number of people in Japan infected with HIV as a result of injecting drugs is also comparatively negligible.

In marked contrast, since 1991 the number of HIV cases attributable to sexual transmission has grown at an accelerated rate (Kitamura, 1994). The main (reported) route of transmission is heterosexual contact (predominantly male-to-female), with male–male sexual contact the third most frequent cause of infection, accounting for approximately one-third of all nonhemophilic cases reported in Japan. Rather surprisingly, the second most common risk category is "Other/Unknown." Because this category includes some men who had sex with both men and women, official statistics for men infected via "homosexual transmission" underestimate the actual number of men infected via this route. Furthermore, because of the residual stigma attached to homosexual activities, it is likely that some HIV-infected men who have sex with men have dishonestly or incorrectly attributed transmission to heterosexual contact. In any case, the relatively large proportion of cases in the catch-all "Other/Unknown" category testifies to Japanese reticence about confronting the HIV/AIDS crisis openly.

Of course, reticence is to be expected in a Japanese society that considers it shameful to be HIV-infected, physically disabled, or chronically ill. In Japan, where wheelchair accessibility is essentially a nonissue, "the disabled live in their own version of apartheid — a world that gives an insight into what people with AIDS, a far worse stigma, are encountering" (Sesser, 1994, p. 63). In a racially and culturally homogenous country such as Japan, difference breeds contempt and misunderstanding. To be noticeably different in Japan is to be "the nail that sticks up," a nail which, not surprisingly, "gets hammered down" (Sesser, 1994, p. 64). The fear of social ostracism is so complete that as of 1995 only four HIV-infected people had publicly proclaimed their seropositivity: two hemophiliacs and two self-identified gay men (Ikeda, 1995).

Beyond the possible loss of emotional support from loved ones, including friends and family, public disclosure of an HIV-positive diagnosis can precipitate loss of employment, insurance, and medical coverage (Ikeda, 1995) and discrimination in housing, schools, and jobs (Feldman & Yonemoto, 1992). Because of this, some HIV-positive Japanese elect to pay medical costs themselves, rather than admit to their insurance companies and employers that they are infected. Familial ostracism, on the other hand, may be necessary to protect the family from the communitywide censure that in Japan often accompanies the shame of having an HIV-infected relative (in much the same fashion, the descendants of survivors of the nuclear attacks on Hiroshima and Nagasaki remain socially stigmatized).

Ignorance and discrimination extend to the medical profession as well. Many Japanese healthcare professionals have a very limited understanding of HIV infection and AIDS [in one study, conducted in 1990, almost half of the nurses interviewed believed that HIV was transmissible by mosquitoes and small amounts of saliva, and a similar proportion worried that they themselves might be infected (Kawahara et al., 1994)]. Many physicians are unwilling to treat AIDS patients, who may also be turned away from public hospitals [only 15 percent of the hospitals responding to a 1994 survey admitted that they accepted HIV-positive and AIDS patients (Hoshino, 1995)]. As a consequence of widespread social opprobrium, hospitals that treat HIV-positive patients often do so clandestinely, lest they frighten away their noninfected customers, who fear both the risk of contagion and the possibility of being labeled, by association, as HIV-positive themselves (Hoshino, 1995; Sesser, 1994). In an attempt to reassure skittish patients, one public hospital posted a notice insisting that it had no HIV-positive patients (Ikeda, 1995).

In Japan, fears of social ostracism and financial ruin discourage people from getting tested for the presence of HIV antibodies. This problem was exacerbated by the 1989 passage of the so-called AIDS Prevention Law ("The Law Concerning Prevention of Acquired Immunodeficiency Syndrome"), which requires healthcare professionals to report within 7 days every HIV-positive blood test to the local prefecture, which in turn reports to the AIDS Surveillance Committee (Miyazaki & Naemura, 1994). By law, the physician must report any seropositive patient's age, gender, nationality/ethnicity, and the putative route of infection. [The reporting requirements do not apply to people infected through the receipt of tainted blood, however. This exception arose as a concession meant to mollify vocal hemophiliac groups displeased by a preliminary draft of the legislation, which was "leaked" to the media (Feldman & Yonemoto, 1992).] Although neither the patient's name nor any other identifying information are required in most cases, a physician is obligated to report both the patient's name and address if he or she believes the patient will ignore doctor's orders. The law also empowers prefectural governors to interview and subsequently order the compulsory HIV antibody testing of suspected "HIV carriers" (Swinbanks, 1987). Fortunately, many of the more intrusive provisions of the AIDS Prevention Law have never been enforced (Nakagawa & Morino, 1994).

However well-intentioned, this level of scrutiny may, in fact, be epidemiologically counterproductive. As Eriko Ikeda, chief director of the cultural programs section at Japan Broadcasting Corporation argues, "when there is little incentive for people to want to be tested for AIDS in the first place, it is extremely doubtful that surveillance by the government will change their minds, especially when all they can hope for after a trip to the clinic is to be treated like an untouchable" (Ikeda, 1995, p. 24). Suggestive evidence that testing is not reaching the populations most in need was obtained by Gen Ohi and colleagues, who surveyed students, office workers, self-identified homosexual men, and prostitutes about their willingness to be tested under the provisions of the AIDS Prevention Law, which had recently been proposed but was not yet passed by the Diet. The results revealed an inverse relationship between self-perceived risk of infection and willingness to be tested, with prostitutes and gay men the least willing to undergo HIV antibody testing (Ohi et al., 1988).

The consequences of a positive test are so feared that some Japanese fly thousands of miles to be confidentially tested in Hawaii (Sesser, 1994). Many others simply forego testing, despite behaviors that place them at risk of infection. At the other extreme, profound ignorance of transmission mechanisms causes men and women at little or no risk to anxiously flood AIDS hotlines with phone calls seeking reassurance. Fear is especially high among self-identified gay men, regardless of the objective risk of infection. For example, according to Megumi Baba, head of the Waikiki Health Center's Japanese testing and counseling program, some of the gay men who travel to Hawaii to get tested have never even had sex (Sesser, 1994). Just being gay, they believe, puts them at risk. Although this notion may seem incredibly naive, it is not uncommon in Japan, where AIDS is often still perceived as a "gay disease" — especially a disease of gay foreigners. The persistence of such attitudes can be explained, in part, by the paucity of sexuality and AIDS education sanctioned by the government. Moreover, efforts to heighten AIDS awareness and increase knowledge of the particulars of this disease are handcuffed by Japanese reticence to openly discuss sexuality in the schools. Commenting upon the Ministry of Education's guidelines for HIV/AIDS education in the public schools, the Japanese sexuality educator, Kyoko Kitazawa, suggests that the Ministry "intends that teachers should teach HIV/AIDS prevention to students without mentioning sexual intercourse" (Kitazawa, 1993/94, p. 11).

The group most often blamed for the introduction and maintenance of HIV infection in Japan are "foreigners" (*gaijin*) — originally gay tourists, but later extended to include foreign-born commercial sex workers. Prejudice against foreigners is prevalent within the

Japanese gay community as well. Foreigners are *persona non grata* at many (but certainly not all) gay Japanese establishments, including some bath houses, bars, and "love hotels." In most cases the discrimination is open. For example, several listings in *Spartacus*, the international guide for gay travelers, include admonishments warning foreign visitors that "Only Japanese [are] Welcome." Such attitudes reflect both longstanding cultural beliefs that foreigners are "dirty" and contact with them potentially "polluting" (Hendry, 1987), as well as a somewhat realistic appraisal of the relatively greater proportion of foreign gay men who are infected with HIV and with whom, consequently, sexual activity poses an elevated risk of HIV transmission.

The widespread Japanese perception of AIDS as a disease of foreigners and foreign countries (especially America) is also evident in the reporting requirements of the AIDS Prevention Law, which mandates not only the reporting of the suspected mode of transmission, but also the country where transmission is believed to have occurred. It is, of course, patently absurd to suppose it possible in all cases to pinpoint the exact occasion of HIV transmission, especially after a lapse of up to 10 years (as noted earlier, in Japan relatively few cases of HIV infection are detected prior to the onset of AIDS). Nevertheless, with the exception of a few ambiguous cases, the AIDS Surveillance Committee has managed to assign every known case of HIV infection to either the "Within Japan" or the "Outside Japan" category (Miyazaki & Naemura, 1994). The majority of heterosexually infected people, it is claimed, were infected overseas, whereas domestic transmission is blamed in most cases of homosexual infection.

Physical attacks on gays ("gay-bashing") are fortunately rather rare in Japan, where laws against violence tend to be respected (Paxton, 1991). Nevertheless, homophobia remains a tangible problem for the country's openly gay men and women. As discussed previously, for a Japanese man to enjoy the physical attractions of another man is one thing; to turn his back on family — including ancestors, extant relatives, and future descendants — by failing to reproduce is quite another. Thus, exclusive homosexuality remains taboo. The exclusively homosexual man or woman occupies the fringes of Japanese society, shamed by his or her identity, stigmatized by difference, and threatened by societal ignorance. The association of homosexuality with AIDS in the minds of many Japanese has only made the gay Japanese struggle for basic human rights and dignity more difficult.

One striking example of anti-gay discrimination took place in 1990 at a public youth center in Tokyo. In this now famous case, a small group of self-identified gay and lesbian youth known as OCCUR (Association for the Lesbian and Gay Movement) was forbidden access by the municipal government to a publicly funded facility, the Fuchu Youth House, after openly proclaiming their sexual orientation. The group, whose main organizational objectives include disseminating accurate information about homosexuality to the Japanese public and providing AIDS education to the gay community, has about 300 members and is one of Japan's most visible gay and lesbian organizations (Sesser, 1994). The Tokyo Board of Education, which manages Fuchu Youth House, explained their decision to deny OCCUR use of the facility by suggesting that "if homosexuals use the center, this will cause a bad influence on the education of youth" (Nakagawa, Morino, & Kazama, 1994, p. 64). Likewise the director of the center maintained that, "Fuchu Youth House has a duty to promote the sound development of young people" (Paxton, 1991, p. 56), implying that information about homosexuality and AIDS, and interactions with gay and lesbian youth would have a detrimental effect on the moral development of other young Japanese.

Soon thereafter, OCCUR filed a lawsuit — the first ever gay rights suit in Japan — charging the Tokyo Board of Education with illegal discrimination. In a landmark legal decision handed down in 1994, a Tokyo district court ruled in favor of the plaintiffs, Takashi Kazawa, Masanori Kanda, and Masahi Nagata, finding that the municipal government acted in a discriminatory manner, and awarded them $2600 in compensation. The court further determined that the discrimination and harassment of lesbians and gays should not be allowed and, according to OCCUR, recognized homosexuality as a valid sexual orientation.

Although the OCCUR decision has been hailed as a major victory for gay and lesbian rights in Japan, the blatant anti-gay bias evinced by the Tokyo government (and other more subtle forms of homophobia) persists. This is especially troubling in light of the ignorance that surrounds both homosexuality and AIDS in Japan. The OCCUR decision coincides with a growing awareness in the international AIDS prevention community of the epidemiological importance of ensuring basic human and civil rights (Mann et al., 1995). Globally, the primary weapons against AIDS and HIV infection are knowledge and understanding. The substantial behavioral changes made by gay men in large American and European cities in the 1980s provides powerful testimony to the effectiveness of knowledge and community unity in combating infection. But the organizational and educational activities necessary to increase AIDS awareness in the community cannot be conducted in the shadows, under a thick veil of homophobia, as Tokyo's Board of Education would have it. The OCCUR case thus has implications beyond the immediacy of establishing basic human and civil rights for Japanese gays; it may also serve as the cornerstone of a nascent campaign against HIV/AIDS in the Japanese gay community.

CONCLUSION

Historically, Japanese society has demonstrated comparatively tolerant attitudes toward homosexuality, provided that social constraints of moderation, propriety, and duty to one's family were respected. Homosexuality was thus typically expressed within a context of bisexuality, regardless of whether this duality in sexual personae was necessarily consonant with the core identity of the Japanese men and women in question. However, recently more and more Japanese are self-identifying as gay or lesbian. The adoption of an exclusively gay or lesbian identity, especially when openly and publicly expressed, challenges traditional Japanese notions of the proper role of same-sex behaviors in the sociosexual economy, elevating these behaviors from mere diversions to possible barriers to familial continuity.

Temporally coincident with this challenge comes an equally potent attack from without — the very real threat of a widely disseminated AIDS epidemic. Condom use with casual partners remains quite low for both heterosexual and homosexual activities (Munakata & Tajima, 1996), which is especially troubling in a country in which visiting prostitutes rivals baseball in popular imagination (among men) and in which bisexuality is more socially acceptable than exclusive homosexuality. Many of Japan's prostitutes and other commercial sex workers are immigrants from counties such as Thailand and the Philippines in which the prevalence of HIV is staggeringly high. Moreover, the risky practice of traveling to foreign countries on "sex junkets" remains popular with gay and straight Japanese alike (including women). Bisexuality, as practiced in Japan, poses an additional threat by providing uninterrupted chains of transmission, from female to male, male to male, and male to female. Combined with the widespread ignorance of HIV transmission routes that exists in Japan, these several factors could foretell a potentially devastating AIDS epidemic (Munakata & Tajima, 1996). [Existing high levels of infection with other sexually transmitted diseases among homosexual and bisexual Japanese men (Isomura & Mizogami, 1992) demonstrates the potential for rapid dissemination of HIV once established.]

There is a danger, of course, that fear about AIDS and a naive association of AIDS with homosexual behavior might lead to further discrimination against gay men and women. In Japan, there are no laws protecting people from employment, housing, or other discrimination based on perceived sexual orientation. As suggested in this chapter, traditional tolerance for same-sex relationships could wilt under the combined stress of association with a potentially fatal disease and violation of the social compact that places reproduction above personal self-fulfillment. The AIDS Prevention Law, which contains several clauses of a discriminatory nature, suggests the potential for restrictive legislation targeting gay Japanese and others affected by AIDS. However, this potential is lessened somewhat by the Japanese propensity for compromise. Moreover, if the OCCUR case can be generalized, there is reason to hope that the Japanese courts would be negatively disposed toward further discriminatory actions or legislation. Thus, it is likely that Japan's long-standing legal tolerance of homosexuality can withstand the combined onslaught of AIDS and the reconstruction of homosexuality as an identity rather than a behavior. Moreover, as emphasized throughout this chapter, the "legal" way has never been the Japanese way.

Acknowledgments

We thank Jim Senter of the UCLA Law Library and Alan Hauth of the Center for AIDS Intervention Research for providing bibliographic assistance. Thanks are also due to Rocky Koga, Gary Leupp, and Constance Penley for their thoughtful comments on a preliminary draft of the paper. This research was supported, in part, by grant P30-MH52776 from the National Institute of Mental Health.

REFERENCES

Abramson, P. R. (1986). The cultural context of Japanese sexuality: An American perspective. *Psychologia — An International Journal of Psychology in the Orient, 29*, 1–9.

Abramson, P. R., & Hayashi, H. (1984). Pornography in Japan. In N. M. Malamuth & E. Donnerstein (Eds.), *Pornography and sexual aggression* (pp. 173–183). New York: Academic Press.

Abramson, P. R., & Pinkerton, S. D. (1995). *With pleasure: Thoughts on the nature of human sexuality.* New York: Oxford University Press.

Allison, A. (1996). *Permitted and prohibited desires: Mothers, comics, and censorship in Japan.* Chicago: Westview Press.

Audet, B. (1994). Government struggles to develop action plan as concern about AIDS grows in Japan. *Canadian Journal of Medicine, 151*, 351–352.

Baruma, I. (1984). *Behind the mask: On sexual demons, sacred mothers, transvestites, gangsters, drifters, and other Japanese cultural heroes.* New York: Pantheon.

Beer, L. W. (1984). *Freedom of expression in Japan: A study in comparative law, politics and society.* Tokyo: Kodansha International Ltd.

Benedict, R. (1946). *The chrysanthemum and the sword: patterns of Japanese culture.* Boston: Houghton Mifflin.

Bolz, H. F. (1980). Judicial review in Japan: The strategy of restraint. *Hastings International and Comparative Law Review, 87,* 77–83.

Bornoff, N. (1991). *Pink samurai: Love, marriage & sex in contemporary Japan.* New York: Pocket Books.

Bowers, F. (1974). *Japanese theater.* Tokyo: Tuttle.

Brown, R. G. (1979). Emerging judicial restraints on constitutional guarantees of freedom of expression. In L. Gray & G. Whitmore (Eds.), *Current studies in Japanese law* (Occasional paper 12, pp. 24–38). University of Michigan: Center for Japanese Studies.

Conner, R. P., & Donaldson, S. (1990). Buddhism. In W. R. Dynes (Ed.), *Encyclopedia of homosexuality* (pp. 168–171). New York: Garland.

DeVos, G. A. (1973). *Socialization for achievement.* Berkeley: University of California Press.

Feldman, E. A., & Yonemoto, S. (1992). Japan: AIDS as a "non-issue." In D. L. Kipp & R. Bayer (Eds.), *AIDS in the industrialized democracies* (pp. 339–360). New Brunswick, NJ: Rutgers University Press.

Guest, R. (1995). Japan proposes settlement for tainted blood. *British Medical Journal, 311,* 1044–1045.

Haley, J. O. (1982). Sheathing the sword of justice in Japan: An essay on law without sanctions. *Journal of Japanese Studies, 2,* 265–274.

Haley, J. O. (1984). Introduction: Legal vs. social controls. *Law in Japan: An Annual, 17,* 1–6.

Hendry, J. (1987). *Understanding Japanese society.* London: Routledge.

Hoshii, I. (1987). *The world of sex, vol. 4: Sex in ethics and law.* Woodchurch, England: Paul Norbury.

Hoshino, K. (1995). HIV+/AIDS-related bioethical issues in Japan. *Bioethics, 9,* 303–308.

Ikeda, E. (1995). Society and AIDS. *Japan Quarterly, 42,* 21–32.

Isomura, S., & Mizogami, M. (1992). The low rate of HIV infection in Japanese homosexual and bisexual men: An analysis of HIV seroprevalence and behavioural risk factors. *AIDS, 6,* 501–503.

Kamiya, M. (1987). Freedom of expression. Kyoto American Studies Seminar, Specialists Conference, Section II: Judicial Protection of Civil Liberties — A Comparison of American and Japanese Constitutional Law. *Law in Japan, 20,* 12–39.

Kawabata, Y. (1964). *Beauty and sadness.* Tokyo: Tuttle.

Kawahara, N., Hashizume, E., Murashima, S., Tanaka, H., Nagami, K., Mizutani, S., Morishita, T., Tomita, Y., Minami, N., & Deguchi, K. (1994). Changes in knowledge and attitudes about AIDS among nurses in Mie Prefecture, Japan (abstract no. PD0062). *Tenth International Conference on AIDS, 10*(1), 364.

Kawashima, Y. (1983). Americanization of Japanese family law, 1945–1975. *Law in Japan: An Annual, 16,* 54–68.

Kitamura, T. (1994). Summary of the epidemiology of HIV/AIDS in Japan. *AIDS, 8*(Suppl. 2), 95–97.

Kitazawa, K. (1993/94). Sexuality issues in Japan: A view from the front on HIV/AIDS and sexuality education. *SIECUS Report, December 1993/January 1994,* 7–11.

Leupp, G. P. (1995). *Male colors: The construction of homosexuality in Tokugawa Japan.* Berkeley: University of California Press.

Mann, J. M., Gostin, L., Gruskin, S., Brennan, T., Lazzarini, Z., & Fineberg, H. V. (1995). Health and human rights. *Health and Human Rights, 1,* 7–23.

Masami, I. (1963). The rule of law: Constitutional development. In V. Mehren & A. Taylor (Eds.), *Law in Japan: The legal order in a changing society* (pp. 69–91). Cambridge, MA: Harvard University Press.

Miller, N. (1992). *Out in the world: Gay and lesbian life from Buenos Aries to Bangkok.* New York: Vintage.

Mishima, Y. (1968). *Forbidden colors.* New York: Knopf.

Miyazaki, M., & Naemura, M. (1994). Epidemiological characteristics on human immunodeficiency virus infection and acquired immunodeficiency syndrome in Japan. *International Journal of STD & AIDS, 5,* 273–278.

Miyazaki, M., O'Brien, T. R., & Naemura, M. (1995). Surveillance for the acquired immunodeficiency syndrome in Japan. *Journal of Acquired Immunodeficiency Syndromes and Human Retrovirology, 9,* 312–313.

Munakata, T., & Tajima, K. (1996). Japanese risk behaviors and their HIV/AIDS-preventive behaviors. *AIDS Education and Prevention, 8,* 115–133.

Nakagawa, S., Morino, Y., & Kazama, H. (1994). "The AIDS prevention law" in Japan: Has it been preventive or promotive? (abstract no. PD0269). *Tenth International Conference on AIDS, 10*(1), 415.

Ohi, G., Terao, H., Hasegawa, T., Hirano, W., Kai, I., Kobayashi, Y., Inaba, Y., Muranatsu, Y., Miyama, T., Ashizawa, M., Kamakura, M., Uemura, I., & Niimi, T. (1988). Notification of HIV carriers: Possible effect on uptake of AIDS testing. *Lancet, 2,* 947–949.

Oppler, A. C. (1949). The reform of Japan's legal and judicial system under allied occupation. *Washington Law Review, 24,* 293.

Paxton, M. (1991). Out of the closet in Japan. *World Press Review, 38,* 56.

Ramseyer, J. M. (1995). Oko v. Sako: Kyogen and litigation in medieval Japan. *Law in Japan: An Annual, 25,* 135–140.

Ross, C. (1995). Way paved for HIV settlement talks in Japan. *Lancet, 346,* 1091.

Schalow, P. G. (1990a). Japan. In W. R. Dynes (Ed.), *Encyclopedia of homosexuality* (pp. 632–636). New York: Garland.

Schalow, P. G. (1990b). Samurai. In W. R. Dynes (Ed.), *Encyclopedia of homosexuality* (pp. 1149–1150). New York: Garland.

Seidensticker, E. C. (Trans.). (1976). *The tale of Genji.* New York: Knopf.

Sesser, S. (1994). Hidden death. *New Yorker, 70*(37), 62–64, 66–68, 87–88, 90.

Swinbanks, D. (1987). AIDS becomes a notifiable disease in Japan despite protests. *Nature, 326,* 232.

Takayanagi, K. (1967). The conceptual background of the constitutional revision debate in the Constitution Investigation Commission. *Law in Japan: An Annual, 7,* 1–24.

Yamada, K. (1992). Pathological status and therapy of HIV-infected hemophiliacs in Japan. *Southeast Asian Journal of Tropical Medicine and Public Health, 23*(Suppl. 2), 127–130.

5

Mexico

JUAN LUIS ÁLVAREZ-GAYOU JURGENSON

Introduction

Mexico is a federal, democratic republic of 31 states and a federal district, with the federal executive at Mexico City. The population of Mexico exceeds 91 million and is predominantly *mestizo* (mixed race), derived from the original pre-Colombian inhabitants and the European colonials, mainly Spanish and French. Indians from numerous and distinct cultures (Paz, 1961) make up a substantial minority, especially in the south, totaling about 10 million. The population is youthful, growing, and becoming increasingly urbanized. In 1992, 58.5 percent were under 24, 55.2 percent were classed as economically active, and 57.4 percent were living in towns with populations of more than 15,000 (Instituto Nacional de Geografía, 1995). The predominant religion is Roman Catholic.

Mexico has had a turbulent history. The colonial period lasted from the year 1520 for 300 years until revolution achieved independence. Thereafter, for most of the nineteenth century, save for a period of relative calm under the presidency of Porfirio Diaz (1876–1910), the country was in a perpetual state of civil war, in addition to war with the United States and invasion by France. When Diaz was overthrown in another revolution a further period of military-dominated governments and intermittent strife followed. Only in the last 70 years has there been substantial peace.

The country remains politically very unsettled. Only in recent times has a true opposition to one-party rule been established. A conflict in Chiapas, where the mainly Indian Zapatista Liberation Army started an armed movement, has given impetus to the transition to a more democratic system. Popular discontent with modern republican governments centers on complaints of financial corruption, which many believe has been the cause of impoverishment in the population. Elections for Congress are due in 1997 and for president in 2000, and there is a strong possibility that the highly conservative Partidó Acción Nacional (PAN) will win important positions. This party has extremely conservative views on sexual issues such as abortion and gay liberation. For example, the mayor of the large city of Guadalajara, where this party is in power, tried to ban the wearing of mini-skirts by women employees in government offices. It has been established that this party is linked financially to very powerful ultra-right-wing groups (González, 1994). A peculiarity of the Mexican situation is the strong link between political conflicts and the resulting economic backlashes that adversely affect the lower and middle classes especially.

JUAN LUIS ÁLVAREZ-GAYOU JURGENSON • Mexican Institute of Sexology, Del. Cuauhtémoc, México, D.F. CP 06760, Mexico.

Sociolegal Control of Homosexuality, edited by West and Green, Plenum Press, New York, 1997.

CULTURE AND VIEWS ON HOMOSEXUALITY

Although the majority of the population is *mestizo*, as a result of interbreeding of indigenes and immigrants, the culture, due to early Spanish occupation, is strongly influenced by Judeo-Christian ideology, which, among other things, strongly censures and seeks to suppress any form of nonreproductive sexual activity.

In examining the shaping of attitudes toward homosexuality, one must consider some of the values that are believed to have prevailed among the indigenous population. There is evidence of sex between persons of the same gender being severely punished by the Aztecs and of women who engaged in lesbian acts being garotted (Requena, 1979). The Aztecs are thought to have penalized particularly severely the *cuiloni*, that is, the passive, effeminate partners in intermale sex (Novo, 1972). Nevertheless, attitudes appear to have differed among some of the native peoples. Some indigenous groups accepted or practiced male homosexuality more freely, as in the region of Juchitan in the state of Oaxaca, among the Huastecos and Totonacos in the state of Veracruz, and among the Huichol and Cora Indians of the state of Nayarit (Lumsden, 1991). Reports of widely prevalent homosexual behavior among the natives of the state of Veracruz are referred to by Bernal Diaz del Castillo and Hernán Cortez (Requena, 1979).

Research by Italian anthropologist Miano-Borruso (1996) among inhabitants of the Tehuantepec Isthmus who are of Zapotec origin has found that the male homosexual has a recognized place in that society. Known as *muxe* or *mampo*, he is usually considered by the mother as the best of her sons. Whereas women work outside, he stays and looks after the home and, unlike other sons who leave to marry, stays to care for the parents in their old age. As Miano-Borruso notes, "The Zapotec culture has found family and social spaces for them and has assigned functions that allow them to integrate with dignity to normal life" (1996).

Although generalizations are problematic in such a large and varied country, in modern Mexico homosexuality attracts wide social disapproval. It is considered by many to be a deviance, a vice, and a sign of decadence or mental disease. Most of the population are poorly informed on sexual matters, and a great amount of myth prevails, such as the idea that male homosexuals are sexually aggressive, liable to commit the most cruel crimes or to seek to overpower any male that crosses their path; that any teacher who is homosexual will be a child abuser and convert children to this "vicious behavior"; or that male homosexuals wish to be women.

Family tradition is strong in Mexico, and men remain in the parental home until they marry. Most families would be deeply shamed to have an overtly homosexual son. Some families maintain a conspiracy of silence to avoid confrontation with what they do not want to have to acknowledge. Many young gay men take pains to keep their homosexual contacts covert and preserve a front of heterosexual masculinity. They are helped in doing so by the fact that only effeminate males, *maricónes*, are readily identified as deviants. Consequently, only a minority of the men who have frequent same-sex contacts, many of whom marry and have families of their own, mix freely in overtly gay circles or cohabit with a lover (Carrier, 1995). Reputations are saved by a macho stance, presumed adherence to the active role in anal intercourse, and a choice of submissive, effeminate partners who can be regarded as substitutes for women.

The Law

The constitution of Mexico grants its citizens individual freedom in all respects that do not transgress the rights of others. On the other hand, every state has its own penal code that establishes which behaviors amount to criminal offenses and sets the punishment for them. None of the state penal codes considers homosexual contact in itself a criminal offense. A noticeable exception occurs in the penal code of the Federal District (site of Mexico City), in which, in Article 201, imprisonment of 3–8 years applies to anyone

> who facilitates or procures the corruption of a minor under 18 years of age,... [by] inducing to the practice of begging, alcoholism, to the consumption of narcotic drugs, to the practice of prostitution, homosexualism, to be part of an organized delinquent group or to commit any crime.... When by means of the repeated practice of the corrupted acts the under age or incapacitated [individual] acquires the habits of alcoholism, drug dependence, prostitution, homosexuality or to be part of a delinquent group the punishment will be an imprisonment of 5 to 10 years. (Penal Code, 1995)

The law thus places homosexuality on a level with alcohol abuse, illicit drug use, prostitution, and other behaviors that people regard as "vices." This seems to reflect the generally prevalent, uneducated idea of homosexuality. Even though, apart from this exception, homosexuality does not feature in the criminal law, the larger cities have bylaws and police rulings that are frequently used by corrupt officers to prey upon homosexuals. For instance, these rulings give police the right to "arrest anyone who behaves and uses language that contravenes public decency" or "anyone who makes gestures that are offensive to other people ... who disturbs public order ... who invites, permits or engages in prostitution or carnal commerce" (Asamblea de Representantes, 1995). The main factor that determines the decision to arrest is the judgment of uneducated, underpaid, and corrupt policemen. Anything they choose can be used by police officers to arrest someone, especially a "gay attitude." Their real purpose is to threaten, blackmail, and finally obtain money for letting the gay man go free. A contributing factor to this is the hierarchical system whereby senior police officers receive money from those under them, thereby creating a vicious circle of corruption that obliges the policeman on the street to extort money in any possible way. A majority of gay men in Mexico City have reportedly experienced police extortion.

City authorities also can show intolerance. Periodically, the city authorities enforce raids in certain areas, mainly where there are a great number of bars. They are meant to be looking for weapons or drugs, but there are always men in these bars who are detained for no other reason than because they are homosexual and can be made to pay to be set free. In 1991 Mexico was the chosen venue for the Annual Conference of the International Gay and Lesbian Association (ILGA), which was scheduled to take place in Guadalajara; the municipal authorities, with no real cause other than the supposed need to safeguard public morality, refused to allow the event to take place in the city, and the conference had to be moved to the Port of Acapulco.

In contrast to the attitudes of the authorities toward male homosexuality, in general, an absolute silence is preserved regarding lesbianism. This fact could stem from Judeo-Christian ideology, wherein an important consideration is to avoid waste of the male breeding cells. When men ejaculate outside a vagina, whether in masturbatory activity or in homosexual acts or even in zoophilic activity, the reproductive waste is evident, whereas a female never "loses" ova by masturbating or having a lesbian encounter.

THE MEDIA

Books, Newspapers, and Magazines

Although it does not compare with activity in the most developed countries, the publishing industry in Mexico is stronger than in other Latin American countries and has shown greater interest in publishing books concerned with sexual matters, both by local authors and by foreign authors in translation. Books dealing with homosexuality, however, are highly exceptional, and the few that have appeared have been the work of small, noncommercial outlets.

The main national circulation newspapers are published in Mexico City, although many States have their own local papers. Recently, an influential newspaper from the industrialized state of Nuevo Leon has started daily publication of an affiliate in Mexico City called *Reforma*. The rightwing conservative newspapers do not usually have articles on sexuality. When it started, *Reforma* had a weekend section on the subject, but this has ceased.

Liberal papers like *La Jornada* or *Uno mas Uno* are strongly pro-feminist, pro-gay liberation, anti-sexual violence, and pro-decriminalization of abortion. It is estimated that close to 2 million clandestine and illegal abortions are performed in Mexico every year, creating severe health problems for many women.

For some years *El Nacional*, a newspaper owned and operated by the government, published a weekend supplement on HIV/AIDS that dealt openly with gay and bisexual matters as well as preventive or safe-sex procedures. It was discontinued without explanation at the beginning of 1995.

There are a great number of magazines published on a great variety of subjects and with a diversity of prices and printing quality. Those dealing with sexuality could be rated as soft-porn and are exclusively heterosexual. For many years a local subsidiary of *Playboy* magazine has been published, but its price is too high for the majority of the population.

Specialist Gay Magazines

For about 5 years a magazine for gay men called *Macho Tips* was published and sold in newsstands. It had articles by known figures of the gay scene as well as some written by sexologists and other authors. It included somewhat explicit color photographs of nude men, but these men were never engaged in sexual activity. Probably more for financial reasons than anything else it was discontinued. *Hermes*, another gay magazine, has also ceased recently after circulating for 2 or 3 years.

Currently only two mainly gay magazines are published in Mexico. One is popular and inexpensive, under $1 U.S. and entitled *Efebos, los hombres mas bellos* [Ephoebus, the most beautiful men]. It features explicit pictures of poor photographic quality, mostly monochrome, showing young nude males, some with an erection and in apparent masturbatory activity. It includes short articles, a news section, and a readers' letter section giving names and addresses. The second magazine, *Boys and Toys*, is larger and of better quality, costing over $3 U.S. The editor is a very well-known transvestite actor and gay liberation activist, Tito Vasconcelos. The magazine combines serious political articles and news concerning gay liberation matters with male fashion, a guide to the gay bars of several cities, interviews with theatrical personalities, and a substantial classified announcement section listed state-by-state for 26 of the 31 states of the Mexican Republic. Most of the announcements are requesting or offering contact. A few advertisers state that they are married and the great majority ask for a letter with a picture. There is a short international section, with many entries from Cuba, some from Europe and some from other South American countries — Argentina, Colombia, Peru, Ecuador, and Panama. The pages devoted to nude color photographs of male models repeat the printed message "safe sex — only with a condom."

Other gay magazines on sale in newsstands are mainly imported from Spain. In addition, noncommercial pamphlets are published by many gay groups. An example is *Ser gay*, which is distributed in bars and gathering places, with information on what to do, where to go — bars, discos, cultural activities, and more — and advertisements directed to gay men. Another is *El Arca de Noé* [Noah's Ark], which has only a classified section and advertisements.

Television

Two private channels compete in providing national coverage, Televisa and Azteca. Matters of sexuality are presented occasionally, mainly on talk shows or journalistic programs. Mexican networks have a strong self-censuring attitude, and therefore homosexuality is usually not dealt with unless the program deals with HIV/AIDS. Preventive messages from the official government AIDS agency, Consejo Nacional Para el Sindrome De Immuno Deficiencia Adquirida (CONASIDA), concerning AIDS, were being aired, but because the mention of the use of condoms attracted pressure from ultra-right-wing groups, these messages have been discontinued. However, in connection with child sexual molestation, Televisa has sustained for a good number of years messages aimed at advising children of their right to say no to anyone who approaches them.

Radio

Unlike television, radio has had a recent plethora of programs related to sexuality. All aspects, including male homosexuality and lesbianism, are spoken about openly. In Mexico City, at least three broadcasting companies that have national coverage have had programs on sexuality for at least 2 years. Many other stations also feature the same, but sometimes the quality and accuracy can be questionable. One station, with no national coverage, has an exclusively gay program conducted by the aforementioned actor Tito Vasconcelos. The weekly program deals with interviews, gossip, music, and news of the gay community. Its noncommercial transmitting station belongs to the Ministry of Education, which has been known to be quite liberal despite its governmental origin. Another weekly program, transmitted via a station owned by Televisa, deals exclusively with gay matters and is presented by gay men. Both programs aim at providing a service to the gay community rather than educating the general public.

The medium of radio has the best opportunity to put out gay issues. With the exception of the two specialized programs cited, however, there is clearly a tendency to link the material with HIV/AIDS and not with gay rights.

THE GAY MALE SCENE

Large-scale gay communities such as those that exist in San Francisco and other places in the United States are not to be found in Mexico, but most of the larger cities do have gay bars, which are listed in the magazine *Boys and Toys*. Mexico City has nearly 30 identified bars and discos, many of them featuring transvestite shows. Some of the bars in Mexico City, notably El Taller [The Workshop] and El Vaquero [The Cowboy], have operated for a decade or more; for many years, the latter has included a sex shop with explicit gay material. It is generally supposed that these bars operate freely, not because of an open attitude on the part of the regulatory authorities and officials, but more likely through the payment of fixed unofficial fees.

At least in Mexico City, a fair number of clothing shops and a few sex shops target the homosexual community in some of their displays. General businesses, such as travel agencies, sometimes advertise in the gay magazines. Rendezvous sites — "cruising areas" — are not much in evidence in Mexico City, save for the gay bars and some well known cafés, but the subway is frequented for this purpose. Young male transvestite prostitutes can be seen on the streets in Mexico City and some other large towns. Whether the fair number of clients they seem to attract are all aware of their true sex is doubtful. A popular Miss Mexico contest for transvestites is scheduled every year.

Some prominent intellectuals, writers, actors, and sculptors are part of the gay scene. A quantity of gay literature, poetry, and novels is published by commercial firms and sells well. An example is *El Vampiro de la Colonia Roma* by Luis Zapata. There are plays by openly gay writers, and Mexico City is said to have more gay theater and literature than any other Spanish-speaking city in Latin America (Lumsden, 1991). One gay author, founder of the group Guerilla Gay, Xabier Lizárraga, is also one of the founders of the Mexican Institute of Sexology, a private organization dedicated to education and research on all sexual issues, not just those related to homosexuality.

With the support of a cultural museum belonging to the prestigious National Autonomous University (UNAM), a Semana Cultural Lésbica Gay [Lesbian Gay Cultural Week] is held annually. In 1995 the event was dedicated to Sor. Juana Inés de la Cruz, the highly reputed nun, poet, and writer who lived 100 years ago. The motto of the week was "Against intolerance, our presence." In 1996, the cultural week will be in honor of the laureate French writer Marguerite Yourcenar and the Italian filmmaker Pier Paolo Pasolini.

In most of their activities the gay and lesbian communities remain separated, but for some purposes, mainly cultural enterprises, they act together. One example is the cultural week organized by the Circulo Cultural Gay, in which both genders participate. For the last 23 years the Parade of Gay and Lesbian Pride has taken place each June in Mexico City, crossing the main streets of the city center. The press and the media cover the parade, but mostly with a somewhat mocking tone, particularly aroused by the transvestites in the parade. Some participants in the parade tend to be verbally aggressive toward bystanders, and others shout imaginative and comic slogans. Within the gay community opinions differ; some criticize the presence of transvestites, and some consider the parade as political and defend the gay, festive atmosphere as freedom of expression. The inclusion of the lesbian movement in this parade as well as in the cultural week is a development of the 1990s.

There are many gay groups, such as Ser Humano and Ave de México, working for AIDS prevention, education, and assistance to afflicted persons. Other groups, such as Colectivo Sol, also work strongly for gay rights and human rights and have very clear political positions. Many groups are formed but maintain a low profile and are sometimes short-lived. In many cities in the Mexican states there are groups working actively, but they are obliged to do so clandestinely for fear of official repression or to avoid the social stigma in their communities that would attach itself to them and their families. Groups can afford to be more open only in the big towns, such as Mexico City, Guadalajara, Monterrey, Xalapa, and a few others. Some groups have been at work for many years, such as Guerrilla Gay and Colectivo Sol in Mexico City, the Grupo Homosexual de Liberación (GOHL) in Guadalajara (which some years ago was far more active and influential than any of the groups in Mexico City), and Xochiquetzal in the city of Xalapa, named after the Aztec goddess who, with Xochipilli, protected "illicit" sexual relations and even prostitution (Quezada, 1989). A recently formed Jewish group of gay males called Shalom Amigos is especially noteworthy, as the Jewish community in Mexico traditionally has been extremely conservative regarding sexual matters and very opposed to homosexuality.

Gay groups locally and in Mexico City have taken a strong political stand and have mobilized human rights campaigners against the murder, persecution, and incarceration of gay transvestite prostitutes in the dissident state of Chiapas in 1995 and 1996. They demand the protection of human rights and the release of those affected. There have been references to this in foreign media, but such matters receive scant coverage in Mexico.

For the religiously inclined in the gay community, there is an ecumenical church, La Iglesia de la Comunidad Metropolitana [The Church of the Metropolitan Community], which was originally founded in Los Angeles in 1968 by Rev. Troy Perry. It claims to have 200 chapters in 11 countries. Other than the chapter in Mexico City, the church has chapters in Cuernavaca and Guadalajara and may soon have others in Monterrey and Veracruz. The church advertises in *Boys and Toys* magazine.

THE LESBIAN SCENE

In Mexico, the lesbian scene has a relatively low profile. Although there are some active groups, because of their lack of confidence in divulging information, even when given anonymously, it proved much more difficult to obtain knowledge about them than about gay men's groups. The first organized group of lesbians was established in Mexico in 1977. Since then many others have emerged and disappeared, such as Lesbos and Oikabeth, the latter lasting for 7 years until its disappearance in 1984. The lesbian movement has always been closely related to feminism and political issues, much more so than the male gay movement. For instance, in 1978 Oikabeth aligned with the National Front for the Liberation of Woman (FENALIDEM) and also joined up with the National Front Against Repression. When the lesbian groups dissolved, many of their members continued to participate actively in political and feminist activities. Also in that year, Oikabeth, the

Lambda group (a mixed gay and lesbian group), and Fhar put forward three lesbians and three gay men as candidates in the elections for Congress.

In 1984 lesbians separated from the mixed group GOHL in Guadalajara and set up the specifically lesbian group Patlatonalli, although they still worked together for cultural and other activities. In 1985, groups emerged that started working in the field of HIV/AIDS among lesbians and gay men, thus beginning a diversification of purpose among the organizations.

Other lesbian groups have formed and later disappeared or fragmented. Several groups jointly organized the First National Lesbian Encounter in Guadalajara in 1988, but following a second Encounter in Mexico City in 1990 there was considerable disintegration and many women moved into the wider feminist movement. In 1992 El Closet de Sor Juana was started. Sor Juana is the previously mentioned nun-poet who presumably lived in a cloister, hence the word "closet" in the group's title. The organization offers workshops, video debates, a coffee shop, a documentation center, and organized parties. Additional currently active lesbian groups are Tasexma in Mexico City, Patlatonalli and Oasis in Guadalajara, La Fortaleza (for mature lesbians) in Xalapa, and the Lesbian Group of Tijuana.

The groups have two main functions. The first is consciousness-raising through groups that foster reflection; consideration of human, sexual, and reproductive rights; questioning of sexual roles; and discussion of violence toward women from a feminist perspective. The second is to encourage social action to promote recognition of the existence of lesbianism by participation in activities such as round tables and radio and TV programs aimed at increasing public visibility. Lesbian groups also work with gay men to oppose police raids and discrimination and sensationalism in the media. Lesbian groups have prevailed upon the Revolutionary Workers Party to nominate lesbian women as candidates for Congress in two elections.

Lesbians feel that they have only limited recognition among the larger women's groups and political parties. Violence against lesbian groups has not occurred in Mexico, but lesbians feel oppressed through the denial of their existence and the repressive action at family and legal levels. Their groups have to contend with severe financial problems. They have fewer sources of income in comparison with the male gay community, which benefits from male earning power as well as from bars, publications, stores, sex shops, massage parlors, and transvestite prostitution, all of which provide opportunity for commercial activity.

CONCLUDING THOUGHTS

"The meaning attached to homosexuality and the identities of those men who have sex with other men in contemporary Mexico varies across the country. For to be sure Mexico is an incredibly diverse country" (Lumsden, 1991, p. 5). Thus any generalization on the subject for the whole of Mexico will have flaws. Nevertheless, a few general comments can be made.

Lesbian groups, more than gay male groups, tend to focus on internal and self-reflective work as well as political and social activities, even though at the unorganized level there are bars and meeting spaces that cater mainly to lesbians. The sociopolitical agenda of the organized lesbian movement is well expressed in a document by Patria Jiménez Flóres (1994a) in which she puts forth a series of social demands, including the following:

- A general law against discrimination in which discrimination based on sexual orientation is penalized.
- The explicit right of homosexuals to adopt with equal rights of jurisdiction over children with no discrimination related to sexual orientation.
- The prohibition of any attempt to apply any sort of therapy to lesbians and homosexuals with the aim of changing their sexual orientation.
- The right of all heterosexual, bisexual, and homosexual individuals to receive effective, complete, and equal nondiscriminatory attention to reproductive health.

This clear political stand is expressed through lesbian participation in the Consejo Nacional de Representantes de la Convención Nacional Democrática (a meeting called by the Zapatista rebel movement in Chiapas) and with "the demand for a legitimate and democratic government." Lesbian groups from Mexico also participated actively in the Womens' World Conference in Beijing in 1995 (Jiménez & Careaga, 1994b, p. 7).

The future of gay rights, of sex education, and of all issues of sexuality in Mexico is quite uncertain, mainly due to the probability of increased access to higher levels of government by the conservative PAN. Nevertheless, educational programs should aim to separate homosexuality from AIDS in order to direct education in prevention toward the whole population. There is also a need for education on tolerance and human rights, the equality of genders, and the recognition and acceptance of the existence of lesbianism. This requires that education have a predominantly attitudinal ingredient that enhances respect for diversity, for minorities, and for any nonreproductive expression of sexuality that does not harm anyone. This, in my view, can only be achieved through a strong and well-thought-out educational program concentrated on children. They are, after all, the most receptive members of society, and they hold the key to any nation's liberty in the future.

Acknowledgments

Much appreciation is due to the Mexican pioneers, men and women, who for many years have written, researched, and taught about the right of male homosexuals and lesbians to be accepted in society and to enjoy the human right to live and express their diversity.

I thank those who have contributed information and suggestions and have made this chapter possible. They include Gloria Careaga and Patria Jiménez from El Closet de Sor Juana, José Luis Carrasco, and many who did not wish to be mentioned, as well as the many lesbian and gay friends who have enriched my personal and professional life over many years.

REFERENCES

Asamblea de Representantes (Chamber of Representatives of Mexico City). (1995). *Reglamento de policía y buen gobierno de la Ciudad de México*. México City: Edit. Porrúa.

Carrier, J. (1995). *De los otros: Intimacy and homosexuality among Mexican men*. New York: Columbia University Press.

Congreso de la Unión (Chamber of Representatives). (1995). *Código penal del Distrito y territorios federales (Penal Code)*. México City: Edit. Porrúa.

González, E. (1994). *Conservadurismo y sexualidad en México*. México City: Edit. Rayuela.

Instituto Nacional de Geografía, Estadística e Informática [National Census Office] (1996). México City: Official publication.

Jiménez Flores, P. (1994a). *Demandas, propuestas y acciones*. Unpublished manuscript.

Jiménez Flores, P., & Careaga, G. (1994b). *Diagnóstico nacional sobre la participación de las lesbianas de América Latina y El Caribe en la Conferencia Mundial de Mujeres*. Unpublished manuscript.

Lumsden, I. (1991). *Homosexuality, society and the state in Mexico*. México City: Solediciones.

Miano Borruso, M. (1996). Homosexualidad en el Istmo Zapoteco (Homosexuality in the Mexican Zapotec Isthmus). *Archivos Hispanoamericanos de Sexología, II*(2), pp. 83–99.

Novo, S. (1972). *Las locas, el sexo, los burdeles*. México City: Edit. Novaro.

Paz, O. (1961). *The labrynth of solitude*. New York: Grove Press.

Quezada, N. (1989). *Amor y magia amorosa entre los Aztecas*. México City: Universidad Nacional Autónoma de México.

Requena, A. (1979). Sodomy among Native American peoples. *Gay Sunshine, Summer/Fall*, p. 37.

Zapata, L. (1996). El vampiro de la Colonia Roma. México City: Grijalbo.

6

BOLIVIA
Developing a Gay Community— Homosexuality and AIDS

TIMOTHY WRIGHT AND RICHARD WRIGHT

INTRODUCTION

Before AIDS, there was no gay community in Bolivia. To be sure, there were men who had sex with other men, but their relationships rested on a fictionalized notion that one of the partners was a woman. The participants in such encounters could enact this fiction with little difficulty because, for them, anatomy per se did not define gender. Members of this subculture referred to themselves as *gente de ambiente*, which literally means "people of the atmosphere." These people shared a special understanding of the world—an understanding diametrically opposed to the confrontational Anglo-European conception of "being gay," which idealized personal acceptance and public acknowledgment of one's sexual orientation. By contrast, *ambiente* understanding was characterized by a precarious strategy of heterosexual emulation constructed so as not to disturb the status quo.[1]

The social milieu of homosexual men in Bolivia—even in the most cosmopolitan urban centers—continues to be dominated by the *ambiente*. But the coming of AIDS already has changed this milieu and promises to disrupt it further still. Concomitantly, a new understanding of homosexuality influenced by a variety of outside sources is beginning to emerge. These changes have profound implications for the legal and social mechanisms that traditionally have served to regulate homosexual behavior in Bolivia.

ELEMENTS OF THE *AMBIENTE* SUBCULTURE

The *ambiente* subculture in Bolivia is composed of three analytically distinct groups of actors: *travestis*, *camuflados*, and *hombres*. These groups are not mutually exclusive; there is some movement between them, but they coexist uneasily and regard one another with considerable ambivalence. In this sense, it is misleading to equate the *ambiente* with what is commonly understood as a gay community. Nevertheless, shared cultural assumptions about gender and sexuality dictate the way the three groups define themselves and map out their social and sexual geography.

---

[1]For an intriguing discussion of the *ambiente* subculture in another Latin American country, see Taylor (1986).

TIMOTHY WRIGHT • Formerly of Collaborative Program for the Prevention and Control of STDs and AIDS, Santa Cruz, Bolivia.   RICHARD WRIGHT • Department of Criminology and Criminal Justice, University of Missouri–St. Louis, St. Louis, Missouri 63121.

Sociolegal Control of Homosexuality, edited by West and Green, Plenum Press, New York, 1997.

Travestis

In colloquial terms, *travestis* [transvestites] are almost universally defined within Bolivian culture as "easy women in the rough part of town." *Travestis* view themselves as victims of a calamity of nature; only their genitalia and the effects of testosterone challenge their identity as biological women. The solution to this calamity, as they see it, is to adopt a female appearance. Their strategies for achieving this goal vary but, in general, include using heavy make-up and wearing clothing that is culturally charged with connotations of sexual availability. In fact, at times *travestis* are seen by the general public simply as female prostitutes. The public gathering places of *travestis* are restricted to seedy establishments located in the marginal zones of urban areas. These are usually dance halls open all night on weekends where *travestis* can socialize with each other and meet *hombres* [men] for sexual liaisons.

Although not the group with the most numbers within the *ambiente* subculture, only *travestis* fit the Bolivian stereotype of what are commonly called "homosexuals" and are popularly disapproved of as scandalous deviants. Moreover, they do not find universal acceptance within the *ambiente* itself. *Camuflados*, in particular, criticize them as trouble-makers who give all homosexuals a bad name. By contrast, *travestis* see *camuflados* as "traumatized" and "hypocritical" for disguising their "true female nature"; a disguise that is not inconsequential for *travestis* since it leaves the burden of societal rejection squarely on their shoulders.

Camuflados

The term *camuflados* [camouflaged] provides a subtle indication of how homosexuality is understood in Bolivia; homosexuals are "female" males — in essence, fake women. *Camuflados*, unlike *travestis*, do not see themselves as women trapped in men's bodies, but define their "femaleness" in terms of a single sexual practice — the insertee role in anal intercourse. This taboo act is contrary to the Bolivian conception of manliness, but the conventional male appearance of *camuflados* does not betray their deviance.

Camuflados divide themselves into high and low status groups — *jailonas* and *bagres* — according to their socioeconomic position. The perceived naturalness of this division is apparent in the fact that neither group has a specific label for itself. However, each is referred to by members of the other in a pejorative manner. *Jailonas* translates approximately as "snooty, snobby rich girls," while the term *bagres* equates poor camuflados with catfish, scavengers who live off the dregs.[2]

As a camouflaged subgroup among the *ambiente*, *bagres* ironically conspire to escape the scorn reserved for identifiable homosexuals by congregating to socialize in the most public places: plazas, parks, open markets, and principal avenues. This is achieved using coded communication embedded in a veneer of expected male conduct. The public violation of this conduct is staunchly criticized as *quemante* [burning], because it can reveal homosexuality to outsiders. On the other hand, since it is common in Bolivia for men to spend much social time together and since one's presence in such locations lends itself to all sorts of convenient explanations, public areas afford surprisingly invisible and

[2]In Cochabamba, Bolivia's third-largest city, rich *camuflados* are called *hamburgesas* [hamburgers], and poor *camuflados* are called *salchipapas* [french fries with cheap sausage].

(importantly) cost-free opportunities for *bagres* to gather. Dance halls often serve a similar function; being heterogeneous public establishments, *bagres* can congregate there with little difficulty rather than seeking out a "gay bar."

Jailonas, in contrast, seek privacy in its more literal sense. They prefer to congregate among themselves behind closed doors and thus patronize the Anglo-European "gay bar clones" that emerge from time to time in Bolivia's largest cities.[3] Alternatively, they meet in private homes. Because of their privileged economic position, at least some *jailonas* live apart from their families — in general, a rare occurrence in Bolivia.

Camuflados (both *jailonas* and *bagres*) must develop strategies to initiate contacts and establish liaisons with desirable *hombres*. The *camuflados'* dilemma in this process hinges on the social requirement that they adhere to gender-specific rules, while simultaneously revealing to select persons that this adherence is, in fact, a disguise. Communication is achieved when the *hombre* understands that beneath the camouflage resides an individual who functions as a woman in sexual practice. Messages skillfully charged with double entendres and subtle nuances embedded in casual conversation between a *camuflado* and an *hombre* epitomize this communicative process. *Camuflados* employ effeminate gestures and offer *hombres* the opportunity to join a table, have a drink, or smoke a cigarette as a means of conveying their erotically charged intentions.

Bagres encounter little difficulty in finding sexual partners because they carry out their social lives in open, heterogeneous social settings frequented by *hombres*. *Jailonas*, however, must more consciously attract *hombres* while operating behind closed doors. Typically, they attempt to do this by issuing appealing invitations to social events such as barbecues or swimming pool parties. *Hombres* frequently are motivated to please *jailonas* because this may lead to a further invitation and hence another chance to live like the rich for a brief period of time. In short, *jailonas* often depend on their economic advantage to structure the sexual and social behaviors of *hombres*.

A less common strategy among *jailonas* for finding sexual partners hinges on a flexible understanding of the *hombre* category. This flexibility allows them to have sex with one another by agreeing on who will play the *hombre* in any given sexual encounter. In this sense, *jailonas* are the *ambiente* subgroup most similar to the Anglo-European gay cultures that they sometimes idealize.

Camuflados, be they *jailonas* or *bagres*, escape societal scorn to the extent that they manage to affect the behaviors associated with "normal" male conduct. Doing so, however, leaves them anxiously trapped in an ongoing set of conflicts. Achieving erotic gratification must therefore be understood contextually as a double victory; without compromising their social identity, they have successfully managed to negotiate a sexual encounter with an *hombre*.

Hombres

Hombres do not see themselves as homosexuals, nor are they seen as such within or beyond the *ambiente*'s boundaries. Although in recent years the term "bisexual" has entered into limited usage in Bolivia, it has little or no meaning in popular conceptions of sexuality. *Hombres* are viewed, very simply, as "normal" men. Within the *ambiente*'s

[3]As of this writing, there was a total of three so-called gay bars in Bolivia, two in LaPaz and one in Santa Cruz.

tenuous categorization system of in-group players, *hombres* are defined by three behavioral manifestations. First, they display typical male attitudes and stances as revealed by comments that indicate an erotic attraction to women and an on-the-prowl posture toward sex, an interest in sports and drinking alcohol, and a general bravado in social conduct. Second, in sexual practice *hombres* must be penetrators, men known or assumed to have performed as insertors in vaginal or anal intercourse.

In *ambiente* understanding, an *hombre* who conforms to the above two standards is not considered a homosexual, and thus becomes a legitimate sexual target for those members of the *ambiente* who do see themselves in such terms. However, a third criterion must yet be met before other members of the *ambiente* are willing to discount fully the possibility that the *hombre* is simply an outsider. To be of the *ambiente*, an *hombre* must demonstrate in attitude — and ultimately in behavior — that he is an *entendido* [one who understands]. If he rejects, or is indifferent to, repeated approaches made by a *marica* [sissy — a term widely used by *hombres*], he clearly is not an *entendido*. The mere fact that an *hombre* responds to an approach, however, does not settle the issue. The true definition of the *hombre-de-ambiente* centers on his compliance with the unspoken code of conduct of the *ambiente*, including the rules of give-and-take. Although highly ambiguous, variable, and temporally bound by social context, it is generally understood by *hombres* that accepting an invitation from a *marica* entails a sexual obligation. Fulfillment of this obligation makes the hombre an "insider," at least for the time being. *Hombres*, unlike *camuflados* and *travestis*, enjoy unrestricted movement across the borders of the *ambiente*.

SOCIOLEGAL CONTROL OF THE *AMBIENTE*

Although *travestis*, *camuflados*, and *hombres* are distinct groups within the *ambiente*, they are influenced — albeit in different ways — by four common social factors that, taken together, serve to limit the behavioral options open to them. The first of these factors is the negative attitude toward homosexuality held by most Bolivians; homosexuals are widely seen as pathetic failures who are inadequate as men, yet not really women. Under this rubric, homosexual men may be regarded with pity or as a fruitful source of jokes. More severe critics, however, may associate them with immorality or criminal behavior.

The second social factor that circumscribes the day-to-day activities of all homosexual men in Bolivia concerns gender relations and the role of machismo (a strong emphasis on the masculinity of men).[4] Men are expected to be aggressive in their pursuit of sexual pleasure with women, who in turn are expected to steadfastly resist their advances. This inherent tension in gender relations is reduced through social arrangements that function to segregate men from women. Throughout their lives — even after marriage — men spend much of their free time socializing among themselves.

The third social factor bearing on the daily lives of Bolivian homosexuals is the primacy of the family. As does almost everyone in Bolivia, the majority of *gente de ambiente* reside with their nuclear and extended families for their entire lives. To do otherwise would risk being perceived as a family reject — a rogue — a label that few Bolivians would wish to

---

[4]For an excellent discussion of the relationship between machismo and homosexual behavior in a Nicaraguan context, see Lancaster (1988, 1995).

cultivate. At stake is more than emotional well-being. Membership in a family is the very foundation of economic security in Bolivia — a serious consideration in a country with high unemployment and underemployment, low wages, and an all but nonexistent social welfare system.

The final — and perhaps most important — social factor that influences the way in which homosexuals may conduct their affairs centers on the fact that Bolivia is South America's poorest nation. Widespread poverty shapes the *ambiente* in two important ways. First, in-group players must perpetually manipulate their economic strengths and weaknesses to their best advantage in seeking sexual gratification. Second, the police view the *ambiente* with keen economic interest, ever hoping to spot an opportunity to supplement their abysmal salaries through extortion or blackmail.[5] The Bolivian penal code is silent on the issue of homosexuality,[6] but homosexuals are not free from illicit police actions that have the effect of controlling their behavior. Bolivian police officers operate largely outside of the formal law, idiosyncratically dispensing a rough-and-ready — and often self-serving — form of street justice. Thus, suspected homosexuals may be detained for questioning on any number of trumped-up charges, such as theft or drug possession. In these cases, both parties understand that the "real crime" at issue is homosexuality and that the suspect is expected to compensate the arresting officers in return for their silence about this matter.

Travestis

Travestis are far and away the *ambiente*'s most easily recognizable social group. As such, they are the group most likely to be subjected to overt and recurring social control efforts. The limited social geography open to *travestis* follows the contours of transitional urban zones associated with criminality; in consequence, *travestis* often are stigmatized as criminals. Further, their appearance as street prostitutes associates them in the popular mind with wickedness; hence, they also are stigmatized frequently as immoral. Both of these popular images of *travestis* leave them vulnerable to — and virtually defenseless against — abuses at the hands of the police. Morality campaigns, bolstered by a newspaper corps anxious to increase circulation, fuel sporadic *batidas* [police raids] of dance halls frequented by *travestis*. Those apprehended during these *batidas* often must pay off the police in order to escape a lengthy period of detention; typically, the sums involved are quite small by Anglo-European standards,[7] but are not inconsequential to the parties concerned. Police impoverishment and the low status of *travestis* synergistically interact in the "vulnerability to abuse" equation. In practice, however, most *travestis* are as poor or poorer than the police, and this helps to discourage police extortion by undermining its utility.

[5]A typical Bolivian police constable earns approximately 200 Bolivianos a month (about $40 U.S.). By contrast, maids, construction workers, and cab drivers usually make 300 Bolivianos a month.

[6]By any reckoning, Bolivian law is notably underdeveloped; the entire set of laws regulating *all* forms of sexual conduct — both consensual and nonconsensual — occupies just two pages of the country's penal code, *Codigo Penal* (Serrano, 1972). That code sets the age of consent at 17, with violations punishable by up to 5 years' imprisonment.

[7]During a recent *batida* in Santa Cruz, for example, a number of *travestis* were detained by the police until each of them agreed to contribute 40 Bolivianos (about $8 U.S.) allegedly to be used to purchase "a bag of cement to repair the station's courtyard" — an infrastructural improvement that was never made.

Camuflados

It is part of our commonsense wisdom that the rich are less subject than the poor to illicit police actions. In the case of *camuflados*, this wisdom holds true; *bagres* — the impoverished *camuflados* — suffer disproportionately from such actions when compared to their more affluent counterparts, the *jailonas*. But this is not to suggest that *jailonas* are wholly immune from police interference. While *jailonas* typically are not readily identifiable as homosexuals, their dress and demeanor set them apart as *la gente buena* [the rich people]. This leaves them especially vulnerable to extortion by the police because, to preserve their privileged socioeconomic status, many feel compelled to keep their homosexuality secret. Ironically, however, the same social position that makes *jailonas* targets for police extortion also sometimes protects them; few law enforcement officials in Bolivia are willing to risk incurring the ire of the rich and powerful.

Jailonas are more likely than any other homosexual group to patronize the few gay bar clones located in Bolivia's major urban centers. While these establishments are attractive to *jailonas* for the privacy they afford, they also are easy marks for the police. Bribes paid by the owners of these bars keep the police at bay most of the time, but *batidas* still occur. When that happens, the relationship between *jailonas* and the police becomes a contest of fear. The police, aware that *jailonas* are anxious to keep their deviance undercover, attempt to extort money from them in return for silence. But doing so entails a degree of risk for the police, as *jailonas* evoke fear simply by exalting their elite social class membership. Put simply, the police are asking themselves, "How much money can I demand without getting into trouble?" and the *jailonas* are asking themselves, "How much money will it take to get me out of this mess?" In a situation already fraught with anxiety, the two groups must find a mutually tolerable answer to these questions. Intermittent police intrusions, coupled with the *jailonas'* general disdain for mixing with the few *bagres* who may show up at any given gay bar clone, sharply restricts their attendance at such establishments and helps to explain why so few places exist.

Similarly, bars established specifically for homosexually identified men have scant appeal to the largest *ambiente* subgroup, the *bagres*. Socializing in heterogeneous settings allows them to pass as *ordinarios* [common folk], invisible to and protected from police harassment, without denying them the social milieu needed to pursue sexual encounters with *hombres*. Their on-again, off-again invisibility appears to offer them many concrete advantages in going about their day-to-day lives. *Bagres*, however, are not always able to manipulate the switch that controls their invisibility. Living at home with their families and perennially short of cash, they often have difficulty finding places to have sex with their *levantes* [pick-ups]. Walls behind dance halls, bushes in neighborhood fields, alleyways, construction sites, or bathrooms in movie theaters may facilitate a sexual encounter, but in such isolated settings the *hombre* may also attack or rob the *bagre*. In these cases, *bagres* cannot turn to the police without disclosing their own "deviance" and thereby setting themselves up for extortion. Needless to say, few of them select this option. In fact, crimes committed by *hombres* against *bagres* appear to be infrequent and are usually petty. *Bagres* develop a protective form of "urban smarts" they call being *zorra* [a female fox]. Furthermore, their unremarkable social and economic standing, advantageous in other ways as well, seems to provide them with some protection from crime.

Hombres

Hombres float in and out of the *ambiente* as suits their momentary financial needs and sexual desires. They are privileged members in that they are desired and pampered by all of the other players in the *ambiente*, yet they are largely invulnerable to being sanctioned for their behavior. In police roundups of homosexuals, for instance, *hombres* are generally not taken in. Similarly, if they are caught in a compromising encounter with a *travesti, jailona*, or *bagre* they can argue that they were victimized by the homosexual's aggressiveness and can fully expect to be "understood." To avoid social sanctions, *hombres* merely need to stick to their strict presentation of themselves as normal males. This excludes any expressed solidarity or identification with homosexuals. On the contrary, *hombres* are cued to view such people as objects of exploitation and as second rate, ersatz women. Their personal, one-on-one relationships with individual homosexuals vary enormously in their depth of emotional involvement but, as we shall see later in this chapter, the stance culturally expected of them diminishes the chances of forming a "gay community" in Bolivia.

AIDS AND THE EMERGENCE OF THE "GAY COMMUNITY"

AIDS made its official debut in Bolivia in 1985 when the first Ministry of Health-recognized case was diagnosed. As if coupled with this alien disease, the concept of the "gay community" arrived in the country at approximately the same time. For most Bolivians, these strangers from far away were difficult to understand; hence, they drew little attention. For the *gente de ambiente*, however, this baffling duo proved to be both scary and intriguing; one half — AIDS — was feared as a murderer, while the other half — the concept of the gay community — was cautiously welcomed as a liberator. Together, these powerful foreign imports began inexorably to twist, mold, and reshape the traditional configuration of the *ambiente*.[8]

The first indication that the traditional Bolivian understanding of homosexuality was beginning to change was the appearance of a new vocabulary in the nation's newspapers. The word "gay," which resisted translation into Spanish, began to appear in print about 1985 linked to such unimaginable notions as *el movimiento gay* [the gay movement] and *discriminacion contra los gay* [discrimination against gays]. *Bisexualidad* [bisexuality] competed with *orientacion sexual* [sexual orientation] as the most incomprehensible and un-Bolivian of concepts the newspaper boy could deliver to the family's living room. But these were not the only newfangled linguistic challenges to the traditional Bolivian lexicon of homosexuality; the daily arrival of translated stories from foreign wire services such as Reuters and United Press International ensured a steady flow of "up-to-date," and "modern" ways of conceiving same-sex relationships.

It was largely through newspaper stories and word of mouth that members of the *ambiente* — especially *travestis* and *camuflados* — became increasingly aware of the fact that *organizaciones gay* [gay organizations] had established a firm foothold in many Latin American countries. And while they could easily dismiss Mexico as being far away and

---

[8]Strikingly similar processes have been documented in, among other places, Mexico (Carrier, 1995), Brazil (Parker, 1993), and the Philippines (Tan, 1995).

Brazil as being sexually liberal, the dawning realization that such organizations existed in Argentina, Uruguay, Chile, and Ecuador provoked considerable discussion within the *ambiente*. However, it was probably the example of the Movimiento Homosexual de Lima (MHOL) in Peru that served most directly to convince Bolivian homosexuals that some sort of gay organization might succeed in their own country; after all, Bolivia and Peru are cultural siblings.[9]

What the *gente de ambiente* did not realize was that many of the gay organizations in the countries surrounding Bolivia, including MHOL, only partially reflected indigenous movements. Many of these organizations received substantial economic support and logistic guidance from international development agencies of U.S. or European origin; it was only a matter of time before one of these would turn its attention toward homosexuals and homosexuality in Bolivia. But another international institution, the Roman Catholic church, also would play an important, if unofficial, part in the formation of a Bolivian gay community.

Ironically, the first formal gay organization in Bolivia was established in Cochabamba, one of the country's most socially conservative urban centers. Known as Dignidad [Dignity],[10] this organization — which continues to exist — has a board of directors, a post office box, a newsletter, stated goals and objectives, and a stable meeting place. The founding of this organization is closely associated with the inspiration and support of a Roman Catholic priest from the United States. This priest sought to alleviate the emotional, social and legal difficulties faced by the *gente de ambiente*, and, as his knowledge about these difficulties increased, he became more and more committed to forming some sort of gay organization for mutual support. Operating since the late 1980s, the experience of Dignidad demonstrates the inherent difficulty of forging a gay community in the face of the traditional Bolivian conception of homosexuality. *Hombres*, for example, do not participate in the organization at all because, in Bolivian understanding, they have no place in a group of homosexuals. Nor do the few *travestis* who live in Cochabamba; these individuals feel unwelcome by the *bagres* who make up the majority of the organization's membership. *Jailonas* (or *hamburgesas*), who are anxious to appear fashionable and sophisticated, are attracted to Dignidad because the very idea of a gay organization seems Anglo-European and therefore desirable. But their participation is self-limited to that of paternalistic patrons because more direct involvement would bring them into frequent contact with *bagres* (or *salchipapas*), who they see as lowering the tone of the group. Similarly, *bagres* dislike *jailonas* (even while they envy them), but tolerate their presence because they need the material and financial resources that such individuals can provide. In short, two of the three elements of the traditional *ambiente* play little or no part in Dignidad, while subtle rivalries between the rich and poor *camuflados* complicate the organization's efforts to achieve its aims of promoting unity, solidarity, and friendship among homosexuals in Bolivia. Nevertheless, Dignidad is regarded as an important and progressive development by many Bolivian homosexuals, especially those in Cochabamba.

Over time, Dignidad has come to enjoy a degree of acceptance and influence un-

[9]In the colonial period, the area now called Bolivia was known as Alto Peru [Upper Peru]. Even before that time, the Incas ruled over "Tawantinsuyu," an empire that covered much of the territory currently occupied by the two countries.

[10]Not affiliated with the U.S. Catholic gay organization that operates under the same name.

imaginable in Bolivia prior to the AIDS epidemic. In 1994, for instance, a Bolivian psychologist affiliated with the Pan-American Health Organization recruited 40 of its members for a 4-day AIDS prevention workshop. Significantly, several regional Ministry of Health officials agreed to speak at this workshop. Although the workshop was tense — the Ministry of Health officials made degrading comments about their audience and thereby discouraged constructive dialogue — the mere fact that it took place indicates that the Bolivian government is beginning to take homosexuals and homosexuality seriously.[11] In fact, the directors of Dignidad have been invited to speak at a workshop in La Paz attended by relatives of high-ranking government officials and other representatives of Bolivia's ruling class. As a result, the members of Dignidad increasingly are coming to see advantages in belonging to a "gay community"; they can speak about the unspeakable and, in doing so, can begin to air their concerns before people with the power — if not yet the inclination — to bring about real change.

At about the same time that Dignidad was founded, a U.S.-funded AIDS prevention project began operation in Bolivia. Initially, this project focused on improving laboratory procedures for sexually transmitted disease testing and educating the country's state-registered female prostitutes[12] about AIDS. In 1993, however, the project expanded its prevention strategy to incorporate gay men's outreach — Alcance Gay — coordinated by an American public health worker based in Santa Cruz. The coordinator designed an outreach approach to promote *sexo mas seguro* [safer sex, another newfangled linguistic challenge to Bolivian sensibilities] among the players of the *ambiente*. As originally envisioned, this approach would not involve the formation of a gay organization because, in the coordinator's words, "not all homosexually active males in Bolivia see themselves as gay" (Wright, 1993, p. 29).

Nevertheless, the bureaucratic culture characteristic of U.S.-funded development projects worldwide is geared toward process and outcome evaluations that involve site visits to specific facilities to verify that work is in progress, coupled with quantitatively based judgments regarding such things as the number of clients served. Obviously, the geographically amorphous and often chaotic nature of true outreach work did not fit neatly into this evaluative framework. While the general concept of non-gay identified men who have sex with men was familiar to the project's leadership, in practice they evidenced a strong preference for a fixed site facility targeted at so-called gay men — never mind that this could jeopardize the project's ability to reach non-gay identified members of the *ambiente* subculture (see, e.g., Parker, 1992). By March, 1994 — 1 year after the founding of Alcance Gay — the organization had rented a small room in Santa Cruz to serve as a center for AIDS prevention education, condom distribution, and healthcare referral. This facility attracted a small group of homosexuals who, under the guidance of the American coordinator of Alcance Gay, formed themselves into what might loosely be described as a gay support group. Known as Unidos en la Lucha por la Dignidad y la Salud [United in the Struggle for Dignity and Health], or UNELDYS, the organization incorporated the name of Co-

[11]Further evidence that the Bolivian government is beginning to take homosexuals and homosexuality seriously can be found in Melgar, Andrade, and Navarro (1994).

[12]Prostitution is illegal in Bolivia. Despite this fact, prostitutes are required to register with the state in order to receive a permit to operate. Most of the country's female prostitutes are unregistered; to our knowledge, none of Bolivia's male prostitutes are registered.

chabamba's gay group and simultaneously acknowledged that its economic well-being was linked inextricably to the threat of AIDS.

By 1994, it was becoming increasingly obvious in Bolivia that the words "gay" and "AIDS," while not synonyms, were at least linguistic first cousins. The country's first Gay Day celebration — held that year — clearly demonstrated this to be so. Gay Day commemorates the 1969 Stonewall Riots in New York City, a historical event virtually unknown to most UNELDYS participants in Santa Cruz. Nevertheless, the American coordinator of Alcance Gay seized on the idea of a Bolivian Gay Day celebration as a means of increasing awareness of AIDS in the *ambiente* subculture. The Gay Day concept generated a great deal of enthusiasm among the players of the *ambiente*, especially among the bagre subgroup, from which the majority of UNELDYS participants were drawn.[13]

Needless to say, the proposed Gay Day celebration had to pass through some uniquely Bolivian bureaucratic and cultural filters before coming to fruition. For example, all large public gatherings in Bolivia require prior approval from the cultural affairs director of the city in which the event is to take place. The cultural affairs director in Santa Cruz, however, was initially reluctant to issue a permit for the Gay Day celebration because she deemed it far too controversial. After 3 days of tense negotiations between the director and the American coordinator of Alcance Gay, a permit was approved. The approval sent shockwaves through the ranks of the *ambiente*; it seemed nothing short of incredible that the city authorities would allow such a celebration.

Likewise, the traditional Bolivian understanding of homosexuality quickly surfaced during discussions about the *way* in which Gay Day should be celebrated. UNELDYS participants responsible for planning the event were unanimous; the centerpiece of the celebration should be the election of Miss Gay Bolivia,[14] chosen from among contestants representing each of the country's nine departments. No other method of celebrating the day received serious consideration.

On June 25, 1994, Santa Cruz's *gente de ambiente* became gays — at least for the night — as the Miss Gay Bolivia contestants, dressed in drag, answered questions about AIDS and AIDS prevention before 500 people at the Eclipse dance hall (see Serrano, 1994). Interestingly, the person posing these questions was an American public health worker. Observing this event, one of the police officers assigned to control the crowd was overheard to remark: "If it weren't for the fact that this show has government approval — and I still can't figure out how it got it — this would be a great opportunity to rake in a bundle!"[15] Clearly, the traditional Bolivian understanding of homosexuality was beginning to give way, however slightly, to the brave new world of gay politics.

CONCLUSION

What will all of this mean for the day-to-day lives of homosexual men in Bolivia? Prediction has never been social science's strong suit, but the following general observations seem warranted. At the most basic level, the difference between the traditional

---

[13]Indeed, this event increased the number of homosexuals participating in UNELDYS to a point where the organization required larger premises; a UNELDYS house was established in Santa Cruz in late 1994.

[14]Significantly, the proposed election was for "Miss Gay Bolivia," *not* the Spanish language equivalent.

[15]This remark has been translated from the Spanish.

Bolivian *ambiente* subculture and the Anglo-European gay community resides in the sphere of individual cognition. The *ambiente* is an ethereal place — an abstract notion — that resists precise definition. Thus, it is easy for people to float in and out of this subculture with little cognitive dissonance. The gay community, by contrast, is a concrete social and political entity with a sharply defined and self-identified homosexual membership. There is no ambiguity about "being gay." For the foreseeable future, the social milieu of homosexual men in Bolivia almost certainly will continue to be dominated by the *ambiente*. If nothing else, Bolivian society's strongly negative attitude toward homosexuality will see to that.

In the longer term, however, it is equally certain that an identifiable gay community will continue to grow and expand in Bolivia. For one thing, Bolivia is highly dependent on foreign development assistance, and homosexuals, because of AIDS, suddenly have become an important social resource to attract such assistance. Easy access to this resource demands the recognition of a gay community. What is more, foreign donors often are committed to the idea of developing a gay community, if for no other reason than this serves to facilitate their AIDS prevention efforts. For another thing, AIDS itself is likely to encourage the expansion of the gay community concept in Bolivia by gradually destroying the "invisibility" of the *ambiente*. The ethereal quality of this subculture will be difficult to maintain in the face of increasing AIDS-related deaths. Finally, some members of the *ambiente* subculture will be drawn to the idea of a gay liberation movement as a way of improving their individual circumstances.

Experience to date suggests that *bagres* — the poor *camuflados* — are the *ambiente* subgroup most receptive to the notion of forming a gay community. As a needy population, they view such a community as holding some promise for providing them with tangible benefits (e.g., official meeting places, recognized social events). Moreover, they have little to lose by openly identifying themselves as homosexuals. Or do they? Certainly, membership in a gay community will make the *bagres* more readily identifiable as homosexuals to the police and thus perhaps more vulnerable to extortion. Conversely, the fact that they have banded together into a more cohesive community may help to protect them from police corruption. Only time will tell which of these two possible scenarios is correct. But given the historically low levels of compensation for police officers in Bolivia, things do not look hopeful on this front.

Similarly, it is unclear whether the social world of *bagres* will be changed for better or worse by the development of a gay community. For example, where will *hombres* — their traditional sexual partners — fit into this new community? And how will their families react to a gay community? Remember that membership in a family is virtually the only social security that anyone has in Bolivia and that almost all Bolivians live with their nuclear an extended families throughout their entire lives. Can a gay community successful coexist — or compete — with these arrangements? There simply are no easy answers to su questions.

REFERENCES

Carrier, J. (1995). *De los otros: Intimacy and homosexuality among Mexican men.* New York: Columbia ersity Press.

Lancaster, R. (1988). Subject honor and object shame: The construction of male homosexuality and stigma in Nicaragua. *Ethnology, 27,* 111–125.

Lancaster, R. (1995). That we should all turn queer? Homosexual stigma in the making of manhood and the breaking of a revolution in Nicaragua. In R. Parker & J. Gagnon (Eds.), *Conceiving sexuality: Approaches to sex research in a postmodern world* (pp. 135–156). New York: Routledge.

Melgar, M., Andrade, R., & Navarro, F. (1994). *Plan a Mediano Plazo para la vigilancia y prevencion del VIH/SIDA.* La Paz, Boliva: Secretaria Nacional De Salud.

Parker, R. (1992). *Bisexual behavior and AIDS in Brazil.* Baltimore: Academy for Educational Development.

Parker, R. (1993). Within four walls: Brazilian sexual culture and HIV/AIDS. In H. Daniel & R. Parker (Eds.), *Sexuality, politics and AIDS in Brazil* (pp. 65–84). Washington, DC: Falmer Press.

Serrano, R. (1994). Una noche al margin. *Reflejos de la Semana, 388,* 16–17.

Serrano, S. (1972). *Codigo penal.* Cochabamba, Bolivia: Editorial Serrano.

Tan, M. (1995) From bakla to gay: Shifting gender identities and sexual behaviors in the Philippines. In R. Parker & J. Gagnon (Eds.), *Conceiving sexuality: Approaches to sex research in a postmodern world* (pp. 85–96). New York: Routledge.

Taylor, C. (1986). Mexican male homosexual interaction in public contexts. In E. Blackwood (Ed.), *The many faces of homosexuality: Anthropological approaches to homosexual behavior* (pp. 117–136). Binghamton, New York: Harrington Park Press.

Wright, T. (1993). *Male homosexuality and AIDS in Santa Cruz, Bolivia: Sexual culture and public health policy.* Unpublished report submitted to the United States Agency for International Development.

7

Islam

PETER AVERY

The Word "Homosexuality": Human Judgmentalism

In the matter of homosexuality, the Orient was formerly more tolerant than certain Western peoples tended to be, especially before the Reformation, with which the strong inculcation of morality, as judged by man, donned the mantle of religion, replacing a formerly predominant faith and acquiescence in what were believed to be the judgments of God. In the post-reformation era, man became judge, to the detriment both of tolerance and of the acceptance of God as the supreme judge. Human notions of morality usurped the role of religion as the guide to conduct. Before the effects of the Reformation came fully into play, a more benign attitude toward homosexuality may be perceived in the literature of the Elizabethan period. Poets such as Shakespeare and Robert and Philip Sidney[1] benignly and unselfconsciously spoke, to a by no means necessarily exclusively elite audience, in terms remembered from the courtly love of an earlier age and influenced by Marsilio Ficino's commentary of 1469 on Plato's *Symposium* known as the *De Amore* ['*Concerning Love*'].

In Muslim society God to this day has remained in theory the only judge, and man is as He made him, which leaves room for predestinarian ideas. Such thinking was displayed when the *Qází* [judge] of Hamadán was arraigned for being "head over heels" in love with a blacksmith's boy and threatened with one of the penalties prescribed for sodomy in Islam, being thrown from a high place. He burst into verse to the effect that

> Two things have incited me to sin:
> *Unhappy fate* and deficient intellect.

The king of the day in the end pardoned the judge, thus the story ended with the couplet

> Whoever sees his own faults
> Impugns not the faults of others[2]

a sentiment typical of the more tolerant Islam that preceded "Westernization," and the aping of an alien morality. Part of the problem is that, due to mass education tending to cater to the lowest common denominator, refinement has declined to the point where sophisticated ways of coping with and keeping beautiful the passion of love — with under-

---

[1]Robert Sidney's poems have recently been identified; see *The Poems of Robert Sidney* (P. J. Croft, Ed.), Oxford University Press, Oxford, England, 1984.

[2]From the *Gulistán* [*Rose Garden*], a collection of moral tales in prose and verse written in 1258 by the great Shírází poet Shaikh Sa'dí (d. 1292). The quotations, based on an old manuscript of the work, come from Chapter V, Story 19, on "Love and Youth" (italics added).

PETER AVERY • King's College, Cambridge CB2 1ST, England, United Kingdom.

Sociolegal Control of Homosexuality, edited by West and Green, Plenum Press, New York, 1997.

standing of its various forms of expression — have been lost. Even worse: witch-hunting and prurience have taken their place, while, with disregard of religious values, the concept of love itself has become obscured.

Islamic religion originated in Arabia and, with, in particular, Iranian and Byzantine influences, became the core of a great world culture. The irony is that, until the establishment of a largely northwestern European hegemony over Middle Eastern key areas, Islam was host to no such category as "homosexuality." Nor, for that matter, was Europe when Napoleon invaded Egypt in 1798 and set the stage for European infiltration into North Africa and lands east of the Levant. The word homosexuality came into use in English in 1897, 11 years after Krafft-Ebing published *Psychopathia Sexualis*. St. Paul and other Epistle writers of the New Testament, such as Jude, used for nonprocreative sex a word that translates as "fornication." The Arabic word is *líwát*, generally translated as "sodomy." Its derivation is associated with the name Lot, Arabic *Lút*.

SCRIPTURAL BACKGROUND

Before discussing Koranic references to sodomy, as they occur in the context of the story of Lot, the New Testament Epistles must again be mentioned for the reason that nothing specific is said in them about "sodomy." This is very much in keeping with how Muslim legal texts, and the Koran itself, treat the question of what is assumed to be sodomy, i.e., "fornication." They treat it as they do adultery, for which the penalties laid down in medieval Muslim manuals are the same. St. Paul, writing from Rome to the Galatians, lists the two together with a number of other sins. "Now the works of the flesh are manifest; which are these; Adultery, fornication, uncleanness, lasciviousness." Jealousy, witchcraft, idolatry, anger, "drinking bouts," and orgies are also on the list, but the New English Bible leaves out "adultery." "Fornication" probably covered it, as it is taken to in this discussion.[3] What is of interest is that in the scriptures referred to, all these vices appear to be treated as of the same degree of evil. Modern interrogators of candidates for professional and vocational posts should perhaps be mindful, when asking people if they are homosexual, of the extent to which in our time homosexuality has been allowed to assume a special cachet of its own. In Pauline terms, they should also enquire whether they are envious, proud, greedy, seditious, revellers, "and such like."

In one place, St. Paul states that fornication should be fled from because other sins are "without the body," but fornication sins against what is the "temple of the Holy Ghost":[4] It defiles the body. With this exception, the juxtaposition of other misdemeanors alongside fornication implies that what was seen as socially disruptive and therefore evil *sexual* behavior was not in the Christian-Judaic tradition originally seen as a sin distinct from others, though not the less evil for this, although in Leviticus (20:13) the punishment is death for two men engaged in the "abomination" of intercourse with each other "as with a woman," but so is it for intercourse between a man and his daughter-in-law (20:12). Nevertheless, awareness of homosexuality as something requiring special attention and

---

[3]St. Paul's Epistle to the Galatians (5:19–21).

[4]I Corinthians (6:18–19). The concept of the human body as the *temple* of the divine is alien to Islam, which, however, sees Man as created in God's image and man's purpose in having been created to realize that image in himself.

treatment seems to have been absent; contrast this with Western society today, in which homosexuality is commonly regarded as a personality trait, often as a "disorder." Until Islamic countries fell under Western influence, they too missed the modern differentiation of homosexuality from other sins. In one of the only three places in the Koran in which the sin of men "approaching" or "penetrating" men is unambiguously mentioned, it is juxtaposed with "cutting the road," i.e., highway robbery, and with behaving disreputably in assemblies. Further, in several other of the approximately 17 allusions to Lot and the destruction of the "cities of the Plain," also mentioned are matters such as shortcomings in the decent dispensing of hospitality.[5]

ISLAMIC HISTORICAL AND LEGISLATIVE DEVELOPMENT

For the purpose of this discussion, mention of the Koran is essential. It is the foundation of Islamic law and the ultimate sanction for human acts, including the prescribing of punishment. In addition to precluding any individual being responsible for the execution, the fact that punishment for adultery and sodomy should be stoning to death might, indeed, be attributable to the Koran's statement that the punishment of the Cities of the Plains included their being deluged by gravel or lumps of "baked clay." Similarly, another punishment for sodomy, the culprit being crushed beneath a wall, might have been suggested by the walls of Sodom crumbling to rubble in chastisement for its people's wickedness. In either instance, the aim surely was the elimination of the culprit by depriving him of any semblance of a human form and returning him to dust.

In addition to the Koran, another pillar of Islamic law is the dicta and example of the Prophet, his Companions, and, especially in the case of the Shí'í sect in Islam, descendants of his daughter, Fátima, by Muhammad's cousin and son-in-law, 'Alí, who was one of the Companions. This basis of law is known as *hadíth* (plural *ahádíth*) [traditions]. These traditions and the Prophet's *sunna* [custom] supplement the Koran, which did not cover every contingency. Nor was it proven adequate for the conditions obtaining once Islam, in which no distinction was made between the temporal and spiritual, the political and the divine, found itself a religion that was also an imperialism over regions formerly dominated by Byzantium and Iran and far from primitive. It is in the *hadíth* that draconian directions for punishing sexual delinquency are found; in one report, the Imám 'Alí himself is credited with ordering a person taken in sodomy to be stoned to death and then cremated in a pit. In *hadíth* it was ruled that, as with adultery, both guilty parties should be punished, even to death, although modifications were admissible on such grounds as age, marital state, and mental health. Equally severe penalties were applicable to false witnesses, a matter that, doubtless because of the risk of calumny, was given as much attention as the

---

[5]From the Koran, Surah XXIX, 28, in which "barring the way" is mentioned and which translators have generally taken to refer to highway robbery, although Bell (1937/1960, p. 387, fn. 1) suggests it might allude to the effect of sodomy, as barring the way of offspring. The other two explicit references to men "coming to men" in all the Koran, where the matter is always, by inference or clearly, associated with the story of Lot and the destruction of his city, are at XXVII, 56 — "Do you come to men in lust instead of women?" — which is followed by the assertion, "You are a people ignorant"; word for "ignorant," however, also carries the sense of being without faith, or pagan. The second reference is at VII, 79, to the same effect, except that here the question is answered by the assertion, "You are an intemperate [or wasteful] people."

crime itself. In the eighth and ninth centuries came the schools of law, named after their founders, Malikite, Hanbalite, Hanafite, and Shafi'ite. In the codification and sophistication of Muslim law they accomplished a major development, as did the authorities who sifted and authenticated the *ahádíth*, some two centuries after the Prophet's death and, significantly, also after Muslim conquests from Central Asia to Spain, from Damascus to Aden.

Running an empire made clarification of the law necessary in order to meet wider and more complicated contingencies than those arising in Bedouin desert society. In the latter, as it was in pre-Islamic times, and as will be noted later in this chapter, evidence is lacking of intercourse between persons of the same sex being a problem or threat to society. At the same time, Islamic law's meticulous concern with commercial and contractual matters does reflect the fact that the Prophet's cities of Mecca and Medina, more his milieu than the surrounding desert, were trade centers that furnished pack animals for trans-Arabian caravans, in which their denizens intensely participated. That this law, the *sharí'a*, should include provisions against illicit sex and that these provisions should become an increasingly important article of the law after the completion of the conquests — notably after the establishment of the 'Abbássid Caliphate of Baghdad in 750 AD — can be attributed to Muslim legislators' encounter with practices more prevalent in the conquered lands than in the Arabian peninsula. S. D. Goitein (1979) introduces an interesting aspect of this encounter. While he finds no significant incidence of homosexuality in pre-Islamic Arabia, Goitein is of the opinion that its "immense spread in early Islamic times has … little to do with Islam as a religion or with the Arabs as a race. It was the outcome of the superimposition of a caste of warlike conquerors over a vast defenseless population…. Any conqueror, whether Arab, (or later) Turk, or Mongol could take what he liked" (p. 47).

To this explanation it might be added that peoples who feel insecure and under threat have been noted to be prone to homosexuality. The people of the failing Byzantine and Sasanid Empires must have felt so in the seventh century, as their empires crumbled before the forces of Islam. Arabs, although they also included the Greeks in the charge, have been apt to follow Herodotus in ascribing the introduction of pederasty among them to the Persians. Franz Rosenthal cites an Arab author, Al-Jáhiz (d. 868–869), for the view that "homosexuality spread in the Muslim world owing to the army life of the [Persian] Khorásánians who brought the 'Abbássids into power." Thus when the great and highly erotic poet of 'Abbássid Baghdad, Abú Nuwás (d. circa 813 or later), spoke of relations with boys in the boldest and most anatomically detailed fashion and averred that they were to be preferred to girls because they neither menstruated nor got pregnant and were purer, he was reflecting "changed political and social circumstances" (Rosenthal, 1979, p. 19). He was also most likely a first- or second-generation Muslim convert and Iranian in origin; in Iran there had anciently been a tradition, associated with the tending of the sacred fire in the Zoroastrian Fire Temples, that preadolescent boys were those pure enough to rearrange the ashes, but it must be remembered that, as a religion of fertility, it was decidedly homophobic.

A reference to the use of military slaves, which began with 'Abbássid Caliphs' recruitment of Turkish slaves and survived until the Ottoman Sultan Mahmúd II destroyed the celibate Janissary Corps in 1826, brings matters to times nearer the present. So, too, does reference to the still, in several important Islamic lands, observed custom of segregating the sexes, which has probably had as much, if not more, to do with homosexuality in Islam as anything else. Daniel Pipes (1981) links homosexuality with the use of slave soldiers kept in their barracks segregated from women, which, as he observes, made military slavery capable of "benefitting the leaders by supplying them with a pool of subservient men available for sexual relations ... the young recruits offered a choice of 'beardless ones,'" and, on good grounds, he suggests that favoritism related to homosexual leanings was a factor in ensuring slave soldiers' frequent attainment of high government positions (p. 99). But in alluding, as Pipes does, to the celebrated love between the Sultan Mahmúd of Ghazna (who reigned 998–1030) and his slave, Ayáz, an account of this affair given by the twelfth century Persian author Nizámí the Prosodist of Samarqand must not be overlooked. It shows what should not be surprising: the orthodox Muslim prince's pious desire not to break the law; the delicacy, except in the more bawdy poetry, with which such a love could be treated; and the overriding sense of honor, not to be dissociated from that of shame, which is a strong feature of the society under discussion. The account, as translated by E. G. Browne, is as follows:

> The love borne by Sultán ... Mahmúd to Ayáz the Turk is well-known and famous.... Now [the Sultán] was a pious and God-fearing man, and he wrestled much with his love for Ayáz so that he should not diverge by so much as a single step from the Path of the Law and the Way of Honour. One night, however, at a carousal, when the wine had begun to affect him and love to stir within him, he looked at the curls of Ayáz, and saw, as it were, ambergris rolling over the face of the moon, hyacinths twisted about the visage of the sun, ringlet upon ringlet like a coat of mail; link upon link like a chain; in every ringlet a thousand hearts and under every lock a hundred thousand souls. Thereupon love plucked the reins of self-restraint from the hands of his endurance, and lover-like he drew him to himself. But the watchman of *"Hath not God forbidden you to transgress against Him?"* thrust forth his head from the collar of the Law, stood before [the] Sultán, and said, "O Mahmúd, mingle not sin with love, nor mix the false with the true, for such a slip will raise the Realm of Love in revolt against thee, and like thy first father thou wilt fall from Love's Paradise, and remain afflicted in the world of sin."[6]

More down to earth are two pieces of advice given by a father to his son in a *Mirror for Princes*, a didactic manual on how great men ought to conduct themselves. The *Qábús Náma* [*The Record of Qábús*], written by a minor Iranian ruler in 1082 AD, counsels the young man not to grant his favors to one sex only, but to enjoy both young men and women in order not to incur the hostility of either sex (Levy, 1951). Later in the same chapter the royal son is instructed to desire young men during the summer and women in the winter, but, instead of explaining this, the writer closes the chapter with the remark that he has to be brief on such (potentially lust-enflaming) topics, and "May we be forgiven!"[7]

Muslim poets and prose writers of the Classical Age of Islamic literature in Arabic and Persian frequently made their graceful compositions serve an ethical purpose; it is possible that an anecdote like that about Mahúd and Ayáz was composed as much with an eye to public morality as to fact. It is also reminiscent of that ideal of Platonic love mentioned at the outset of this Chapter, and it introduces the "Collar of the Law."

[6]From *Revised Translation of the Chahár Maqála ("Four Discourses") of Nizámí-i-'Arúzi.* London: Cambridge University Press for E. J. W. Gibb Memorial Series, 1921, p. 37.

[7]From Levy (1951, p. 78). For the relation of the hot and cold humors to sexual inclinations, see Franz Rosenthal on Ar-Rází in *Asian Homosexuality* (W. R. D. Dynes and S. Donaldson, Eds.), New York, Garland, 1992, pp. 45–174.

For either anal or, as stated in an important manual[8] respecting Shí'í law, (that pertaining to Islam's second great sect, the Shí'í in contrast to the Sunni or "Orthodox" majority division), intercrural intercourse between men, the death penalty is in effect mandatory. This needs to be interpreted in conjunction with that part of Muslim law termed *hadd* (plural, *hudúd*), literally "limit" or "boundary." In the Koran (II, 229), *hudúd* are mentioned as the "limits set by Alláh." There are seven Koranic references to *hadd*. Several of them concern not infringing the limits of the repudiated wife's dowry rights in divorce. Here is evidence of the manner in which marriage was regarded as a contract covering the transfer and sharing of property. One reference in the Koran (IX, 97), is interesting and of more general application, for it shows how keeping within limits was linked in men's mind with faith in what God revealed to His apostle. It refers, by implication, to the maintenance of proper order and the warding off of chaos, which was a supreme preoccupation of ancient man: "Bedouins [desert Arabs] are more apt not to know the limits of what Alláh has sent down on His Messenger, because they are strong in unbelief and hypocrisy."

Capital offenses are *hadd* offenses, but, given certain specific circumstances, punishment can be mitigated to *ta'zír*, chastisement that generally takes the form of public whipping with a regulated number of lashes. It is much resorted to today by either legal authorities or illicit vigilantes in Iran. In valid Islamic law, the difference between *hadd* sentencing and *ta'zír* is that the former is mandatory, and the latter is at a judge's or magistrate's discretion.

These two categories of law aside, since the *sharí'a*, rather than a legal system, is a divinely revealed code of conduct designed for the preservation and cohesion of a world community, even, or more particularly, in the area of applications of *hadd*, there are devices for inhibiting recourse to law and the call to inflict the severest penalties. In a manual of Hanbalite law, that of the school originating with Ahmad ibn Hanbal (d. 855 AD) and considered the most rigorously puritanical of all, in the context of punishment of adultery and sodomy by death there is the reminder of the tradition to the effect that that it is preferable for an Imám[9] to forgive rather than err in his judgment. But a most potent deterrent to conviction for an act such as males consorting with each other anally reposes in the legal requirement that no less than four witnesses, men of proven integrity and good standing in society, must be able to swear to having seen the act committed. As is explained in the Chapter on Pakistan in this work (Chapter 8), such a provision tends to nullify the law, and reference has already been made to the crime of *qadhf*, giving false witness, for which the penalties are dauntingly harsh. Further, a person charged with the sexual crime in question has the option of confessing, but doing so four times and with the warning of what conviction would entail. However, if he sincerely repents before conviction, he is acquitted, for, as the manuals never cease to recall, in the words of the Koran, "Alláh is forgiving." It was with points such as these in mind that this Chapter opened with a reference to tolerance in the context of classical Islamic law.

---

[8]See A. Querry, *Droit musulman: receuil des lois concernant les musulmans shyites*, Paris: Imprimorie Nationale, 1871–1872, pp. 496 ff, where it is also stated that a woman convicted of tribadism will be subject to 100 lashes whatever her condition, free or servile, single or married, and whatever her religion, but if thrice convicted, on the fourth conviction, the woman will be subject to the death sentence. She will be pardoned if she sincerely repents prior to conviction. Only one party to the act is mentioned as subject to punishment.

[9]A religious leader who, in a religion that is law as much as theology, is also juridically empowered.

Law as a Code of Society-Preserving Conduct

Taking the *sharí'a* as a code of societal conduct, two assumptions arise. First, that the preservation of social order is cardinal for a society to be effective and lasting. The great North African Arab philosopher and social historian Ibn Khaldún (d. 1382), discussing the things that corrupt "sedentary culture," cites adultery and homosexuality as leading to "the destruction of the (human) species." Adultery is included because it results in "confusion concerning ... descent," so that the natural compassion for his children felt by a father, and hence the all important cohesion of the family, are lost. Homosexuality is cited because, more directly than adultery, it leads to the destruction of humankind: It prevents the production of offspring. Therefore, he adds, the school of law under which he lived, the Malikite, is correct in punishing homosexuality with lapidation. This, he concludes, shows understanding of "the intentions of the religious law and their bearing upon the (public) interest" (Khaldún, 1958, pp. 295–296). The preoccupation with the prevention of chaos and preservation of the race alluded to earlier is expressed in the dread entertained by Muslims of the classical period, of *fitna*, the exceedingly evocative word carrying the burden of "disorder," "dissension," the threatened breakdown of society, and hence the Koranic statement (II, 188) that "dissension, *fitna*, is more calamitous than killing." It was the maintenance and continuation of God's creation in His Community of Believers that were at stake, and the approach in classical Islamic law was ethical and, above all, pragmatic.

Modern Times

Islam's modern manifestations cannot be said to include the legal clarity on issues of sexuality and privacy that is characteristic of classical Islam. The Koran is explicit on not entering other people's houses unless a "friendly interview" is sought and the inmates treated with civility (XXIV, 27 & 28): "Do not enter until permission is given you, and if you are told to go away, go away." Interestingly, Khomeini's decree of December 1982 included emphasis on the safeguarding of people's privacy and the prohibition of entering homes and prying into private sources of pleasure therein. That Khomeini found it necessary to issue injunctions of this sort indicates the extent to which, in the Islamic Republic of Iran, certain Muslim principles were apparently being violated.

As for sodomy, under a law ratified by the Iranian Parliament in December 1991, both partners, provided they are mature, sane, and acting of their own volition, are subject to the same punishment — which is execution — as those who sodomize a minor; the passive partner is subject to the *ta'zír* punishment of 74 lashes unless he acted under duress. It appears that even if the perpetrator chooses the option of confessing four times, he will be the one to be punished. According to Article 117, the rule requiring four "righteous" male witnesses is still invoked, with the safeguards against false testimony, *qadhf*. Female testimony is inadmissable. Contrary to the Shí'í law manual cited earlier, under the 1991 Iranian law punishment for intercrural or buttock *frottage*, *tafhíz* shall be, not execution, but, if committed "without entry," 100 lashes for each man. If the doer is non-Muslim and the recipient Muslim, the doer will be condemned to death. One bizarre provision is Article 123, according to which two men not blood relations found lying naked under the same coverlet "without any necessity" will receive *ta'zír* punishment of up to 99 lashes. Proof of lesbianism, *musáhiqa* [rubbing], is the same as for homosexuality between males, but the death penalty will only be enforced after the act has been repeated four times, and punishment is quashed if a lesbian repents before the witnesses give their evidence. There are also provisions against pimping for fornication, *ziná*, or homosexual satisfaction. Two witnesses are required, or twice repeated confession, and the punishment comprises lashes and exile from the guilty party's place of abode.

Laws have, it is reported, been passed against overtly sexual kissing, and visitors to Iran indicate a high degree of oppression in sexual, as in other, aspects of life, even in what in normal societies would be regarded as innocent flirtation. Charges of homosexuality, often coupled with those related to drug abuse or trafficking, appear in certain known instances to have been levelled against persons, an elderly writer for example, who are regarded as politically dangerous to the regime. The issue of homosexuality has become politicized and, as has been seen in other, including European totalitarian, states, can be used to crush those regarded as political malcontents. Recent informants have spoken of how in Iranian cities sexual frustration is creating a highly charged atmosphere, and, of course, the veiling and segregation of women are rigorously applied, so the frustration is increased. This atmosphere could eventually have political consequences the details of which, save to say that frustration of male sexuality through female segregation has often seemed to be one of the causes of volatile political activity in Islamic nations, would be beyond the scope of this chapter.

SEX AND ECONOMICS: THE SHAME FACTOR AND HUMOR

In countries where the Code Napoléon has been a moderating influence, such as it has been in Syria, Lebanon, and North Africa, and where, in the postcolonial period, police and, more especially, vigilante operations, are less prominent than they are under the present oppressive Iranian regime, there is considerable scope for homosexual encounters. In these encounters, however, the economic factor, police corruption, and even policemen's penchant for such contacts, as well as for levying blackmail, often intrude. Such was the case in bombed-out and occupied German cities in the immediate aftermath of World War II. Great poverty provides a hunting ground for the homosexual. The kind of trade alluded to here is notable in Muslim lands in North Africa, although not by any means taken up, particularly in Egyptian cities, solely for gain and without desire for mutual pleasure. Nonetheless, in a place like Tangiers, its prevalence and practice by young lads is directly to be related, as such boys have themselves been heard to say, to their need to take something home "to mother" for the family budget and not, as they are apt to tell their non-Arabic speaking foreign clients, for money "to go to the cinema." Iranians are a sardonic and often, with good reason, pessimistic people, for all their undoubted verbal wit and agility, whereas Egyptians are humorous, and full of fun, a factor that makes a difference in attitudes toward homosexuality. Same-sex sexual play has for centuries been the subject of jokes all over the Islamic world. These jokes have been enshrined in poems and prose, and lewd stories are also whispered in Iran, for example, about vaseline and condoms. In one story, the purchaser of the former, asked how much he required, told the pharmacist, "Enough to do one arse." That he said this out loud to the perturbation of the chemist and male and female customers in his shop elicited the rebuke that he was behaving with unpardonable shamelessness. As alluded to earlier, shame is a vital factor in Islamic lands, and some authorities have been of the opinion that anything goes provided it is not flaunted, a fact not unrelated to what has been said about the sacredness of privacy. But while the shame factor is of very ancient origin, in the context of modern Muslim attitudes toward unprocreative sexual activities it must be seen to have taken on a new dimension: the shamefulness of indulgences considered examples of imported Western corruption. The harshness of post-revolution Iranian law in this regard is part of a virulent anti-Western, anti-corruption drive, and this in a land where not only is corruption rife, but where it has also always been the practice to attribute domestic ills to outside influences.

PORNOGRAPHY

In Islamic countries, until fairly recently, although there were always dancing girls and boys, there has been hardly any notion of pictorial pornography.[10] Poetic literary images of beautiful, adored ones of the male or indeterminate sex, far from being pornographic (except in deliberately obscene verse or on a certain type of nineteenth-century privately used lacquered playing cards), have been used to extol what could be interpreted as images of the Divine. Much of the "erotic" poetry that excited the interest of nineteenth-century European dilettantes is in reality the expression of mystical intimations and is no more "erotic" in a sexual sense than the verses of St. John of the Cross.

ENVIRONMENTAL EFFECTS AND SOUTHEAST ASIA

The problem with looking at the culture of sexuality or ethos is complicated by, especially in the case of such an all-pervasive a religion as Islam, the risk of insufficient attention being paid to influences both external and ancient. In this instance, pre-Islamic influences have molded the peoples concerned. In fact there are more Muslims in southeast Asia and the Pacific region than in the Middle East and North Africa, but it seems that pre-Islamic culture and mores in, for example, Malaysia, the Philippines, and Indonesia have left an indelible mark on the present-day Muslims of the area. Environment, too, has to be taken into consideration: Where the environs are far more lush than in the little-watered countries of western Asia and North Africa, it makes for a naturally tolerant, lackadaisical people. Times might be changing in, for instance, Malaysia, where there is evidence of increasing propaganda on behalf of "Fundamentalist" Islam. Yet these same villages into which fanatical mullas are finding their way to preach their uncompromising dogma formerly recognized a respected *pundam*, the village's favorite transsexual transvestite. As any reader of *The Arabian Nights* knows, transvestism was also a phenomenon of the heartlands of Islam, where in Baghdad and other cities women prostitutes sometimes resorted to male attire to make themselves attractive to males who might have preferred

---

[10]Until recently, because it is reported that in commercial centers in Saudi Arabia, a country where the law is well known for its rigor, but doubtless also elsewhere in the region of the Persian Gulf and Levant, trade has become brisk in the importation of pornographic, but not specifically homosexual, videos. If this is so, it is surely a new development in the Islamic world, which is of a religion that condemns images of living creatures. Their abuse for sexual gratification would mark a serious departure from Muslim norms and could, indeed, be regarded as a Western-originated "corruption"—but so could (and in some circles are) Western films.

boys. But it seems that in the southeast Asian regions mentioned in this chapter, anal intercourse has not been nearly so common as is intercrural intercourse, at which the youths are reported to be expert. It has been suggested that this might account for a comparatively low incidence of AIDS prevailing in the region until recently, except on the perimeters of U.S. bases in the Philippines. It has been reported that in the last few decades in Indonesia the Islamic authorities, presumably in reaction to Western criticism, have become less tolerant of homosexual practices, but that popular acceptance of them, untrammelled by hypocrisy, seems hardly to have diminished. Transvestism continues, and there is also evidence of an incipient androphilic subculture, but of course in southeast Asia Islam has been superimposed on substrata of very ancient cultures, such as Buddhism and Hinduism, which differ a great deal from the Islamic in their treatment of sexuality.

Acknowledgments

In the preparation of this chapter, I have been much helped and encouraged by John Cooper of the Cambridge University Oriental Studies Faculty and by Basim Musallam, also of the faculty and a Fellow of King's College.

REFERENCES

Arberry, A. J. (1963/1982). *The Koran*. Oxford, England: World's Classics.
Bell, R. (1937/1960). *The Koran*. Edinburgh: T & T Clark.
Goiten, S. D. (1979). The sexual mores of the common people. In A. S. Marsot (Ed.), *Society and the sexes in medieval Islam* (Sixth Giorgia Levi Della Vide Bienneial Conference, p. 47). Malibu, CA: Undena.
Khaldún, I. (1958). *The Muqaddimah, an introduction to history* (Bollingen Series XLII, vol. 2) (F. Rosenthal, Trans.). New York: Pantheon Books.
Levy, R. (Trans.). (1951). *A mirror for princes*. London: Cresset Press.
Pickthall, M. (1992). *The Koran*. London: Everyman's Library 105.
Pipes, D. (1981). *Slave soldiers and Islam: The genesis of a military system*. New Haven, CT: Yale University Press.
Rosenthal, F. (1979). Sex and society in medieval Islam. *Bollingen Series XLIII*(2), p. 19.

SELECT BIBLIOGRAPHY

Bouhdiba, A. (1985). *Sexuality in Islam* (A. Sheridan, trans.). London: Routledge and Kegan Paul.
Dunne, B. W. (1990). Homosexuality in the Middle East: An agenda for historical research. *Arab Studies Quarterly, 12,* 55–82.
Dynes, W. R. D., & Donaldson, S. (Eds.). (1992). *Asian homosexuality*. New York: Garland.
International Gay and Lesbian Human Rights Commission. (1996). *Asylum claims: Islamic world: Iran*. San Francisco: Author.
Irwin, R. (1994). *The Arabian knights: A companion*. London: Allen Lane, Penguin.
Musallam, B. F. (1981). Birth control and Middle Eastern history: Evidence and hypotheses. In A. L. Udovitch (Ed.), *The Islamic East, 700–1900: Studies in economic and social history*. Princeton, NJ: Darwin Press.
Sayyid Marsot, A. L. al. (1979). *Society and the sexes in medieval Islam*. (6th Giorgio Levi della Vida Biennial Conference). Malibu, CA: Undena.
Schmitt, A., & Sofer, J. (Eds.). (1992). *Sexuality and eroticism among males in Moslem society*. Binghamton, NY: Harrington Park Press.

8

Pakistan

STEPHEN O. MURRAY AND BADRUDDIN KHAN

Introduction

The Islamic Republic of Pakistan was founded when British colonial rule of the Indian subcontinent ended in 1947. The basis for the division into the countries of India and Pakistan was the fundamental religious differences between Hindus and Muslims that had persisted and sharpened over the centuries since the Mughal conquests of India. Muslims and Hindus worked together to oust the British, and educated Muslims successfully lobbied for Pakistan to be carved out from predominantly Muslim areas of the subcontinent. Thus, they would escape discrimination as second-class citizens. While religion was the defining distinction between the two groups, it was also clear to the professional class of Muslims that they would be considered inferior in a Hindu India, even one that was nominally secular. Islam became central to the definition of this new country (which then included two Muslim non-India components — what was East Pakistan broke loose in a bloody revolt in 1971 to become Bangladesh) and to the identity of its population, which is more than 97 percent Muslim.

Pakistan has stumbled unevenly (and, so far, with limited success) toward an ordered and democratic system of government. Today, the law-and-order situation in Karachi is precarious. In this congested and polluted industrial headquarters of more than 12 million, people live in constant fear of political murders, kidnappings, and shootings, in the midst of what seems to have become chronic low-grade civil war based in ethnic strife. Much of the original post-colonial elite was Mohajir (those journeying to a new land, i.e., not from the Sindh). This includes the founder of Pakistan, Mohammed Ali Jinnah (1876–1948), a Bombay lawyer who had spent a considerable amount of time in self-exile in England, designing the blueprint for the country and later negotiating the specifics with the other political parties, and who died shortly after his dream of Pakistan had become a reality. Many of these Mohajirs came from provinces in what is now India and were not natives of Karachi or the Sindh province in which the city is located. Native Sindhis greatly resent the success of Mohajirs, and this has become a basis for ethnic conflict in recent years of political devolution and increasingly rigorist religious revivalisms.

Although, clearly, waves of puritanism rose and fell before contemporary "fundamentalism," traditional and modern Islamic states (with the exception of contemporary Iran) have not attempted to extirpate homosexual behavior or its recurrent practitioners from

STEPHEN O. MURRAY AND BADRUDDIN KHAN • El Instituto Obregón, San Francisco, California 94107-3239.

Sociolegal Control of Homosexuality, edited by West and Green, Plenum Press, New York, 1997.

society.[1] The Islamic Republic of Pakistan has a penal code, and Section 377 of it prohibits "carnal intercourse against the order of nature with any man," with a punishment of up to 100 lashes and from 2 years' to life imprisonment. Arrests and trials do not occur for such infractions. As elsewhere with unenforced sodomy proscriptions, the existence of the law is a threat — a threat conducive to blackmail.

While the law is largely irrelevant to life in Pakistan, those acting in its name are not. Paying off policemen is a cost of doing many kinds of business in Pakistan, and especially clandestine ones such as prostitution. Police recurrently take money and/or sex from those they know to be involved in same-sex sex (commercial or not). Before discussing police and male prostitution, we shall discuss how the basic organization of the society precludes "gay" homosexuality.

THE PATRIARCHAL FAMILY: THE GREEDIEST OF GREEDY INSTITUTIONS

There is no "gay life" in Karachi, in the Western sense of the word: no bars, no newspapers, no organizations, and few instances of lovers living together (see Khan, 1997). Just as predictably, sex between men occurs often, and committed and emotional "friend-ships" develop. However, the paramount institution of Pakistani society is the biological family. The purpose that gives meaning to life is to enhance the family — increasing its size and resources, protecting its honor, and improving its status. While there is probably no society in which these are not valued,[2] in Pakistan these are the clear and unswerving raisons d'être for life itself, and they supersede individual desires and differences if or when there is any conflict.

Children live with their parents until they get married. It is virtually unheard of for an unmarried son to live in the same city as his biological family but apart from it. Single men and women may live with their parents (even without economic need) through middle age and beyond. Even separate households function as social satellites, linked inexorably by social and biological bonds to the family center.

There is a very practical foundation to this focus on the closed corporate community of the patriarchal family. The family establishes one's station in life, which in turn sets boundaries for the aspirations of individuals. Individuals may somewhat exceed these boundaries, but "social status" is virtually impossible to change in just a generation or two and does not naturally follow material success.

[1]Traditionally, Islamic courts have admitted testimony only by adult Muslim male eyewitnesses. To establish that sodomy was committed requires four trustworthy Muslim men to testify that they saw penetration ("the key entering the key hole"), or someone must confess four times. Punishment for unproved accusation is severe, further discouraging testimony. Usually in Arab and other Islamic societies, everyone successfully avoids public recognition (let alone discussion) of deviations from normative standards — sexual or other (see Murray, 1997c).
[2]Attempts to manufacture exceptions include the Mamlūk military elite, purchased anew in each generation from the steppes of Eurasia, who ruled Egypt and Syria from 1249 (when they defeated an invading army of Crusaders led by St. Louis, until the mass army of Napoleon defeated them in 1799); a similarly recruited Ottoman elite; celibate Roman Catholic priests and Buddhist monks; and eunuchs in many societies. However, even those precluded from producing heirs have found ways to favor family members, even from considerable geographic distances. And the Mamlūks found ways to provide for children who could inherit their Mamlūk status or any of the wealth they accumulated (see Murray, 1997b).

Producing and nurturing male heirs is the paramount responsibility of sons and the wives that are incorporated to produce and care for them. Families devote themselves selflessly to caring for their young (and not so young), with a devotion that seems pathological in the West. Rather than temporary breeding grounds for children to grow up in before they move on to independence, families are like organisms that extend themselves by absorbing their young, and they grow stronger or weaker based on the contributions of the new entrants. This is not just one model of life in Pakistan; it is not a choice: It is the *only* way of life. Only in the context of this environment is individual love recognized, and it is supported only if it furthers the family's interests. This applies to marriages, which are usually arranged. Whether husband and wife get along with each other is far less important than whether they breed well. If a husband takes care of his family's security needs and bears many children, what he does for personal sexual satisfaction is uninteresting to everyone involved, so long as he is discreet and does not squander excessive resources. It is certainly not discussed, and it simply does not matter. It can be said to be "tolerated," insofar as total obliteration of recognition and total lack of valuing is tolerance.

"Moral issues" of two men having sex, as in the Christian West, do not arise. The tolerance of covert extramarital homosexual liaisons does not mean that there is ready, good-humored indulgence in this regard. To the contrary, homosexual behavior is derided in public discourse. Pragmatic accommodations to individual tastes must necessarily be worked out discreetly. From the standpoint of "family," it is less risky for males to have affairs with males than with females whose bodies — in particular, their reproductive capacities — belong to others. The Qur'an proscribes homosexual behavior, although it prescribes more severe penalties for infidelity with a woman.

In this environment, homosexual sex is uninteresting, since it does not create children, nor does it add the potential for children to the family's resource base (except to supplement the income of lower-class hustlers). In fact, sex in general is interesting primarily because of its impact on family, rather than its potential for individual pleasure or carnal fulfillment.

This interdependence between individuals and family is further exacerbated by the lack of widespread health insurance and social security benefits. The public health system is very poor, and private hospitals are expensive. While some companies pay for employee health coverage, the individual without a steady job and without family ties finds himself precariously alone and unprotected. In Pakistan, family support is literally a matter of life and death — not just "social existence," but the only insurance against illness and disability.[3] Sexual releases are of the "pragmatic" variety, which assumes that the male (as a sexual animal) needs release before (or in addition to) marriage. Some women and mullahs regret that such needs exist, but even they tacitly accept such "outlets." (Kinsey's term is particularly apt here.) Boys may jokingly use the term *gandu* [a man attracted through the *gand*, i.e., the anus], but there is an undercurrent of sexual tension; it is accepted within the framework of reality that men derive satisfaction through "buggering the *gand*," preferably of younger men or boys (older men yearning for youthful flesh are a not uncommon sight in parks and other public pick-up places). The normal spectrum of desire can be seen, irrespective of age, although social convention makes it easier to understand the notion of the older sodomizing the younger, in the context of the exercise of power and the release of

[3]See Murray [1992; 1995, pp. 33–48] for some comparative instances.

sexual tension. It is understood that such acts are a loathsome necessity to some, but not heinous or necessarily predatory. They are within the natural framework of sexual couplings and carry with them the risk that the physical act may plant seeds of emotion. There is unspoken consensus that this risk is reasonable, when balanced against the alternative that single young men in heat may breach the restraints of virgin daughters or learn other bad habits through consorting with prostitutes. What is totally unacceptable is for these outlets to act as a long-term substitute for the duty to bear children. Similarly, everyone expects male–male emotional relations to occur — much classic verse and song celebrates male–male love[4] — but such special feeling must not preclude marriage and siring children. Even if "everyone knows," it is still likely that no one will say anything about what is known, either about the general pattern or such instances that are known but not acknowledged. Protection of the public sphere from acknowledgment of even (or especially) rampant homoeroticism sustains stigmatization, strangling any possible challenge to conventional contempt.

"Gay" implies a legitimation of a relationship that runs counter to family, and therefore gay life does not exist in Pakistan, or in other Muslim societies.[5] From a practical standpoint, two lovers would find themselves without any social context. There *is* no threat to family: Other kinds of relationships are simply irrelevant. At worst, there is ridicule; at best, there is willful blindness to the situation. The most successful gay relationships in urban Pakistan are never the most important relationship for either partner; the family necessarily occupies that position.

Furthermore, the lack of privacy in most living situations makes a personal relationship that is outside the norm impossible to maintain. Occupants in poorer households share what little space they have. In wealthier families, servants provide a very effective monitoring system, and it is impossible to maintain secrecy. Any secrecy that anyone crafts is so isolating that its maintenance corrodes the very relationship it was intended to protect.

Preventing "shame" or otherwise embarrassing the family is the most basic requirement for respectability. Respectability is the basic requirement for social acceptance, and social acceptance is the oxygen without which life ceases to exist in any meaningful way.

AGE-STRATIFIED MALE–MALE SEX

At least since early 'Abbasid time (i.e., 750 AD), sexual receptivity has been assumed to be a "natural" part of male beauty in the abode of Islam. In anal intercourse, the inserter tends to be older, the "man," while the insertee tends to be younger, or an available *gandu* or a rented *malshi* [masseur]. In some encounters, kissing is unacceptable. In yet other encounters, a boy will willingly offer himself for anal penetration, but shyly refuse to allow

[4]The high status awarded to love between men is a continuation of Moghul and Sufi traditions of Islamic mysticism (see Naim, 1979; Schimmel, 1975). These traditions have been diluted by Hindu and, in recent decades, Western influence in Pakistan, including psychiatric medicalization.

[5]Turkey and Indonesia provide incipient exceptions, with small organizations of persons identifying themselves as "gay" and pressing for protection against police depredations and effective education about HIV transmission that explicitly acknowledges male–male sexual contact (see Tapinc, 1992; Yüzgün, 1986). In that penetrator and receptor roles are dichotomized by status (primarily age, secondarily gender), Muslim male–male sex is also "non-gay."

the inserter to see or stimulate his genitals or to kiss him. Generally, the receptive partner finds anal intercourse more acceptable than fellating the man. This is in part due to the special significance of rules of cleanliness that are part of the Muslim tradition; the genitals are "unclean," and defiling to "clean" mouths.

Although pederasty has not been the only form of homosexuality in Islamic cultures (especially in the eastern reaches of Islam, where flamboyant gender-crossing roles have been attested, see Murray, 1997a), it has long been the idealized form. Age-stratified male–male sexual relations in Islamic societies have lacked the pedagogical warrant (rationalization) exemplified in ancient Greece and, until recently, New Guinea, in which the boy "graduates" through sexual service into recognition of his full development to adult manhood (see Herdt, 1984). The pleasure of the man was and is the justification for Muslims anally penetrating boys. The culturally appropriate basis for desiring boys is their beauty, not their incipient masculinity. There is disagreement (both within and between Islamic cultures) about whether sexual relations with older boys or men are harmful to the development of the masculinity of those penetrated. Even where such behavior is not seen as permanently stigmatizing or traumatic, no one claims that homosexual receptivity masculinizes the boy and prepares him for manhood. For no Islamic society is there any attestation of a conception of insemination as necessary for maturation like that recorded for some highland New Guinea societies, in which homosexual receptivity is a necessary part of all boys' initiation into manhood. Being inseminated as a boy is a hindrance, if not always a bar to attaining adult masculinity. Nor is sexual involvement with a man an advantage to one's public reputation or individual self-conception as masculine. The boy in such sexual exchanges is quite clearly feminized, whether permanently or only temporarily, by being "used as a woman."

Of all the societies in which age-stratified homosexuality has been described in some detail (including Greece, Melanesia, Japan, and Sudanic tribes), Islamic ones seem least to expect that the sexually used boy will grow up to be a man. Boys in Islamic societies may outgrow being sexually used, but the assertion that they are junior warriors, which existed in feudal Japan as well as in ancient Greece and in Highland New Guinea until its recent pacification, is (and has been) missing in the pederasty of Islamic societies (outside military training schools).[6] In all these non-Islamic instances, however, the cultural expectation was for the boy to outgrow sexual receptivity, not to enjoy it so much that he would continue. Whether regularly penetrated boys will later become masculine is believed to be a matter of fate in Islamic societies. Although not aided, adult masculinity also is not precluded by childhood and adolescent sexual receptivity. Some pretty boys "graduate" to being husbands and fathers. In the native view, others are fated to want to continue being penetrated by men, in some cases depilating to simulate the beauty of youths.

MALE PROSTITUTES, THEIR FAMILIES, AND THE POLICE

Placing a price on lovemaking, as is becoming increasingly common (including after-the-act extortions as well as what was known in advance to be a commercial exchange),

---

[6]No one seems to have inquired about what happened to the *zun'i-sufuri* [young caravan wives] of Central Asia (especially on the Silk Road) when they became adults.

transforms it into an economic transaction and removes all semblance of play or tenderness. This section considers Pakistan's "rent boys."[7]

Males seeking males for sex drive around, if they have an automobile or motorbike, or visit certain restaurants, cinemas, hotel lobbies, video game shops, parks, or railroad stations. Many of those stalking paying customers prefer to "conduct business" in the back seats of clients' cars or to go to hotel rooms rather than to run the risk of being assaulted or robbed by someone taking them home (if they have a home with any privacy for sexual liaisons). Turning tricks in cars and hotels also allows boys to get back and connect with another customer sooner.

A large number of the full-time male prostitutes operating in Pakistani cities are runaways. However, there are also many part-time prostitutes — especially schoolboys and those working in hotels and garages — who prostitute themselves on the side for extra money, for clothes and gifts, or for other jobs (especially the promises of television or cinema roles). Most range in age from 15 to 25. It is a short career in which the product's market value generally declines rapidly.

Male prostitutes and their clients vary in ethnic origin, including natives of all four provinces as well as refugees from Afghanistan and Iran. Most have had little or no education. Average earnings are in the range of 5000–7000 rupees a month, although those whose clients are foreign tourists, sailors, and marines earn considerably more. The lowest stratum of prostitutes is composed of those from poor families renting their bodies to other low-income men. Some lower-class boys function as "wives" of poor men who cannot afford to get married.

Assaulting boys and then photographing them in the nude is a common way of trapping boys "into the life" of prostitution. Many were sexually abused at an early stage in their lives. Mutjaba (1997) estimates every ninth or tenth boy in school or even at work is sexually molested. The boy never reports this to his parents out of fear that they will blame him rather than the perpetrator.[8]

Some families turn a blind eye to their son's profession because they are dependent on income from his trade. This is especially the case of the son who has migrated to a city and is supporting the family by sending them monthly money orders. Generally, families of male prostitutes are blissfully ignorant of their profession, because the boys take great care to

---

[7]This entire section, not just what is directly attributed in the text to him, is mostly based on the research of Mutjaba (1997).

[8]As in other Islamic societies, anyone who is known to have been penetrated has greater difficulty warding off others who want to use him sexually. Once a Muslim boy's anus is known to have been opened by someone, others press to open it again. As Tony Duvert (1976) wrote, specifically in reference to Muslim North Africa:

> A penetrated anus attracts the bachelors of the community like a pot of honey draws flies. One is known to be available and talked about. Everyone goes to him to relieve their need, sometimes by force. It would be shocking if he refused once he had been breached.... A proper [obéissant] boy keeps his asshole sealed tight. The one whose is open[ed] becomes the whore [le putain] of the other boys and thereby helps save theirs.... One will be the bottom for all. The first who relaxes [his guard] is fucked [pédé]. (pp. 77–78; translation by S.M.)

There is also a widespread view that being penetrated is pleasurable, so that the penetrated become addicted to the pleasure. The cultural corollary is that the only safe way to avoid becoming a receptacle for every horny male around is not to "submit" even to one. See Murray (1997c; 1995, pp. 59–64) for elaboration and comparison to similar Latin American beliefs of the dangers of being anally penetrated.

avoid discovery. Indeed, acquiescing to the demands of someone threatening to expose something discrediting (not always involvement in sex) is a recurrent motif in the accounts of their careers. Mutjaba (1997) provides an example in which a group of policemen terrorized a youth into providing both sex and income from sex with others to them:

> Once Farrukh was apprehended by a group of drunken policeman late at night. They beat him until he told them his name, address, and profession. "Then they took me to their quarters and gang-raped me. Following that they demanded that I 'work' for them or they would throw me behind bars and tell my father."
>
> It was this fear of his father that turned Farrukh into a full-time prostitute.... On average he makes 500 to 600 rupees for three to four hours work an evening. Out of this, 200 rupees go to the police as *bhatta* [a bribe]. Sometimes, he says, he works with the police to blackmail unsuspecting clients. Routinely, the policemen also present him as a "favor" to their homosexual seniors. Police officials also often smuggle boys into various jails across the country to service select inmates. Another boy explains that it is difficult to be independent because "pimps and the hotel owners harass us a great deal and the police are with them, so we don't dare mess with them." (p. 269)

Indeed, a lot of boys are frequently picked up by policemen who use them without payment. In Karachi and Hyderabad many pimps and male prostitutes act as informers for the police and the CIA. Extortion and blackmail by plainclothes police (or those pretending to be police) occur in virtually every area where male prostitution exists.

Maintaining the Invisibility of Any Male–Male Alternative

In recent years, some articles have appeared in the local press about sex between men, often in the context of prostitution or AIDS. This is in part due to the recognition that AIDS is sexually transmitted, but also because the recently freed local press is now analyzing social issues with increasing frequency.

Does this mean that the shadowy gay life that exists in Karachi is now being exposed? To the contrary, male–male sex is still represented as an inferior safety valve. There is no hint in the press, or by even the most daring commentator, that male–male relationships could supplant marriage. Such relationships are seen as symptoms of problems, whether social, economic, or cultural (similar to the decadence shown in Western media). There is still no notion that such relationships could lead to a satisfying life instead of marriage to a woman. Love between men is explained away — whether as platonic and romantic, carnal and expeditious, or decadent and symptomatic of a social problem.

Conclusions

Cultural and religious tradition keeps male–male sexual relationships largely hidden in Pakistan. There is no gay life in the Western sense of the word, and sexual relationships between men must be kept hidden and managed within the context of marriage to a woman. Sex between males is considered irrelevant. This has spawned a population of hustlers, and some men that take boys into relationships as secondary wives. Islamic tradition frowns on but acknowledges male–male sex, and this plays a role in permitting clandestine sex so long as it is not allowed to interfere with family life, which is of paramount importance and continues to be the only stable, enduring institution. Love and sex between men must adapt to the dictates of family, religion, and culture.

The world is shrinking, as satellite television, Internet access, and freer trade open up countries like Pakistan. Individuals emboldened by the short shrift given to their personal identities will find a way to communicate, and through communication communities may emerge. These communities are already forming in India among Muslims and Hindus alike and are maturing in previously sheltered societies like Japan and Thailand and Islamic states such as Indonesia and Malaysia.

REFERENCES

Duvert, T. (1976). *Journal d'un innocent*. Paris: Editions de Minuit.
Herdt, G. H. (1984). *Ritualized homosexuality in Melanesia*. Berkeley: University of California Press.
Khan, B. (1997). Not-so-gay life in Karachi. In S. Murray & W. Roscoe (Eds.), *Islamic homosexualities* (pp. 275–296). New York: New York University Press.
Murray, S. O. (1992). The "underdevelopment" of "gay" homosexuality in Mesoamerica, Peru, and Thailand. In K. Plummer (Ed.), *Modern homosexualities* (pp. 29–38). London: Routledge.
Murray, S. O. (1995). *Latin American male homosexualities*. Albuquerque: University of New Mexico Press.
Murray, S. O. (1997a). Male actresses in Islamic parts of Indonesia and the Southern Philippines. In S. Murray & W. Roscoe (Eds.), *Islamic homosexualities* (pp. 256–261). New York: New York University Press.
Murray, S. O. (1997b). Male homosexuality, inheritance rules, and the status of women in medieval Egypt. In S. Murray & W. Roscoe (Eds.), *Islamic homosexualities*. (pp. 161–173). New York: New York University Press.
Murray, S. O. (1997c). The will not to know: Islamic accommodations of male homosexuality. In S. Murray & W. Roscoe (Eds.), *Islamic homosexualities* (pp. 14–54). New York: New York University Press.
Mutjaba, H. (1997). The other side of midnight: Pakistani male prostitutes. In S. Murray & W. Roscoe (Eds.), *Islamic homosexualities* (pp. 267–274). New York: New York University Press.
Naim, C. M. (1979). The theme of homosexual (pederastic) love in pre-modern Urdu poetry. In U. Memon (Ed.), *Studies in Urdu gazal and prose fiction* (pp. 120–142). Madison: University of Wisconsin Press.
Schimmel, A. (1975). *Mystical dimensions of Islam*. Chapel Hill: University of North Carolina Press.
Tapinc, H. (1992). Masculinity, femininity, and Turkish male homosexuality. In K. Plummer (Ed.), *Modern homosexualities* (pp. 39–49). London: Routledge.
Yüzgün, A. (1986). *Turkiyede escinselik, dün bügün*. Istanbul, Turkey: Hüryüz.

9

Singapore

LAURENCE WAI-TENG LEONG

Introduction

In a survey of the social and legal position of gays and lesbians in 202 countries, Tielman and Hammelburg (1993) observe that English legislation against homosexuality has had a negative impact on the legal status of these groups in former British colonies. For example, the legal infrastructure of India, Malaysia, and Singapore bears the imprint of British colonial administration. In all three countries, the specific section of the penal code that punishes homosexuality is the same (Section 377), and the linguistic particulars of that section are also similar, phrased as "carnal intercourse against the order of nature" and "gross indecency." Even the terms of punishment are the same: a maximum of life imprisonment for sodomy.

It is argued that, if the British legal system is punitive in its philosophical implications and practical applications, then the legal apparatus in Singapore, inherited from the British, can be said to be even more coercive. In the hands of a dominant political party that has been in hegemonic power since the year of self-government in 1959, law has been used as an instrument of social and political control (Hickling, 1992; Tremewan, 1994). Thus, during the colonial period the British used the Preservation of Public Security Ordinance to crush anti-colonial movements. The legacy of this ordinance today is the Internal Security Act, which empowers the state to detain without trial any person who is deemed to be a threat to the security of the nation. This may be for up to 2 years, but is renewable ad infinitum. Since the interpretation of threat is subject to executive powers of the state, those detained under this act have been leaders of opposition parties, political dissenters, and religious leaders, variously labelled "Marxists."

A few examples that otherwise have no relation to sexual offenses are necessary to provide a context for understanding the general climate of law in Singapore. These examples, ranging from trivial to serious, appear disparate, but nevertheless fit into a legal mosaic that reflects the sociolegal status of homosexuality in Singapore.

On the trivial side, law covers the minutia of everyday conduct, with penalties, mostly fines, for matters such as littering, smoking in enclosed spaces like shopping malls, spitting, jaywalking, urinating in public lifts, failing to flush a public toilet after use, having water-logged plants that breed mosquitoes in public housing, and so on. Such laws are actually enforced and administered. Their pettiness is displayed on tourist T-shirts listing all the fines imposed to show that Singapore is indeed a "fine" city. Singapore has been satired in cyberspace as the "land of the rising cane" for the frequency with which flogging is meted

LAURENCE WAI-TENG LEONG • Department of Sociology, National University of Singapore, Singapore 119260, Singapore.

Sociolegal Control of Homosexuality, edited by West and Green, Plenum Press, New York, 1997.

out for a wide range of crimes, such as vandalism, graffiti, possession of fire crackers, robbery, molestation, and gross indecency.

Harsh sentences apply also in less mundane matters like libel and release of economic statistics. In October 1994, an American academic who was teaching in the University of Singapore wrote an opinion piece about Asian repressive regimes that have a "compliant judiciary." Although no reference was made to Singapore or any named persons, he was fined $10,000 for contempt of court and was made subject to a libel suit of $100,000 by the senior minister in Singapore (Lingle, 1996). Also charged were the editor, printer, and distributor of the newspaper, *International Herald Tribune*, which ran the article. The legal system in Singapore over the years has been able not only to restrict speech, but also to apply huge fines to such publications as *Time, Newsweek, Asian Wall Street Journal, Far Eastern Economic Review, Asiaweek* and *The Economist*.

In June 1993, the government prosecuted an editor, a journalist, and three economists under the Official Secrets Act for the leaking and publication of early estimates of the gross domestic product figures a few days before they were officially released. This has a chilling effect on the circulation of information, the Secrets Act being so vague that government has discretion to define any piece of unreleased information as secret. Medical statistics, public housing figures, and economic data are not easily accessible.

From 1974 to 1986 the government published annually a *Statistical Report on Crime in Singapore* that was available in the university library until recently. Access to these reports is now granted only by the Criminal Intelligence Unit of the Criminal Investigation Department on very special grounds, with the added proviso that such figures cannot be published in any form. Lacking access to these reports during the preparation of this chapter, the author has had to rely on newspaper reporting between 1992 and 1996, appeal cases in law reports, and verbal information from interviews.

Strict laws, harsh penalties including corporal and capital punishment, the wide latitude within which petty behaviors are defined as offenses or crimes, and the way information is deemed secret and therefore shielded from access and freedom of circulation all constitute a package within which the proscription of homosexuality is enforced. By and large, criminal and civil laws in Singapore do not allow for any expression of homosexuality.

THE CRIMINAL LAW

"Crime against the Order of Nature"

The law on homosexuality in Singapore follows the tradition in England prior to the decriminalizing Sexual Offences Act 1967, but stops short of the provisions and revisions made in England in 1967 and subsequently. It is immaterial whether acts take place in public or in private, whether there is consent between the males involved, or whether participants have reached an age of adulthood or sexual self-determination. There is no "consenting adults" defense in Singapore, no provision for homosexuality in a zone of privacy, and no "human rights" discourse within which the status of homosexuality might be eligible for legal protection. In short, all homosexual acts in Singapore are punishable.

It appears that homosexual acts are charged under two sections of the Penal Code (Cap. 224):

> Section 377 (Unnatural Offences): Whoever voluntarily has carnal intercourse against the order of nature with any man, woman or animal, shall be punished with imprisonment for life, or with imprisonment for a term which may extend to 10 years, and shall also be liable to fine. Penetration is sufficient to constitute the carnal intercourse necessary to the offence in this section.
>
> Section 377A (Outrages on Decency): Any male person who, in public or private, commits, or abets the commission by any male person, of any act of gross indecency with another male person, shall be punished with imprisonment for a term which may extend to 2 years.

Both sections carry a mandatory punishment of jail. Whereas Section 377A is specifically worded to cover indecent acts with males, Section 377 includes men and women. Indeed, there are more heterosexual than homosexual cases tried under this section. These heterosexual cases appear in the context of male rape of a female victim. For example, in *PP v. Jumahat* (1982), the accused was charged with rape and sodomy of his step-daughter. In *Kanagasuntharam v. PP* (1992), along with a sentence of 14 years and 24 strokes for rape, the accused was given 6 years for the offense of fellatio and 8 years for committing anal intercourse. The three offenses constituted one sexual episode, but the acts were distinguished as discrete units and the sentences meted out accordingly were ordered to run consecutively.

In 1995, two separate cases of heterosexual rape, which were tried in court roughly at the same time, raised the issue of the legal status of oral sex in Singapore. In the first case, *PP v. Victor Rajoo* (1995), the accused was acquitted (though subsequently convicted) of abduction, rape, theft, and robbery and convicted only of having oral sex with a woman. On the basis of weak and inconsistent testimony from the woman the judge ruled that she had probably consented to sexual intercourse, but consent was not an essential element of the oral sex charge. Accordingly, the man was jailed for 6 months and fined $2000 for fellatio. This ruling implied that a person can be charged for having oral sex, even if consent is given and the act is performed between heterosexual adults in privacy. It also implied that, according to Section 377, sexual acts other than vaginal sex are "unnatural" and punishable under the law.

Following this a range of issues were raised (Boon, 1995; "Did You Know?," 1995; Kay, 1995). A high proportion of the population of married couples would have been guilty of a Section 377 offense for having oral sex. Even if they were not tried, what if oral sex was raised as an issue in marital disputes and divorce proceedings? Why would an act, historically embedded in the Chinese custom of "playing the flute," be considered a crime? Section 377 was shown to be itself unnatural, imposed from another cultural tradition and anachronistic in the contemporary setting.

In the second case, in which a man was charged with rape, extortion, and fellatio, the defense lawyer asked the court to rule in the interests of the public whether oral sex between two consenting heterosexual parties is an offense ("Defence Wants Court to Rule," 1995). Justice Lai Kew Chai admitted that oral sex between consenting heterosexual adults, used as "a prelude to natural sex," is not an offense. But when pressed to clarify the statement that oral sex between two consenting adults is not an offense, the judge replied,

"Let's cross that bridge when we come to it." Despite hesitancy, the judge had signalled that oral sex was an integral part of "natural" sex (i.e., vaginal intercourse).

Since married or courting couples have never been convicted for oral sex under Section 377, and only those charged with rape are convicted of oral sex, an apparent contradiction exists. In Section 377 consent is not excusable, but in practice the courts only prosecute cases where there is no consent involved. Thus, in the aforementioned case, Justice Lai sentenced the accused to 5 years imprisonment for forcing the victim to perform oral sex on one occasion and 3 years imprisonment for four other occasions of oral sex. This is an oddity because, without consent from another person, "outraging of modesty" (Section 354 of the Penal Code) would be the proper charge for a person who coaxed another to perform oral sex. That several cases have been prosecuted under Section 377 instead of Section 354 illustrates the confusion, indeterminacy, and contradictions of the Singapore courts when dealing with matters of sexuality. Traditionally, "unnatural offences" in the Penal Code in Commonwealth countries covered sodomy and bestiality, but made no specific references to fellatio or cunninlingus (Gupta, 1984).

"Gross Indecency"

While the framers of the Penal Code intended "unnatural offences" to encompass consensual anal intercourse between man and either man, woman, or animal, in Singapore this section has been applied mostly to heterosexual cases where the male has anal and oral intercourse without the consent of the female. In contrast, Section 377A is applied to homosexual offenses.

In Section 377A, there is a mandatory term of imprisonment for "gross indecency" (read: oral sex, mutual masturbation, or touching of genitals) between two males, either for commission of the act or an attempt at commission, and regardless of location in private or public space. In practice, all the convicted cases of gross indecency had taken place in public settings such as a parked car ("Two Men Caught," 1991), a housing block ("Five Fined," 1991), an open-space park ("Two Men Jailed," 1992), a disco ("Man on Gross Indecency Charge," 1993), toilets in shopping centers ("Guard Caught Two Men," 1994; "Jailed for Sex," 1991; "Two Did Indecent Act," 1994), and a swimming pool ("Two Jailed," 1993).

A man may accuse another male of performing oral sex on him in private settings. In February 1996, a man told a district court that a male lawyer performed oral sex on him while he was asleep in the lawyer's flat ("Man Says," 1996). Justice Lai's earlier vote of confidence in consensual oral sex between adults does not apply to two males. Thus, the lawyer was charged with gross indecency. But such cases tend to be weak because the intentions of the complainant are suspect. In this instance the complainant had earlier demanded $20,000 from the lawyer. The pecuniary motive weakened his testimony and accusation, and the lawyer was acquitted.

Gross indecency charges are successfully prosecuted when incidents take place in public settings, witnessed by a nonparticipant. Thus, among cases cited earlier, a policeman patrolling in the vicinity of a park, a housing block, or a car park caught the men in action. In the remaining cases, security guards at shopping complexes and lifeguards at swimming pools acted as custodial police and complainants.

In 1991–1992 the sentencing norm for gross indecency was 2–3 months, but from

1993 onward it was set at 6 months (*Abdul Malik bin Othman v. PP*, 1993). No explanation has been given for the increase, although it could be related to the fact that punishment for heterosexual *molest*[ation] and rape increased at a time when the general climate of need for law and order in Singapore was contrasted with the apparent lawlessness of America. The magistrate held, in addition, that the length of the sentence would increase with the public visibility of the act and the "degree or moral corruption on the innocent minds of children."

Section 377A refers to males, and only males have been punished by the courts for homosexual acts. There has been no case yet of lesbian acts having been tried. Nevertheless, in principle, certain lesbian acts are punishable under Section 20 of the Miscellaneous Offences (Public Order and Nuisance) Act (Cap. 184), which refers to "riotous, disorderly or indecent behaviour" in a public setting, liable on conviction to a fine not exceeding $1,000 or imprisonment not exceeding 1 month. It was invoked by a journalist who reported two girls kissing and fondling each other in a public swimming pool (Tin, 1993). No police action was taken, however, since the identities of the girls had not been established.

Police Entrapment

In Singapore, the largest number of arrests for homosexual activities is initiated by the police acting as decoys. Contrary to a popular belief that homosexual crimes are tried under Sections 377 or 377A, most are convicted under Section 354 of the Penal Code, known in common language as "molest" or "outrage of modesty." The crime carries a maximum jail sentence of 2 years, a fine, caning, or a combination of any two such punishments.

Typically, the police employ very young male constables dressed in "cruising" attire (tank tops and shorts) to loiter around parks, beaches, toilets, and shopping malls. Making eye contact to signal interest and striking up conversations with "cruisers," these "agents provocateur" arrest their victims the moment they are being touched on the buttocks or genitals. The charge is use of criminal force to outrage the modesty of a person.

When the cruiser does not touch the genitals of the police decoy despite all provocation, the police may rely on Section 19 (soliciting in a public place) of the Miscellaneous Offences (Public Order and Nuisance) Act (Cap. 184). This section covers both prostitution, where money is proposed for the transaction, and soliciting "for any other immoral purpose," where a proposition for sex is made without money being involved. This offense carries a fine of up to $1000, doubling on a subsequent conviction, including a jail term not exceeding 6 months.

If the cruiser uses a symbolic gesture to signal sexual activity with the police decoy, he can be tried under Section 294A of the Penal Code. Originally a section called "obscene songs," it includes the commission of any obscene act in any public place to the annoyance of others. The punishment is a maximum of 3 months jail time, a fine, or both.

Since the late 1980s, police swoops on homosexual haunts have been routine. This was the period of the AIDS panic, and the attempt to arrest the spread of the disease included the strategy of control of homosexuality ("Ban on Homosexuals," 1988). Thus, on July 25, 1989, more than 120 persons were brought to the central police station for questioning. The number arrested was not specified, but the police invoked Section 19 to warn that "loiterers" could be charged for soliciting. Similarly, in Kuala Lumpur, police loaded several military trucks with 260 patrons of a gay bar on the pretext or bringing them to the police station for urine tests for drugs (*ST*, 4 October 1993). Police harassment continues today: Police routinely record the identities of strollers in parks that are known to be gay at night.

Reports of anti-gay operations abound in the press (Chong & Ang, 1992; Yen, 1991; 24 September 1993). Each operation is a labor-intensive enterprise that channels manpower resources to arrests for crimes with no complaining victims. Thus, it took twelve detectives to arrest four men, four police officers acting as bait while the other eight waited at the entrance to a gay beach to arrest the "catch" (Chong & Ang, 1992). On a subsequent day it took fifteen detectives to arrest another four men (Chong, 1992).

The police do not release information about the number of such arrests. Nevertheless, between 1990 and 1994, newspapers reported 67 convictions of homosexuals stemming from police undercover activities. This figure represents the tip of an iceberg, since reporting depends on the exigencies of news collectors (e.g., whether the reporter was at the court, whether other items that day drown out such stories). To avoid the glare of publicity inherent in trials and appeals, the majority of those arrested seek "swift justice" by pleading guilty to escape the attention of the press. These 67 reports are likely to be a minute fraction of the total convicted.

Of the 67 cases reported in the press, 50 were convicted for *molest*[ation] (s. 354), 11 for soliciting (s. 19) and 6 for obscene acts (s. 294A). The sentence given for soliciting was between $200 and $500, for obscene acts $200 to $800. Punishment in molest cases varied over the years. Between 1990 and 1992, men charged with touching the genitals of undercover police were fined $800 to $1000. Then, in 1993, jail sentences of 2–6 months were imposed along with caning — usually three strokes ("12 Men Nabbed," 1993). Since molest constitutes the majority of all convictions, men arrested for homosexual offenses have suffered the harshest of the available penalties.

In April 1994, an appeal decision marked a more lenient approach to cases involving police decoys. The appellant in *Tan Boon Hock v. PP* (1994) pleaded guilty to the charge of touching the genitals of an officer who was participating in a police operation against homosexuals on a gay beach. The magistrate, using the current standard of 9 months imprisonment and caning for heterosexual molest, passed a sentence of 4 months imprisonment and three strokes of the cane. Upon the defendant's appeal, Chief Justice Yong Pung How substituted a fine of $2000 for the jail and caning. This was a surprise decision, given earlier allegations by an exiled academic that the judiciary was a weak arm of an authoritarian and punitive political party (Lingle, 1996) and given well-publicized reports that, under Chief Justice Yong, contesting a ruling would risk a high probability of a much more severe sentence ("Man Jailed," 1996; "Molest Case," 1993; "Molester's Jail Term," 1994; Oorjitham, 1996). Nevertheless, the Chief Justice opined that there was some degree of consent among police officers acting as *agents provocateur* in the arrest of homosexual cruisers. While consent is no defense to a charge of gross indecency (s. 377A) it is a factor in the charge of outrage of modesty (s. 354). The Chief Justice also noted that the sentence of jail was rather inappropriate for homosexuals, who had to bear with an "assortment of male inmates."

This ruling was not an isolated oddity. In *Ng Huat v. PP* (1995), a radiographer was convicted under Section 377A on a charge of touching the penis, chest, nipples, and buttocks of a patient who came in for X-ray examination of his wrist. Chief Justice Yong reversed the lower court's sentence of 10 months imprisonment to 3 months. This was a major concession, as Section 377A prescribes a mandatory punishment of jail with no option of a fine. The Chief Justice opined, "There are varying degrees of gross indecency and I find it difficult to say that the present act was one which was so gravely repugnant as to warrant a very lengthy custodial term.... My other misgiving is that the appellant will be placed in a precarious position by an extended term of imprisonment within a confined male environment, bearing in mind the nature of the offence for which he has been convicted." Aware of the fact that protection of the accused is generally not a principle to be considered in sentencing, he was nevertheless sympathetic to gay men being sent to prison.

The general temper of the Singapore court today reflects a stern attitude toward male harassment of females; the norm of punishment is a jail term, flogging, and, most recently, public shaming via televised court proceedings ("Molester's Hearing," 1995). Although police enticement of homosexuals has never been raised as an issue, the gender of the so-called victim and the element of consent by *agents provocateur* make for qualitative differences between male molest of females and molest of males ("Victim's Gender Matters," 1994), paving the way for a lighter sentence for the latter. Arrest figures for police enticement of homosexuals are not available, but there appears to be fewer cases reported in the press recently. This does not necessarily signify a victory for gays, since the absence of such newspaper reporting may merely reflect editorial policy or the erratic nature of journalistic attention.

After the landmark appeal cases of *Tan Boon Hock* and *Ng Huat* there were only two separate reports of police enticement ("Convicted," 1994; "Man Did Indecent Act," 1994). Instead of charging molest, the police now reverted to charging gross indecency, and these two men were sent to jail. Through my own interviews with members of the gay community and with lawyers, I have learned that cases of police enticement are continuing. Most of the accused do not appeal because of the negative sanctions applied to appellants and because they hope that a speedy trial will absolve them from the glare of relentless newspaper publicity.

CIVIL LAW

Partnership

In America and western Europe, gays have clamored for the right to same-sex marriage and have shifted the meaning of "family" to a wider concept beyond the nuclear unit (Eskridge, 1996; Weston, 1991). In Singapore, as long as homosexual acts are punishable under the law, gay men and lesbians have no official sanction to form partnership unions or free associations, no legal protection against employment discrimination by reason of sexuality or AIDS, and no freedom to circulate information. The criminal law against homosexuality is, in this sense, a determinant of civil law, limiting the life chances and constraining the lifestyles of gays and lesbians.

Singapore recognizes marriage as a legal union between a man and a woman, excluding all other arrangements, such as heterosexual cohabitation, gay and lesbian partnerships, and transgender relationships. The terms man and woman are defined strictly in a biological sense that does not allow for socialization contingencies, psychological developments, postmodern identities, and technologies of gender transformation. In *Lim Ying v. Hiok Kian Ming Eric* (1992), a woman married a man under the provisions of the Women's Charter (Cap. 353) and later discovered that the man was born female, had undergone a sex change operation, and could not consummate the marriage. The court agreed to annul the marriage on the ground that the parties were both female. It gave overwhelming priority to birth certification rather than identity card, to gender attribution at birth and not to later development. A person may change identification documents after sex reassignment surgery, but the law does not recognize the new gender identity.

There is a long but unwritten history of transgender identities in Singapore. Homosexuality has been conflated with effeminacy, transvestism, and transsexuality under the rubric *ah quah*. This colloquial Hokkien term lumped a range of gender and sexual variations into a group to be ridiculed, condemned, and made a spectacle of. Bugis Street was a "society of spectacle" where transsexuals of divergent ethnicities and nationalities attended to the gaze of tourists and the amorous desires of British troops and Australian, New Zealand, and United Kingdom (ANZUK) forces. In 1980, Bugis Street was bulldozed by urban renewal ("Bugis Street," 1980).

Medically, Singapore boasted of advances in sex change operations (Ratnam, 1991). Since 1974, when the first male-to-female operation was performed here, there have been more than 500 sex change operations (Lim, 1990). In view of the large number of transgendered persons, Parliament has recently proposed amendments to the Women's Charter to recognize the identities of those who have undergone reassignment surgery, thus allowing them to marry (Wang, 1996), but the amendment does not make provision for same-sex unions. This rules out the chances of immigration for a foreigner who is the same-sex partner of a Singaporean.

Employment

In the field of employment, there is no antidiscrimination that protects a minority group or an individual. Article 12(2) of the constitution stipulates that "there shall be no discrimination against citizens of Singapore on the ground only of religion, race, descent or place of birth in any law or in the appointment of any office or employment under a public authority." This article does not appear to cover the private sector and categories such as gender and sexual orientation. There are in fact no legal cases of resort to this article to sue for discrimination in the workplace. One reason for this lies in the fact that under the Employment Act (Cap. 91), an employer is not obliged to justify termination of employment if the requisite notice period has been given or if salary equivalent to the notice period has been paid in lieu. The Employment Act merely sets minimum standards of employment, like sick days and hospitalization leave. Moreover, it excludes executive or confidential positions, seamen, domestic maids, civil servants, and quasigovernment employees. By and large the majority of the workforce operates on the basis of common law, where employment is like any other contract. This laissez-faire approach does not confer much bargaining power upon the employee to negotiate the terms of an employment contract.

In the public sector two ministries are known to have employment policies tied to sexual orientation. In the Ministry of Foreign Affairs, self-acknowledged homosexuals are barred from appointments involving access to classified information, while "outed" homosexuals are dismissed or exiled to another ministry. These arrangements range from the top of the hierarchy to the bottom, from diplomats or attachés to the dispatch clerk who handles confidential documents. The grounds for dismissal or refusal to hire stem from the assumption that gays are subject to blackmail because of the secrecy and stigma of their sexual orientation and would, under pressure, leak secrets of state to enemies or foreigners.

Whereas the American military has an antihomosexual policy despite the recent "don't ask, don't tell" compromise under the Clinton administration (Scott & Stanley, 1994; Chapter 10, this volume), the Ministry of Defence does not admit self-acknowledged gay men into the military, notwithstanding a policy that conscripts all able-bodied male citizens of 18 years of age to serve a term of 2½ years in the military or police force. However, the military adopts a medical model of homosexuality in the old European psychiatric tradition. Self-declared gay recruits are subject to medical and psychological examinations and are evaluated on a scale of effeminacy based on mannerisms such as gait and speech patterns. They are relegated to a medical category unfit for combat or commando posts. Thus, self-identified gays serve the army in the capacity of administrative or logistical clerks. They are also relieved of reservist service, which others have to serve for about 3 weeks annually until the age of 40 for noncommissioned officers or 45 for officers.

It is not a crime to be a homosexual, but it *is* a crime to engage in homosexual acts. Similarly, the conscription of self-identified gays into the military implies that it is not against military codes of conduct to be homosexual, but practicing homosexuality in the barracks is a breach of these codes. Homosexual misconduct in the military is normally tried by an internal court and is punishable by demotion of rank and detention for about 40 days, which extends the length of military service accordingly. Among nonconscripts, such as women who join the military voluntarily in pursuit of gainful employment, those found practicing homosexual or lesbian acts in camp are given a discharge and stripped of their rank.

The specter of AIDS has put gay men in a precarious position in terms of job security (Ong, 1993; Lee, 1994). The Singapore National Employers' Federation (SNEF) permits termination of an HIV-positive employee if a large number of colleagues are unwilling to work with this person. It also notes that if employers construe AIDS as a disease contracted through "misconduct," they need not bear the medical expenses for AIDS treatment for the worker. In this way, SNEF passes moral judgment on the worker and, by attributing fault and blame to the individual, deprives the worker of medical welfare and abets the collective stigmatization of the HIV-infected. On June 28, 1992, three major insurance companies drew up a list of "high-risk" jobs — male hair stylist, fashion model, flight attendant, unmarried pilot, male dancer, male fashion designer, tour guide, musician, masseur, sailor — that matched common stereotypes of gay males (Abdullah, 1992).

Access to Goods and Services

There is no antidiscrimination law against landlords refusing tenancies to same-sex couples. In the renting of properties market forces generally predominate, and the ability to pay overrides all other considerations concerning prospective tenants. In matters of residential ownership, the state plays a crucial role in shaping the market to the advantage of heterosexual married couples over unmarried persons. About 88 percent of the population live in state housing, and of these, three-fourths own the properties. Since home ownership is in popular demand, the state, in the guise of the Housing Development Board (HDB), has a scale of allocation that gives preference to extended families, stem families, and nuclear families. Single parents and unmarried persons have lesser priority and must wait longer for public housing. For a long time, unmarried persons were not eligible to purchase HDB apartments except when registered with their aged parents. In recent years, the state's promise to provide universal housing and the increasing supply of HDB units has opened up some opportunities for single persons to purchase public housing. Stringent eligibility criteria and conditions, however, continue to apply. In the "Single Singapore Citizen Scheme," a single person, to be eligible to purchase, must be a citizen and at least 35 years of age and then can only have a small (one- or two-bedroom) resale apartment in locations that tend to be the least desirable in the public housing range. Under the "Joint Singles" scheme, two single people can buy jointly a resale HDB flat, but they must be at least 35 years old. They need not be related, however, and may be of the same or different sex. Singles, in effect, are granted access only to older properties in less than prime locations. Those not qualifying under the various eligibility criteria may turn to the private sector which does not impose conditions except for restrictions on citizen ownership in low-rise housing. Yet, private properties cost three times more than HDB apartments and so may price young singles, gays, and lesbians out of the market.

Freedom of Expression and Circulation of Information

In principle, the constitution, under Article 14 (1)(a), guarantees every citizen "the right to freedom of speech and expression." In practice, national security, defamation, journalistic "responsibility," obscenity, and public morality have been so commonly invoked to constrain speech that there is no tradition or culture of free expression in Singapore.

There are in fact many legal restrictions on the circulation of information, and matters of a homosexual nature fall under these prohibitions. The Indecent Advertisements Act (Cap. 135) prohibits the posting of indecent materials in public areas and punishes persons who circulate such material, written or visual (s. 5, 6). The Undesirable Publications Act (Cap. 338) prohibits the importation, sale, or circulation of certain publications that are periodically gazetted by the Ministry of Information and the Arts (MITA). The Penal Code makes it an offense under Sections 292 and 293 to trade in obscene publications or to circulate them to persons under 20 years of age.

Globalization, rising levels of education, and technological developments in mass reproducibility of materials have compelled the state to adapt to social change. In July 1991, film classification was introduced to permit the screening of films to audiences calibrated according to age. Film classification relaxes the rules of censorship and liberalizes the showing of artistic materials. But different standards apply to different materials. The Censorship Review Committee [Ministry of Information and the Arts (MITA), 1992] adopts a formula of censorship and prohibition based on content and accessibility. Generally, for more accessible mediums, more restrictions are imposed. Conversely, the smaller the audience, the greater the degree of autonomy granted. Thus, films classified as "Restricted/Artistic" (R/A) confine the audience to persons over 21. Theater performances tend to have an elite and generally highly educated clientele; glossy photography books are so high priced that they cater to a small consumer market. Consequently, regulation of the content of these media tends to be less so than the restrictions imposed on videos, print, and broadcasting, all of which cater to an undifferentiated mass audience. This means that what is shown in a cinema under the R/A category will be either unavailable or drastically edited on video. Similarly, gay books written in academic jargon and "serious" mode are available on the shelves of the university's library, but gay books written in informal language and of a chatty style (e.g., Miller, 1992; Nestle & Preston, 1994) are placed among a banned collection.

The censorship rules are more stringent when applied to homosexual materials. The Censorship Committee called for a relaxation of erotic materials, sex manuals, and nudity in the cinema, but argued that "in the light of the sensitivity of homosexuality as an issue, materials encouraging homosexuality should continue to be disallowed" (MITA, 1992, p. 24). Visual representation of homosexual acts is banned, and so are materials that portray homosexuality as a legitimate and acceptable lifestyle. Thus, the gay or lesbian teenager in Singapore grows up with cultural images that either annihilate homosexuals (homosexuality does not exist) or denigrate them (as mad, bad, or sad).

There has been a general trend toward liberalization in the art scene. The last few years have seen the camp performance of Lindsay Kemp from England along with nudity, international plays with gay themes (M. Butterfly), and gay films presented in the annual international film festival. However, such openness is not an institutionalized norm because it is counterbalanced by constant regulation and surveillance. On January 3, 1994, Josef Ng, a performing artist, snipped his pubic hair in a symbolic protest against police entrapment of gays, punishment by flogging and jail sentences for "victimless" crimes, and news media exposure of names and faces of the convicted ("Public Protest," 1994). This 30-second act was performed to a small audience in the early hours after midnight, during which the actor faced the wall with his trunks slightly lowered to reveal only the cleavage of his buttocks to the audience. The small audience consisted mostly of converts and sympathizers. No complaint was filed by any member of the public; it was the press who triggered police action. The actor was fined $1000 for committing an obscene act. The event did not involve any admission fees, but the organizer was fined under the Public Entertainments Act (Cap. 257) for providing public entertainment without a license. To further reinforce the punitive response, the government prohibited the actor from future public performances, barred the performance group from receiving any grant or assistance, and declared a general rule forbidding all performances without fixed scripts. Scriptless performances were said to "pose dangers to public order, security and decency" (Government Acts, 1994). The state now requires the submission of scripts from applicants for public entertainment acts. Scripts enable the state to regulate speech, while refusal to license under the Pubic Entertainment Act serves as "prior restraint" on speech and expression.

Assembly and Association

Article 10 (1)(b) of the constitution guarantees all citizens "the right to assemble peaceably without arms," while Article 10 (1)(c) guarantees citizens "the right to form associations," but both freedoms are subject to restrictions in the name of national security, public order, and morality [Article 10 (2)(c)]. The right of assembly may also be tempered by Section 141 of the Penal Code, whereby the police or courts may designate a group of five or more persons an "unlawful assembly" if it is said to resist the execution of any law or to commit mischief or criminal trespass. Since homosexual acts are offenses, a gathering of gays and lesbians may be construed as unlawful assembly. Section 5 of the Miscellaneous Offences (Public Order and Nuisance) Act (Cap. 184) permits the state to make rules regulating assemblies and public processions. These provisions effectively cap collective action and social protests in general, for whereas most industrial countries have witnessed many union strikes and student movements, the situation here is quiescent.

While opportunities for gays and lesbians to organize for political purposes such as protest, decriminalization, and liberation are precluded, association for recreational purposes may appear feasible by reason of the innocuous nature of leisure activities. In 1993, several gay men met to provide social support, and this session germinated into desultory meetings and then into regular monthly gatherings that mixed topical discussion with ethnic festivities or just general parties. As the number of participants increased and included lesbians and fellow travelers, the informal group named itself People Like Us (PLU). Under the law, PLU is deemed an unlawful society because the Societies Act (Cap. 311) requires all societies to be approved and registered with the state. At least ten names of members must be submitted, but as of May 1996 PLU has been unable to enlist that many persons willing to risk their names and reputations and to undergo other perceived social costs necessary for registration. Even had they succeeded, approval of such a society is uncertain. In April 1995, a journalist, acting on complaints by a mother who had come across the PLU newsletter, decided to do a story about their activities. When this became known, PLU members went underground and suspended all meetings at the community art center that had been their monthly venue for a year. Thus, assembly and association for gays and lesbians in Singapore appear clandestine because of the legal restrictions imposed, not just on societies and the circulation of information in general, but also on homosexuality itself.

Curtailment of association is made evident by the absence of any official gay bars, discos, or saunas in Singapore. In early 1995 PLU applied for a business license under the Companies Act (Cap. 50) to operate a cafeteria, but failed to get approval. There are indeed some bars and discos that have a regular clientele of gays and lesbians (although only two are listed in *Spartacus* gay guide), but these places are subject to constant police harassment. There have been many and persistent police raids on discos with a predominantly gay clientele. All the bars that were raided were closed or no longer have gay clients, including Cheers in 1990, Fire in 1991, Rascals in 1993, Shadows in 1994, and Zouk and the Gate in 1995. Carried out on the pretext of either breach of fire code regulations or drug checks, such raids intimidate clients, who must produce identification papers for police recording. Those without documents are detained in the police precinct until a family member is able to produce the necessary documentation.

Besides identity checks that threaten to expose gays to their immediate families and media coverage, the police may threaten disco owners with closure or refusal to renew their licenses. On February 17, 1988, the Public Entertainment Licensing Unit of the Criminal Investigation Department threatened to revoke the licenses of nightclub owners unless they stopped admitting gays (Chang, 1988). Owners were also barred from featuring all-male fashion shows and promotions like "macho night." On August 3, 1995, the Gate disco was fined under Section 18 of the Public Entertainments Act (Cap. 257) for unlicensed performances in which "men wearing briefs and women wearing brassieres and slacks underneath tattered clothing depicted homosexual and lesbian themes in their dances"

("Disco Fined," 1995). District Judge S. Thyagarajan, finding these performances not only "objectionable, but also disgusting," imposed the maximum penalty of $5000.

THE SOCIAL CONTEXT OF PUBLIC DISAPPROVAL

The Media as Adversary

Beyond the law, the police, and the state, social institutions play a role in the stigmatization of homosexuality in Singapore. The news media, in particular, act as agents of social control, playing an active role in the enforcement of laws, which at normal times remain mostly dormant. Moreover, by publishing the name, occupation, and photograph of an arrested man, the press abets in the commission of public shaming and "outing" of these men as homosexuals.

Given a long history of state control of media, whereby magazines and newspapers have been banned or censored, their editors have been fined heavily for defamation, their journalists have been barred from entry into Singapore, and other strategies of restraint have been invoked (Asia Watch, 1989), the news media in Singapore perform a role drastically different from that in other countries. In America, most journalists perceive themselves as muckrakers or whistle-blowers exposing corruption, political scandals, and unfair monopolies. The press thus assumes an adversarial position against politicians and big corporations. In contrast, the Singapore press tends to take a celebratory position toward public officials. Negative reporting of politicians, policy, or the nation in general is not the order of the day. The laudatory stance towards politicians and national achievements presupposes an attitude of "us" versus "them," where the West is construed as foreign devils and an evil influence on the population, including being responsible for the spread of homosexuality and diseases like AIDS. The news media construct gays and lesbians as "folk devils" (Cohen, 1972). Acting as "moral entrepreneurs" (Becker, 1963), reporters of the *New Paper* informed the police of gay cruising at Fort Road beach. Obligated to respond to a complaint, the police sent a team of *agents provocateur* to make arrests. Reporters and photographers present at the scene were able to *make* news with a story that sells (Chong, 1992, 1993; Chong & Ang, 1992). One of the men whose picture was publicized later committed suicide. It was the *New Paper* that, using pictures and adversarial moralistic cant, alerted the police to the performance of Josef Ng, described earlier, provoking a prosecution for obscenity. It was the *New Paper* that reported on June 22, 1995, risqué dances "of homosexual and sado-masochistic themes" that instigated the police to investigate on the same day and to press charges against the Gate disco ("Disco Fined," 1995). On October 14, 1993, the *New Paper* featured two girls expressing intimacy at a swimming pool, noting that this was a public nuisance and an act of indecency ("Girls Kissing," 1993). On October 12, 1995 the *New Paper* featured a story of a university student who had posed nude for an American gay magazine (Pereira, 1995). No questions were asked about who had access to this magazine or how the papers were able to reprint some of the shots (albeit without genitals). Instead the focus was on the propriety of the student and the reputation of the university. In his fifth year of medical school, the student withdrew from the university.

In the entertainment pages the news media take pleasure in making guesses at the sexual orientation of male Chinese actors and pop stars (Wong, 1991; Lee, 1995). Making an issue out of a performer's alleged homosexuality, the media feed readers' desire for sensationalism and gossip and increases the newsworthiness of gay arrests.

Social Attitudes

In a 1992 survey of 1102 Singaporeans ages 17 and older, 86 percent disapproved of homosexuality and lesbianism as a way of life, 9 percent were indifferent, and only 4 percent expressed positive attitudes ("S'poreans," 1992). Young people and those who had worked abroad were the least disapproving. Among the 86 percent who disapproved, 44 percent cited religious and moral grounds, 25 percent followed the assumed convention that it is just not socially acceptable, 14 percent feared its association with AIDS and sexual diseases, and 10 percent perceived it to be a threat to the nuclear family. Among the 4 percent who approved, 46 percent felt "nothing against it," 29 percent defended the virtue of sexual freedom, and 25 percent argued on biological grounds that an inborn quality should be accepted as a fact of life. On the whole, the survey presented a picture of the average Singaporean as morally conservative and convention abiding. The majority of respondents (90 percent) disapproved of extramarital sex, homosexuality (86 percent), premarital sex (67 percent), and cohabitation (66 percent) as ways of life.

The findings of this survey, however, were skewed by the questions asked and the conduct of the interview. Leading questions on intimate matters of sexuality, asked face-to-face in front of other family members, were bound to produce morally correct answers. The disjunction between attitude and behavior indicates that Singaporeans may be moralistic but not necessarily moral in their conduct. Thus, the large number of respondents who wanted stricter censorship is at odds with the high rates of cinema attendance when R/A movies are shown. In addition, the popular rejection of homosexuality as a legitimate way of life was inconsistent with attitudes toward media depictions of homosexuality. The 46 percent who favored banning print and audio materials that encouraged homosexuality as a way of life were balanced by the 46 percent who wanted some form of access to such materials. Forty-eight percent did not favor visual images of homosexual behavior, but 38 percent were tolerant. On films with gay themes and subplots, 46 percent approved, and 34 percent disapproved (MITA, 1992).

Given the contradictions between attitude and behavior and the conflicting opinions that exist, policymakers tend to play safe and err on the conservative side (MITA, 1992) and do not take controversial positions that would be divisive or alienate the masses. Official policy toward homosexuality is thus resistant to change.

Social Conduct

Beyond surveys of attitudes, behavioral indications reveal the nature and extent of public disapproval of homosexuality. It is rare for two persons of the same gender to be seen expressing intimacying in public, such as kissing or necking. Indeed, this may be classed as a "public nuisance" offense (s. 20, Cap. 184). In 1994, two male diners at Opera Cafe were expelled by the management for affectionate behavior such as hand-holding at the table. Since a considerable proportion of the regular patrons came from the gay and lesbian community, the two males felt comfortable enough to express affection within the enclosed space. But the management engaged in self-policing to avert the possibility of bad publicity and to avoid the risk of losing its liquor license. Hand-holding between two persons of the same sex has been common throughout Asia and is acceptable, particularly between females. However, this tradition has been lost in the context of a bureaucratic, impersonal, and competitively striving society. In Singapore, one can find two males walking hand-in-hand with each other only among the community of guest workers who are mostly of one sex and who come from poorer countries, such as the Sri Lankan laborers of Little India (Serangoon Road), Thai masons at various construction sites, and Filipino maids in Orchard Road.

Although the majority of the local population appear not to tolerate hand-holding between males, they are relatively more tolerant of two males dancing with each other. In discos all over Singapore it is extremely prevalent for males to dance in pairs or in groups to fast beat tunes. Most of these males belong to a younger age category, usually comprising a peer group of military conscripts who are short of female dance partners.

Hate crimes, such as gay-bashing, are rare, but cases of extortion attempts on gay men have been reported ("Man Made Extortion Bid," 1995; "Old Man Conned," 1991; "Police N S Man," 1995). Extortion cases are dealt with severely by a jail term and caning. More common than hate crimes or extortion is ridicule. The Hokkien labels such as *ah quah* [transvestite or transsexual] or *cha boh eng* [girlie] and the Malay equivalent *bapuk* are hurled at effeminate males. Military conscripts and teenage boys are most susceptible to such derogatory mockery and peer bullying. A study of 40 young effeminate males ages 18 and 19 found that they were frequently teased at primary school (Kok, 1991). The authors of this study, four psychiatrists from the university, continue to label homosexuality a "diagnostic disease."

Given a legal system that condemns homosexuality, a medical establishment that classifies homosexuality as a disease, and a society that taunts homosexuals, most gays conceal their sexuality and lifestyles from family members. The age-old patriarchal custom of preserving the male lineage through Chinese associations, male ancestor worship, and pride in generational continuity of surnames exerts pressure on males to procreate. Many gay males feel guilt at not fulfilling their filial duties of marrying and begetting offspring.

Living double lives would have been easier if those lives were compartmentalized by space and time. But space is at a premium in Singapore. Gay men under 35, who are not eligible to purchase a resale HDB flat and who are unlikely to be able to afford private apartments, tend to live with their nuclear families and to learn to practice impression management so that they can conceal their secret. Residing "in the closet" within their own families limits opportunities to develop long-term relationships with a partner. Trying to balance filial obligations, family expectations, and demands of the workplace with the maintenance of a gay relationship outside these realms is an arduous feat few gays have been able to master.

CONCLUSION: SINGAPORE, A LAST FRONTIER

There are rational, moral, and humanitarian arguments for accepting gays and lesbians as human beings, not second-class citizens (West, 1988). Anti-discrimination legislation has been introduced in many European countries (Waaldijk & Clapham, 1993). Asian countries are moving in the direction of greater tolerance. In China there are gay groups in almost every city; there are documentaries, films, photographic albums, and a wealth of publications on gay and lesbian topics. Japan held its first gay parade on August 28, 1994, in which 1000 marched for more than 3 hours through Tokyo streets. Hong Kong decriminalized homosexuality in 1990, now hosts an annual gay and lesbian film festival, and has two grassroots organizations. Thailand has established a gay condominium project for a growing middle-class clientele (Fairclough, 1994). Taiwan, the Philippines, and Indonesia have active gay movements, and a few universities in these nations have for many years offered courses on gay and lesbian studies ("Out of the Closet," 1994).

Singapore appears to be the last frontier in the Asian region for positive gay and lesbian developments. Its leaders boast of economic development, a safe and clean environment, corruption-free government, and material affluence. But the homosexuality laws, a colonial legacy of the British, lag behind. Police tactics, which critics elsewhere recognize as unethical and ineffective, continue to operate. The media treat gays as criminals, perverts, and subjects for gossip and scandal, and the medical establishment still adopts an outmoded model of homosexuality as mental illness.

Rapid economic growth in the Asian region has spawned the *nouveaux riches*, a new middle class that has been in the vanguard of social and political transformation in South Korea, Taiwan, and Thailand (Robinson & Goodman, 1996). Well-educated locally and overseas, many of the new middle class form bodies like nongovernmental organizations and new social movements to protect the environment, minorities, women, and human rights. The rise of gay and lesbian organizations, as well as AIDS activism, in Hong Kong, Taiwan, Indonesia, the Philippines, and Thailand is an instance of this development. Material growth increases options. Thus "guppies," the gay segment of the "yuppie" generation, can pursue an independent lifestyle contrary to tradition.

In Singapore, this middle class is not as liberal as their counterparts in the rest of Asia (Jones & Brown, 1994), because of a weak political culture and a strong state hostile to civil rights (Asia Watch, 1989). However, new technologies and global tendencies can alter this state of affairs. Through the Internet, faxes, and video conferencing, a vast amount of information evades state surveillance. Singaporeans can access gay cybergroups and exchange information. With evaporating borders, globalization facilitates international communication, networking, and overseas travel. As more and more Singaporeans study, work, live, tour, and migrate abroad, they become more aware of gay and lesbian issues. The prospect of legal change for gays and lesbians will ultimately depend on an affluent, educated, informed, and cosmopolitan population.

CITED CASES

Abdul Malik bin Othman v PP, Subordinate Court Magistrate Appeal: 5170–5176 (1993).
Kanagasuntharam v PP, 1 SLR: 81–86 (1992).
Lim Ying v Hiok Kian Ming Eric, 1 SLR: 184–196 (1992).
Ng Huat v PP, 2 SLR: 783–794 (1995).
PP v Jumahat, Singapore High Court Judgments, Vol. 16, 3765–3776 (1992).
PP v Victor Rajoo, 3 SLR: 417–432 (1995).
Tan Boon Hock v PP, 2 SLR: 150–153 (1994).

References

Abdullah, Y. (1992, June 28). Companies cutting risk of insuring AIDS victims. *The Straits Times*.

Asia Watch (1989). *Silencing all critics: Human rights violations in Singapore*. New York: Author.

Ban on homosexuals will force them underground. (1988, March 1). *The Straits Times*.

Becker, H. (1963). *Outsiders*. New York: Free Press.

Boon, Tan Ooi. (1995, August 4). Act was not unnatural, defence lawyer argues. *The Straits Times*.

Bugis Street to be cleared of transvestites. (1980, August 23). *The Straits Times*.

Chong, E. (1995, August 30). Justice Lai clarifies when oral sex is not an offence. *The Straits Times*.

Chong, Gillian Pow. (1988, February 17). Homosexuals banned from night spots. *The Straits Times*.

Chong, Yaw Yan. (1992, March 10). Gay beach: 4 more arrested. *The New Paper*

Chong, Yaw Yan. (1993, September 24). Gays surface again at East Coast beach. *The New Paper*.

Chong, Yaw Yan, & Ang, Dave. (1992, March 9). Ambush on gay beach. *The New Paper*.

Cohen, S. (1972). *Folk devils and moral panics*. London: MacGibbon Kee.

Convicted of gross indecency. (1994, June 19). *The Straits Times*.

Defence wants court to rule on consensual oral sex. (1995, August 19). *The Straits Times*.

Did you know that oral sex, even between consenting adults, is an offence? (1995, July 6). *The Straits Times*.

Disco fined $5,000 for unlicensed live performance. (1995, August 3). *The Straits Times*.

Eskridge, W. Jr. (1996). *The case for same-sex marriage: From sexual liberty to civilized commitment*. New York: Free Press.

Fairclough, G. (1994, August 4) Gay new world. *Far Eastern Economic Review*, p. 60.

Five fined for oral sex offences. (1991, July 22). *The Straits Times*.

Government acts against 5th Passage over performance art. (1994, January 22). *The Straits Times*.

Guard caught two men performing indecent act. (1994, June 1). *The Straits Times*.

Gupta, R. L. (1984). *The medico-legal aspects of sexual offences*. Lucknow, India: Eastern Book.

Hickling, R. H. (1992). *Essays in Singapore law*. Petaling Jaya, Malaysia: Pelanduk Publications.

Jailed for sex through toilet wall hole. (1991, August 11). *The Straits Times*.

Jones, D., & Brown, D. (1994). Singapore and the myth of the liberalizing middle class. *Pacific Review*, 17(1), 79–87.

Kay, Li Man. (1995, July 11). Law implies married people can't have oral sex. *The Straits Times*.

Kok, L. P. (1991). Profile of a homosexual in Singapore. *Singapore Medical Journal*, 32(6), 403–408.

Lee, E. (1994). AIDS and the law. *Singapore Law Review*, 156, 213–243.

Lee, Yin Luen. (1995, August 12). He's blunt on women, but silent on a man. *The Straits Times*.

Lim, S. (1990, December 10). Transsexual counselling others like herself. *The Straits Times*.

Lingle, C. (1996). *Singapore's authoritarian capitalism*. Fairfax, VA: Locke Institute.

A litterbug's mane of shame. (1993, February 22). *The Straits Times*.

Man did indecent act. (1994, June 15). *The Straits Times*.

Man jailed for theft has sentence increased on appeal. (1996, February 16). *The Straits Times*.

Man made extortion bid after oral sex. (1995, October 26). *The Straits Times*.

Man on gross indecency charge. (1993, June 4). *The Straits Times*.

Man says that lawyer performed oral sex on him. (1996, February 6). *The Straits Times*.

Miller, N. (1992). *Out in the world: Gay and lesbian life from Buenos Aires to Bangkok*. New York: Random House.

Ministry of Information and the Arts. (1992). *Censorship Review Committee report*. Singapore, Singapore: Author.

Molest case appeal: Former customs man's term upped. (1993, November 4). *The Straits Times*.

Molester's hearing a first on TV. (1995, March 31). *The Straits Times*.

Molester's jail term increased on appeal. (1994, April 15). *The Straits Times*.

Nestle, J., & Preston, J. (Eds.). (1994). *Sister and brother: Lesbians and gay men write about their lives together*. San Francisco: Harper.

Old man conned by "gay ruse." (1991, September 12). *The Straits Times*.

Ong, W. (1993). AIDS and employment law in Singapore. *The Act*, 4, 9–11.

Oorjitham, S. (1996, February 2). To appeal or not to appeal. *Asiaweek*, p. 5.

Out of the closet: Filipinos debate the relevance of gay literature. (1994, October 5). *Asiaweek*, p. 33.

Pereira, B. (1995, October 12). Is this model an NUS student? *The New Paper*.

Police NS man demanded sex and money from men. (1995, December 20). *The Straits Times*.

Police raid transvestite and homosexual areas. (1989, July 25). *The Straits Times.*

Public protest. (1994, January 3). *The New Paper.*

Ratnam, S. S. (1991). *Cries from within: Transsexualism, gender confusion and sex change.* Singapore, Singapore: Longman.

Robinson, R., & Goodman, D. (Eds.). (1996). *The new rich in Asia.* London: Routledge.

Scott, W., & Stanley, S. (Eds.). (1994). *Gays and lesbians in the military.* New York: Aldine de Gruyter.

S'poreans voice firm "no" to liberal values. (1992, August 4). *The Straits Times.*

39 foreigners among 260 nabbed in anti-vice op. (1993, October 2). *The New Paper.*

Tielman, R., & Hammelburg, H. (1993). World survey on the social and legal position of gays and lesbians. In A. Hendriks (Eds.), *The third pink book: A global view of lesbian and gay liberation and oppression.* Buffalo, New York: Prometheus Books.

Tin, Tang Wai. (1993, October 14). Girls kissing in public pool. *The New Paper.*

Tremewan, C. (1994). *The political economy of social control in Singapore.* New York: St. Martin's.

12 men nabbed in anti-gay operation at Tanjong Rhu. (1993, November 23). *The Straits Times.*

Two did indecent act in toilet. (1994, April 30). *The Straits Times.*

Two jailed for indecent act in pool. (1993, September 30). *The Straits Times.*

Two men caught for indecent act. (1991, June 27). *The Straits Times.*

Two men jailed for indecent act. (1992, January 28). *The Straits Times.*

Victim's gender matters, so molester's sentence reduced. (1994, April 7). *The Straits Times.*

Waaldijk, K., & Clapham, A. (Eds.). (1993). *Homosexuality: A European Community issue.* Dordrecht, the Netherlands: Martin Nijhoff.

Wang, H. L. (1996, January 25). Nod to marriages of sex change persons "practical." (1996, January 25). *The Straits Times.*

West, D. J. (1988). Homosexuality and social policy: The case for a more informed approach. *Law and Contemporary Problems, 51,* 181–199.

Weston, K. (1991). *Families we choose.* New York: Columbia University Press.

Wong, Kim Hoh. (1991, November 21). Waise's queer ambitions. *The Straits Times.*

Yen, Phan Ming. (1991, August 19). Gays stay away from Serangoon Complex. *The Straits Times.*

10

The United States

RICHARD GREEN

Introduction

Surveying American sociolegal control of homosexuality is complicated by the existence of 50 states with individual laws, a federal government with its law, and the substantial cultural diversity between regions of the United States.

This chapter will examine laws prohibiting private, consensual sexual behavior between same-sex persons, employment discrimination based on sexual orientation, the public's opinion on sexual orientation, family law concerns of homosexual parents and partners, homosexual identity, behavior and military service, immigration law, and crimes targeting homosexual victims.

Criminalization

America's history of criminalizing sodomy, the "crime against nature," generally meant to include genital–anal intercourse between two men or between a man and a woman, dates to the time of the original 13 English colonies. All criminalized sodomy as a capital offense (*Bowers v. Hardwick*, 1986; Katz, 1976; Oaks, 1980). As the number of American states increased, criminalization continued. It was unanimous in the 48 states until 1961.

The first state to break formation was Illinois. It followed the American Law Institute's Model Penal Code. This prestigious body of legal scholars proposed that consenting private sexual behavior between same-sex adults should not be of concern to the law (American Law Institute, 1962). Slowly, other states abandoned sodomy laws, but by 1986 these states still constituted a minority.

In 1986 the U.S. Supreme Court considered directly, for the first time, a state's authority to criminalize private, consenting same-sex genital contact. Leading up to that ruling was a series of Supreme Court decisions creating a zone of constitutionally protected sexual privacy. First, married couples and their physicians were protected from prosecution for using or prescribing contraceptives (*Griswold v. Connecticut*, 1965). Then that right extended to unmarried couples (*Eisenstadt v. Baird*, 1972). The right to terminate an early pregnancy was granted to the pregnant woman (*Roe v. Wade*, 1973).

The 1986 test case on sodomy law began with a man being arrested in his bedroom after a police officer gained entry to his house to serve a traffic warrant and observed him

RICHARD GREEN • Institute of Criminology, University of Cambridge, Cambridge CB3 9DT, England, United Kingdom; and Gender Identity Clinic, Charing Cross Hospital, London W6 8RF, England, United Kingdom.

Sociolegal Control of Homosexuality, edited by West and Green, Plenum Press, New York, 1997.

engaged in same-sex fellatio. He challenged the constitutionality of the law even though the state elected not to prosecute. The question eventually answered by the Supreme Court was whether the forbidden conduct was protected as a "fundamental right" so as to require the highest level of state justification for enforcement. By a vote of 5-4, the answer was negative. The court majority found "no connection" between the "earlier sexual privacy cases on the one hand and homosexual activity on the other.... Proscriptions against [sodomy] have ancient roots." The concurring opinion by the Chief Justice pronounced that "condemnation of [these] practices is firmly rooted in Judaeo-Christian moral and ethical standards. [Centuries ago] Blackstone described 'the infamous crime against nature ... a crime not fit to be named'" (*Bowers v. Hardwick*, pp. 190–192, 196, 1986).

In a ringing dissent, Justice Blackman protested:

> Our cases long have recognized that the Constitution embodies a promise that a cer-
> tain private sphere of individual liberty will be kept largely beyond the reach of
> government.... [This] Court ... has refused to recognize ... the fundamental interest all
> individuals have in controlling the nature of their intimate associations with others ...
> the issue raised by this case touches the heart of what makes individuals what they are.
> (*Bowers v. Hardwick*, pp. 203, 206)

Although the federal Supreme Court has not recognized a fundamental right to engage in private consenting homosexual behavior, some state courts have. Before *Hardwick*, in 1978, New Jersey held its sodomy law unconstitutional (*State v. Cuiffini*, 1978), based on the right to privacy enunciated in an earlier case in which I testified. In that case the fornication law was declared unconstitutional (it prohibited consensual intercourse by a man with an unmarried adult woman) (*State v. Saunders*, 1977). Also, pre-*Hardwick*, Pennsylvania in 1980 found that its law failed to meet the "threshold of state power" and that the law forbidding sodomy between unmarried partners was an "irrational distinction based on marital status" (*Commonwealth v. Bonadio*, 1980). New York in 1981 held that criminalizing sodomy infringed on the "right of privacy which is a fundamental right" (*People v. Onofre*, 1980).

In Texas the sodomy law saga has had a tortured and lengthy legal history and continues without resolution. In 1983, a federal trial court held the law to be unconstitutional (*Baker v. Wade*, 1983). However, this ruling was reversed by an appellate panel in 1984 (*Baker v. Wade*, 1984). But then the full federal appellate court overruled that panel in a decision based primarily on religious morality (*Baker v. Wade*, 1985). The U.S. Supreme Court denied review (*Baker v. Wade*, 1986). However, a lower *state* court held that the law violates the right to privacy (*State v. Morales*, 1992) but later on appeal it lacked jurisdiction (*State v. Morales*, 1994), , and in 1993 the state Court of Appeals held that the Dallas police department could not deny employment to a lesbian applicant on the basis of her violating the sodomy law because the law was unconstitutional when applied to consenting behavior in private (*City of Dallas v. England*, 1993). The case has not been granted review by the state Supreme Court; thus there is no ultimate ruling.

A Tennessee lower court held that the state's constitutional right to privacy protects same-sex couples' sexual activity. Thus, the state would have to demonstrate a "compelling reason" to justify the sodomy law, the standard required when a fundamental right, such as privacy, is invoked. That sodomy law (Homosexual Practices Act) was passed after *Hardwick* and reflected Tennessee's concern that sodomy laws could ensnare mixed-gender couples as well as those of the same gender. Then a Court of Appeals held that the sodomy law applying only to same-sex couples was unenforceable (*Campbell v. Sundquist*, 1996a). It held that under the law, the right of privacy was unduly compromised by prohibiting sexual activity taking place "behind closed doors in an individual's home." Turning to the argument that the law reflected a moral choice of the majority of the state, the Court was "unconvinced that the advancement of this moral choice is so compelling as to justify the regulation of private, non-commercial, sexual choices ... simply because those adults happen to be of the same gender." The Tennessee Supreme Court refused the state's appeal (*Campbell v. Sundquist*, 1996b).

In 1996 the Montana sodomy law was enjoined from enforcement by a state lower court because it intruded on the state constitution's protection of privacy (*Gryczan v. State of Montana*, 1996). The law had permitted a prison sentence of up to 10 years for "deviate sexual relations" between two persons of the same sex "or any form of sexual intercourse with an animal." The court agreed that "many Montanans do not approve of homosexual activity." Nevertheless, since the statute was not being enforced, the state was apparently conceding that the individual's expectation of privacy was reasonable. The decision was upheld by the state Supreme Court (ND 96–202, 1997).

The Louisiana sodomy statute (prohibiting unnatural carnal copulation) was nearly overturned. The law has a long history, dating to 1805, when life imprisonment at hard labor was the penalty. But the state Supreme Court overruled a trial court that held the law to be unconstitutional. The suit had been brought on "equal protection" grounds arguing discrimination against same-sex genital contact whether anal or oral, but the court noted that heterosexuals were also covered by the law. Further, the plaintiff's offense was solicitation of oral sex, and this could be prohibited without addressing the constitutionality of a law prohibiting the act under other circumstances (*State v. Baxley*, 1995).

Twenty-two states and the District of Columbia continue to have sodomy laws. Twenty prohibit homosexual and heterosexual sodomy, three only homosexual sodomy. Those that continue to ban only same-sex sodomy are Arkansas, Kansas (under challenge, as noted later in this chapter), and Missouri. States that have decriminalized sodomy include the populous jurisdictions of California, Illinois, New Jersey, New York, Ohio, and Pennsylvania.

At the interface of public and private expression of homosexual sexuality, sodomy laws continue to impact the individual. Rendezvous sites for same-sex liaisons remain concerns of "vice squad" police. Plainclothes officers may patrol gay meeting places and "stake out" public toilets, parks, and beaches where gay men are known to meet. A plainclothes policeman will enter into a conversation about an act of sodomy and then arrest the civilian for "solicitation." Whether or not the sexual act is illegal per se, the stage on which it was to be played may determine that it is not private, and thus solicitation becomes the crime.

Criminal charges brought under such circumstances are typically for solicitation of noncommercial consenting adult sexual conduct, engaging in sexual conduct in a public or quasipublic place, or loitering for the purpose of soliciting or engaging in sexual activity. However, New York held that homosexual solicitation in a car on a public street is private and beyond the reach of the law (*People v. Onofre*, 1980).

The Georgia Supreme Court ruled in 1996 that a man's conviction for soliciting a police officer to a motel for oral sex did not violate its constitution (*Christensen v. State*, 1996). The man had been approached by an undercover police officer wearing a microphone at an interstate highway rest stop. He was sentenced to 12 months probation. Citing

Hardwick, the court wrote, "We hold that the proscription against sodomy is a legitimate and valid exercise of state police power in furtherance of the moral welfare of the public." The court invoked a weak rational basis test of the law's purpose (any seemingly legitimate reason), not strict scrutiny requiring a more exacting standard. The dissent called the majority opinion "pathetic and disgraceful." They stressed that the appropriate standard for review when a privacy right is at issue is strict scrutiny.

A public restroom case in Florida illustrates an unsuccessful police attempt to continue enforcement. A man was arrested for masturbating in a closed toilet stall or cubicle after an officer observed him by peering through a crack between the door and the stall wall. However, the court held that in this setting the man had a reasonable expectation of privacy and further that masturbation was not a crime (*Ward v. State*, 1994).

Legal challenges after solicitation arrests can result in the sodomy law being overturned. In Kentucky, the State Supreme Court struck down its law in a case where a gay man solicited a policeman for oral sex: "Kentucky courts have consistently protected its citizens' right of privacy ... provided the act does not injure or affect the rights, life, security, or property of others." The state was unable to show a compelling reason for the law (*Commonwealth v. Wasson*, 1992).

Although a heterosexual act "solicited" under the same circumstance might not be criminal, that may not provide protection for homosexual behavior. It may, however, provide the basis for a constitutional challenge as a violation of equal protection. The sodomy law in Kansas is under challenge on equal protection grounds after a man was charged with accepting an invitation for oral sex from a plainclothes police officer while sitting in his car and was convicted of solicitation. A similar situation with a man and a woman is not illegal (Topeka artist to challenge solicitation ordinance, 1996, *Lesbian/Gay Law Notes*, January, p. 7).

Whereas the continuing existence of laws criminalizing consenting private homosexual conduct may have relatively little direct impact on most gay or lesbian residents of a state, indirect consequences can be considerable. Accompanying the potential of prosecution (however remote) is the knowledge that the state remains on record as condemning an activity important to an individual's personal identity. Sodomy laws also provide a rationale for discrimination. Employment or housing bias based on sexual orientation can be justified. Child custody can be denied. Seeking police assistance after verbal harassment or physical assault is discouraged by the fear that one's complaint will not be taken seriously. In essence, these laws provide a backdrop for degrading persons with a homosexual orientation.

IMMIGRATION

Homosexual immigrants were first excluded by statute from entry into the United States by the Immigration Act of 1917. The act prohibited the entry of "persons of constitutional psychopathic inferiority" (a psychiatric term of the time). Exclusion was based largely on the "official" American Psychiatric Association designation of homosexuals as mentally ill.

The Public Health Service advised that the diagnosis "psychopathic personality" was sufficient to ban homosexuals because "ordinarily sexual deviation was a manifestation of a psychopathic personality" (H.R. Rep. No. 1365, 82nd Congress, 2nd Session, pp. 46–48, 1952). That term described persons who were "predominantly amoral or antisocial" (American Psychiatric Association, 1957). When a federal court of appeals later held that the diagnosis of psychopathic personality did not include homosexuals, Congress amended the Immigration Act to include "sexual deviates" as an excludable class. The term "psychopathic personality" was no longer considered a medical diagnosis but became a "legal term of art." It was "to be interpreted by what Congress intended as a guide, and not to be left to the vagaries and honest but conflicting theories of psychiatry for determination" (*Boutilier v. Immigration and Naturalization Service*, 1966).

In 1973 the American Psychiatric Association declared that homosexuality was not per se a mental disorder. Then the Public Health Service abandoned its role in effecting homosexual exclusion. It refused to issue medical certificates certifying an alien as afflicted with a medically excludable condition solely based on homosexuality (*Interpreter Releases*, 1979). However, the Immigration Service persisted in exclusion. Until 1990, the Immigration Act continued to ban those afflicted with "psychopathic personality, sexual deviation, or mental deficit" (8 USC Section 1182 a, 4, 1990). Then, a comprehensive reform of US immigration laws deleted exclusion on the basis of homosexuality.

The next wave of immigration case law concerned homosexual aliens seeking political asylum in the U.S. based on persecution in their native country. In 1990 a Cuban was granted asylum on the grounds of homosexuality. The case was an isolated instance without precedent. But in 1994, the U.S. Attorney General issued an order giving it precedential status. The effect is that homosexuals now constitute a "social group" for asylum purposes. Thus their burden in seeking asylum is limited to showing that their group is subject to persecution (Refugee Act of 1980). Homosexuals from Mexico, Brazil, Turkey, Nicaragua, Venezuela, Singapore, Pakistan, and Russia have been granted political asylum.

Still, other forms of immigration discrimination continue against homosexuals. The United States does not recognize same-sex couples under immigration law. Thus, these partnerships can be ruptured when only one partner is permitted entry or citizenship.

The United States has been vigorous in its exclusion of aliens who are HIV-positive or have AIDS. In the late 1980s, HIV-positive attendees at scientific meetings on AIDS, as well as casual visitors, were turned away. In 1990 exceptions were made for those coming to the United States for brief visits to attend a professional, academic, or science congress. An HIV-positive person can also obtain a waiver to visit relatives or receive medical treatment. However, entering the United States with an intent to remain, when knowingly infected with HIV, is grounds for deportation (66 *Interpreter Releases*, June 6, 1989).

EMPLOYMENT

It is not unlawful to discriminate against a homosexual employee unless there is a specific protecting statute. Only nine states prohibit discrimination based on sexual orientation. No federal statute with nationwide application protects homosexual employees against discrimination. Proposed laws, introduced during recent years, have never gathered enough votes in Congress for passage.

Some states have general civil rights laws that should protect homosexuals — California, New York, and Michigan, for example. In some states, specific businesses must serve all persons without discrimination. In California, a state-protected public utility may have special obligations to provide equal treatment to employees (*Gay Law Student's Association v. Pacific Tel & Tel*, 1979).

Title VII is the federal law prohibiting employment discrimination based on race or gender. However, its essentially nonexistent legislative history for gender discrimination (reports and speeches in Congress prior to passage) ordinarily used to demonstrate congressional or legislative intent behind a law, has hampered courts. The gender arm of the antidiscrimination statute was appended to the racial protection body at the last minute in an attempt to defeat it. When the statute passed, the United States had a sex discrimination employment statute with no substantive rationale for courts to interpret.

Expansion of sexual harassment litigation and later of sexual orientation harassment into Title VII gender employment discrimination inevitably inherited the deficit of its sex discrimination parent — no legislative history. Consequently, court decisions have been in disarray. The statute was thought initially to protect female workers from male employers. But because the Supreme Court has protected white workers (the dominant class) from racial discrimination in Title VII actions (reverse discrimination), some federal courts have held that males may seek relief under the gender discrimination law (*Prescott v. Independent Life and Accident Insurance*, 1995). Could the law then protect men or women from men or women based not on their sex, but on their sexual orientation? Some see it as disingenuous to argue that sexual orientation discrimination is not sexual discrimination in that the two are linked — an employer's sexual orientation determines the sex of the employee who would be the object of harassment.

In 1976, a federal court held that sexual harassment could be included as sex discrimination under Title VII (*Williams v. Saxbe*, 1976). The two categories of sexual harassment are "quid pro quo" and "hostile environment." As recognized by the Supreme Court, quid pro quo is when an employer predicates some condition of employment on an employee's submission to unwelcome sexual demands. "Hostile environment" is where verbal or physical conduct of a sexual nature has the purpose or effect of unreasonably interfering with an employee's work performance or creates an intimidating, hostile, or offensive work environment (*Meritor Savings Bank v. Vinson*, 1986).

Another federal appellate court held in 1979 that Title VII does not prohibit hiring discrimination based on sexual orientation (*De Santis v. Pacific Tel & Tel Co.*, 1979). Physical and verbal harassment of an employee in consequence of sexual orientation was held not to be Title VII prohibited discrimination in 1992 (*Dillon v. Frank*, 1992). A year later, in 1993, a federal appeals court held that "harassment by a male supervisor against a male subordinate does not state a claim under Title VII even though the harassment has sexual overtones" (*Giddens v. Shell Oil Co.*, 1993). When male workers claimed a hostile environment from harassment by supervisors and coworkers with writings, drawings, and explicit discussions of homosexual acts, this too was insufficient (*Fox v. Sierra Development Co.*, 1995). The homosexual context was deemed irrelevant: "A work environment saturated with sexual references is potentially abusive to men and women. Nothing here singles out men or women for injury. Thus it is not discriminatory. All persons regardless of sex, gender or sexual orientation might be offended." Those bringing suit had to allege facts indicating that the work environment was hostile to men *qua* men, and not based on sexual orientation.

Recent rulings, however, show a trend toward Title VII coverage. The federal government's Equal Employment Opportunity Commission (EEOC) filed suit in 1995 on behalf of three automobile salesmen who claim they suffered harassment by sexual advances from a male supervisor (*EEOC v. H.J. Nassar Motor Co.*, 1995). Additionally, lower federal courts held in 1996 that males refusing advances and terminated from employment could have a cause of action under Title VII., [e.g., *Ton v. Information Resources*, 1996]. Further, the Washington, D.C., District Court held in a female–female case that allegations of same-gender sexual harassment are actionable under Title VII (*Williams v. District of Columbia*, 1996). The court construed the case as sexual harassment, not sexual orientation harassment.

Allegations of harassment are stronger if they involve a sexual advance and requests for sexual favors, in contrast to "name calling." A worker referred to as a "dick sucker" could not invoke harassment law (*Vandeventer v. Wabash National Corp.*, 1995).

By the end of 1996, there was a split among the federal courts of appeal sitting in different circuits over whether Title VII covered same-sex harassment. To date, the Supreme Court has refused to review this split in authority.

Beyond Title VII, other statutes and governmental agencies can protect against discrimination. Pennsylvania bans sexual orientation employment discrimination in any agency under jurisdiction of the governor. Same-gender harassment may provide a cause of action under California's Fair Employment and Housing Act. The act was invoked to hold a homosexual supervisor personally liable for verbal and physical sexual harassment of a male employee where the allegedly discriminated employee at UCLA Medical Center was heterosexual (*Matthews v. Superior Court of Los Angeles County*, 1995).

Within police departments, antihomosexual employment discrimination is long-standing. A few years after a widely publicized case in which a gay Los Angeles, California, police officer reached a settlement with the police department to implement guidelines for the treatment of gay and lesbian officers, a new lawsuit was filed against the police department by other officers alleging physical and verbal harassment.

Gay lawyers have had mixed results against personal discrimination. An Ohio attorney was dismissed by his firm because of his activities opposing a 1994 Cincinnati voters' referendum rescinding protection of homosexuals' civil rights (see later in this chapter). A lower court found no basis to support a public policy exception that would protect him. The State Supreme Court refused appeal (*Greenwood v. Taft, Stettinius and Hollister*, 1995). By contrast, a Colorado associate with a law firm prevailed in a wrongful discharge case after he revealed to a partner in the firm that he was homosexual. His behavior was lawful off premises, off hours conduct and thus protected by Denver, Colorado, law (*Borquez v. Ozer*, 1995).

The U.S. Supreme Court refused in 1996 to review an appellate decision from Pennsylvania upholding enforcement of a *private* employment contract requiring termination of homosexual employees. The contract provided for automatic discharge based on sexual orientation (*De Muth v. Miller*, 1995).

A 1995 employment case temporarily contained an important new element. A federal appeal court held that a woman's relationship with her female partner is protected by the constitutional right of intimate and expressive association. A female lawyer had accepted employment in the state of Georgia's Law Department. When it was learned that she was to have a religious marriage ceremony with a woman, the job offer was withdrawn. Because Georgia criminalizes sodomy and does not authorize same-sex marriage, the state argued that hiring this attorney would embarrass its policy. The state's appeal to the full appellate court was granted, vacating the earlier decision (*Shahar v. Bowers*, 1995).

The Boy Scouts of America remain steadfastly opposed to gays as scouts or leaders. In a California case in which I served as co-counsel, the issues were (1) whether the Boy Scouts were a "business establishment" and thus subject to state antihomosexual discrimination law and (2), if so, whether there was an overriding defense by the Boy Scouts against enforcement of that law.

An Eagle Boy Scout "came out" as gay in 1980 when he took a male partner to his high school senior prom dance. The local Boy Scout Council then denied his application to be a scout leader. At trial, the court held that the Boy Scouts were a business establishment. However, the organization's First Amendment right of freedom of expression (to discriminate against homosexuals) trumped. On appeal, the scout received an additional setback. The court held that not only did the scouts' constitutional argument prevail, but the Boy Scouts were *not* a business establishment and thus not even subject to the antidiscrimination law (*Curran v. Mt. Diablo Council of the Boy Scouts of America*, 1994). Similarly, in New Jersey a trial court ruled that the Boy Scouts were not a "place of public accommodation" and thus that state's nondiscrimination law does not protect a gay scout leader (*Dale v. Boy Scouts of America*, 1995).

Homosexual public school teachers have not fared well, either. A school guidance counselor was not rehired after she told a coworker she was bisexual. Although she prevailed at trial on a free speech argument, the jury verdict was reversed on appeal. The court's rationale was that "if an employee's expression cannot be fairly considered as relating to any matter of political, social, or other concern to the community," disciplinary action cannot be challenged under the First Amendment. The Supreme Court denied review (*Rowland v. Mad River Local School District*, 1984).

Federal government employees traditionally had not done well fighting employment dismissals based on sexual orientation. Government agencies with the longest-running antihomosexual policies have been the Central Intelligence Agency and the Federal Bureau of Investigation (FBI) (e.g., *Webster v. Doe*, 1988). Government agencies have been notably reluctant to employ homosexuals, especially when there are "security" concerns. Until 1975, homosexuals were denied security clearances per se. Fifteen years later, the Department of Defense's especially elaborate security clearance for homosexuals was upheld by a federal appellate court (*High Tech Gays v. Defense Industrial Security Clearance Office*, 1990).

Major changes to these policies occurred in 1994. The State Department issued a nondiscrimination statement for its diplomatic corps. The Office of Personnel Management, in charge of federal personnel policy, stated that sexual orientation discrimination violates official policies, and the FBI announced that it was adding "sexual orientation" to its official nondiscrimination policy (Law and Society Notes, *Lesbian/Gay Law Notes*, January 1994, p. 7 and February 1994, p. 29).

The U.S. General Accounting Office reported in 1995 that federal government operations requiring security clearances were no longer inquiring about the sexual orientation of applicants. However, concealed homosexuality might raise concerns about potential blackmail (Law and Society Notes, *Lesbian/Gay Law Notes*, April 1995, p. 54). Also, in 1995, President Clinton issued an executive order forbidding discrimination on the basis of sexual orientation in granting access to classified governmental information: "No inference ... may be raised solely on the basis of sexual orientation" (Executive Order 12968, August 7, 1995).

Employment discrimination extends beyond hiring, firing, and harassment. Employment benefits have traditionally been denied same-sex couples (and mixed-sex couples who *choose* not to marry). They include discounts on family coverage for health insurance, family sick leave, and other benefits. But, in the past decade, many employers have granted unmarried partners benefits comparable to those held by married couples. The first to offer an insurance plan covering "domestic partners" was the *Village Voice* newspaper in Greenwich Village, New York City, in 1982.

FAMILY

American family law courts are battlegrounds for child custody or visitation litigation in which at least one parenting figure is homosexual. Early cases involved primarily married mothers who were divorcing their husbands to lead a lesbian lifestyle. Such cases continue, as do the smaller number involving homosexual fathers. A newer variant involves female couples who separate after one partner had borne a child conceived by donor insemination. Additional family law issues are whether two persons of the same sex may adopt a child and whether two persons of the same sex may marry.

One result of my research on children being raised by lesbian mothers is that I have served as an expert witness in child custody cases. Court decisions are widely divergent. In one, a mother was denied custody for not "abstaining" from lesbianism (*Townend v. Townend*, 1975). To the court, "Had the defendant indicated that until her children were reared she would abandon the practice of lesbianism ... the Court might be tempted to experiment with the mother.... But I am struck by the primacy that lesbians, at least the two lesbians who testified here, give to multiple organisms [sic]."

A Massachusetts judge took "judicial notice" of what he considered to be the adverse effects of lesbian motherhood, even though both parents had introduced expert evidence "to the effect that a mother's sexual preference per se is irrelevant to a consideration of her parenting skills" (*Bezio v. Patenaude*, 1980). The appellate court did not see it the same way: "Matters are judicially noticed only when they are indisputably true.... In the total absence of evidence suggesting a correlation between the mother's homosexuality and her fitness as a parent, we believe the judge's finding that a lesbian household would adversely affect the children to be without basis in the record" (*Bezio v. Patenaude*, p. 1216). In contrast, the Supreme Court of North Dakota wrote, "[The mother's] homosexuality may, indeed, be something which is beyond her control. However, living with another person of the same sex in a sexual relationship is not something beyond her control ... concerned parents in many, many instances have made sacrifices of varying degrees for their children" (*Jacobson v. Jacobson*, 1981).

Louisiana in 1995 held that "exposing" a child to a mother's lesbian relationship compromised the child's "best interest" (*Rowan v. Scott*, 1995). In Illinois, also in 1995, a mother's homosexual relationship was also deemed "a proper factor" in determining custody (*Marriage of Martins*, 1995). She lost custody of her two children to their father in a reversal of the trial court.

On the other hand, a Minnesota appellate court wrote in an unpublished case that it is "palpably untrue" that "any contact by children with lesbians or homosexuals is per se harmful to the children's emotional health or development" (*McKay v. Johnson*, 1996). And the South Dakota Supreme Court in 1994 held that awarding primary child custody to a lesbian mother and her partner need not be against the best interests of the child. Circumstances of the case need to be evaluated (*Van Driel v. Van Driel*, 1994).

Courts have been concerned with the stigma attached to the child as a consequence of his or her parents' lifestyle. This often enters into the equation determining the child's "best interests." In Missouri, the court wrote, "We wish to protect the children from peer pressure, teasing and possible ostracizing they may encounter as a result of the 'alternative life style' their mother has chosen…. Such conduct can never be kept private enough to be a neutral factor in the development of a child's values and character. We will not ignore such conduct by a parent which may have an effect on the children's moral development" (*S.E.G. v. R.A.G.*, 1987). In contrast, a New Jersey court wrote, "Hard facts must be faced … there is little to gain by creating an artificial world where the children may dream that life is different than it is…. [The children] will emerge better equipped to search out their own standards of right and wrong, better able to perceive that the majority is not always correct in its moral judgements" (*M.P. v. S.P.*, 1979).

A factual nexus between the parents' sexual orientation and detriment to the child needs to be demonstrated when homosexuality is not a per se disqualification. Some courts, however, have not required showing a nexus of *actual* harm, but will defer to an *assumed* or *potential* harm (*Jacobsen v. Jacobsen*, 1980).

A recent case receiving wide publicity has been the long-running *Bottoms* case in Virginia (*Bottoms v. Bottoms*, 1994). A lesbian mother's mother sought custody of her daughter's child after her daughter revealed her sexual orientation to her. The trial court found that an openly lesbian mother in a relationship with a partner is per se unfit. The court relied in part on the fact that the woman violated the state sodomy law several times a week (oral copulation). Then, the Virginia Court of Appeal reversed and granted custody back to the mother. However, when the case was ultimately heard by the State's Supreme Court, by a 4-3 vote, custody went again to the grandmother. Although the court acknowledged that parental sexual orientation per se is not a basis for determining unfitness, it deferred to the trial court that had found sufficient evidence to determine that this mother was unfit. Of interest to the court was that the mother's sexual conduct "is punishable as a Class 6 felony…. Thus, that conduct is [an] important consideration." Further, living in the home in which there was "active lesbianism" was seen to "impose a burden upon a child by reason of social condemnation" (*Bottoms v. Bottoms*, 1995). The trial court recently reaffirmed its decision of custody to the grandmother because the mother signed a movie contract publicizing their case: "I am less concerned with her lesbianism than [with the boy] being made a poster boy for a cause he could not and did not enlist."

Homosexual fathers have also had mixed results in court. A male scientist who abandoned a prestigious academic career to become director of the National Gay Task Force was the unsuccessful litigant in a landmark New Jersey case. Although the court acknowledged that "the parental rights of a homosexual, like those of a heterosexual, are constitutionally protected," the mother's argument for restricted visitation by the father prevailed, notwithstanding my testimony. The court ordered that, during visitation, the father was "not to be in the presence of his lover" (*J.S and C.*, 1976).

However, a Maine court's judgment that a homosexual father could not have his daughter for overnight stays with a male visitor present was overturned. No evidence had been presented of a possible "deleterious impact" on the children, only "that there *may* be an effect.... [B]ecause there is no showing or finding of effect ... I can only conclude that the Court, rather than focusing on the best interests of the children or the evidence presented, based its decision on its personal dislike of the father's sexual behavior" (*Stone v. Stone*, 1979).

On the other hand, in Virginia, a male couple, in which one partner was the biological father and the two men coparented a girl for 5 years, was condemned by the appellate court. The father's continuous exposure of his child to his "immoral and illicit relationship rendered him an unfit and improper custodian as a matter of law.... The father's unfitness is manifested by his willingness to impose this burden upon her in exchange for his own gratification" (*Roe v. Roe*, 1985).

But, returning to the other hand, a California appellate court invoking the "nexus test" overruled a trial court provision that a father's visitation not be in the presence of any other person "known to be homosexual." This because "no current harm to the child can be attributed to [the father's] sexual orientation. [Further] there is no evidence of future detriment" (*Birdsall v. Birdsall*, 1988). And a North Carolina appellate court similarly overruled a trial court and awarded custody of two boys, 11 and 8, to their homosexual father who was cohabiting with a male. Harm to the children could not be presumed from the father's homosexuality. To the appellate court, the findings of harm to the children in consequence of the father's sexual orientation were "not supported by evidence in the record. [It was] nothing more than the opinion of the trial court.... There must be evidence that the conduct has or will likely have a deleterious effect on the children" (*Pulliam v. Smith*, 1996).

Most states permit homosexuals to foster parent or adopt children. Not Florida. Its statute reads simply, "No person eligible to adopt under this statute may adopt if that person is a homosexual." The Department of Health and Rehabilitative Services, overseeing child placement, has argued in court that homosexuals are law breakers because of the Florida sodomy law (which applies to both heterosexuals and homosexuals). A Florida Court of Appeal upheld the constitutionality of that state's ban against homosexuals as parents in 1993 (*State v. Cox*, 1993). But, the Florida Supreme Court remanded the case for review, holding that argument could proceed invoking the equal protection clause of the state constitution. However, the standard to be applied was "rational basis," not "heightened scrutiny," so that any reasonable state argument would prevail (*Cox v. Florida Department/ Health and Rehabilitative Services*, 1995). By then, the male couple had separated and so dropped their suit. Now, a female-couple case is moving forward.

The governor of California in 1995 overruled a policy on adoptions that had been put in place by the state's social services director. The overturned policy would allow same-sex couples and unmarried persons to adopt children (Law and Society Notes, *Lesbian/Gay Law Notes*, April 1995, p. 55). Nebraska adopted a policy in 1995 prohibiting placement of foster children with homosexual parents or licensing gays or lesbians to be foster parents (Law and Society Notes, *Lesbian/Gay Law Notes*, March 1995, p. 36).

In joint or coparent adoption, both unmarried partners become legal parents. This can protect the child if the couple separates and protect the partner's right to child visitation. The District of Columbia Court of Appeals ruled that unmarried couples, whether of the same or mixed sex, may jointly adopt children (*M.M.D.*, 1995). New York interpreted state adoption law to permit the male domestic partner of a heterosexual birth mother to adopt a child without casting off the birth mother's parental right (*Matter of*

Jacob, 1995) and to permit adoption by the lesbian partner of a child's birth mother [*Matter of Dana (Anonymous); G.M. (Anonymous)*, 1995, *Lesbian/Gay Law Notes*, 1995]. An appellate court in Illinois also upheld an adoption by the lesbian partner of a birth mother (*Petition of K.M. and D.M.*, 1995).

However, a Florida district court held in 1995 that the non-birth mother of a child born to a lesbian couple does not have visitation rights (*Music v. Rachford*, 1995). In California a non-birth mother partner in a lesbian couple can also not assert parental rights (*Nancy S. v. Michelle G.*, 1991; *Curiale v. Reagan*, 1994). But, in 1995, the Wisconsin Supreme Court became the first highest state court to hold that a lesbian copartner could seek visitation after her partnership with the child's biological mother who conceived the child by donor insemination ended (*Custody of H.S.H.-K: Holtzman v. Knott*, 1995): "The origin, nature and quality of the adult–child relationship is to be considered." The relationship had been of 10 years' duration.

Same-sex marriage is prohibited in all 50 states. A few decades ago some adult men petitioned to adopt other adult men to constitute a legal bond between them. A few courts permitted such adoptions, but most took a dim view of this use of adoption laws. (Breaking most state incest laws in consequence of the "father" and "son" continuing a sexual relationship was probably not a risk, as incest generally applies to blood relatives in the immediate family. "Child sexual abuse" of a 30-year-old by the "father" would be even less on target.)

The U.S. Constitution has been interpreted by the Supreme Court as protecting the right to marry as fundamental. Therefore, there must be a compelling state interest to deny it. However, marriage has been interpreted by state courts as a civil status available only between a man and a woman. [In a very early case, before marriage was held to be a fundamental right, the Supreme Court held that the government could forbid marriage between a man and more than one woman concurrently (*Reynolds v. United States*, 1878)].

In 1993, the Hawaii Supreme Court held that the state would be required to issue same-sex couple marriage licenses unless it could prove a compelling justification for its refusal. Although the court held that the due process clause does not provide a fundamental right to marry, the equal protection guarantee could be invoked. A heightened scrutiny analysis was to be the standard to decide the issue, as denial of same-sex marriage could be deemed a form of sex discrimination (*Baehr v. Lewin*, 1993; now *Baehr v. Miike*). In 1995 Hawaii's Commission on Sexual Orientation approved a report recommending that the State's marriage law be amended to permit same-sex couples to marry. In 1996 the Hawaii Senate approved same-sex marriage, contradicting a lower house vote.

On December 3, 1996, in this test case in which I participated in a friend of the court brief regarding the welfare of children raised by same-sex couples, the Hawaii Circuit Court found that the state's prohibition was unconstitutional sex discrimination. The state "failed to present sufficient credible evidence which demonstrates that the public interest in the well-being of children and families or the optimal development of children would be adversely affected by same-sex marriage" (*Baehr v. Miike*, 1996). The state is appealing the decision to the Hawaii Supreme Court.[1]

---

[1]An additional hurdle is a proposal for the general election in 1998. It would ask Hawaii voters if they want to amend their state constitution to permit the legislature to restrict marriage to opposite-sex couples.

If Hawaii permits same-sex marriage, this could create a dilemma for other states regarding whether they would recognize the marriage. Under the Full Faith and Credit Clause of the federal Constitution they would appear required to, but 22 states have passed laws declaring same-sex marriage against public policy and not to be recognized.

Although the U.S. Supreme Court has never ruled directly on an application for marriage by two persons of the same sex, it has refused to take under appeal state court rulings to the contrary. The court's reason for refusing to consider a case of two men denied permission to marry by Minnesota was "want of a federal question" (no federal law or constitutional issue involved) (*Baker v. Nelson*, 1971, *appeal dismissed*, 1972). Thus it will be of considerable interest if the Hawaii Supreme Court permits same-sex marriage and the decision is appealed to the U.S. Supreme Court. When, in a question-and-answer session with the Chief Justice of the Supreme Court William Rehnquist, I asked whether he would speculate on the court's response to such a hypothetical appeal, he demurred that he could not think of a federal question that was involved. However, in 1996, President Clinton signed a federal law forbidding recognition of same-sex marriage (the Defense of Marriage Act). This could alter the requirement of an individual state to recognize the out-of-state same-sex marriage under the Full Faith and Credit Clause. The law will be challenged as a violation of the Constitution.

The definition of what constitutes a family has been considerably expanded in recent years. It may include same-sex couples. A landmark case in New York City involved rights to inherit an economical rent-controlled apartment. Two men had cohabited in the apartment for many years. The lease stated that only immediate family members may continue occupancy upon the death of an occupant. The landlord sought eviction of the survivor. The New York Court held that the male couple constituted family (*Braschi v. Stahl Associates*, 1989).

Domestic partnership is a civil status affording to unmarried couples some of the benefits afforded married couples. Thus insurance benefits, sick leave benefits, hospital visitation rights as "next of kin," and some property transfers can be guaranteed to both partners. Several jurisdictions permit registration of same-sex partners. The city of San Francisco conducted a mass "wedding" ceremony for same-sex couples on March 25, 1996, with the mayor presiding. This was in response to a measure passed by the Board of Supervisors.

MILITARY

Between 1980 and 1990, the military discharged 17,000 men and women for homosexuality. The Navy had the highest rate, with 51% of discharges, but only 27% of the total number of persons in military service (General Accounting Office, 1992).

The military's argument against including homosexual service members is that they impair the accomplishment of the military mission. This stems from security concerns, from promoting a disfavored public image of the military, and from perceived negative impacts on discipline, good order, and morale.

During his successful bid for the presidency in 1992, Bill Clinton promised to reverse the military policy banning homosexuals. However, after his election, that proposal met a firestorm of opposition by the military and the Congress. Hearings were held; studies were conducted.

The Defense Department maintained that "The presence in the Armed Forces of persons who demonstrate a propensity or intent to engage in homosexual acts would create an unacceptable risk to the high standards of morale, good order and discipline, and unit cohesion that are the essence of military capability" (United States Code 10, s. 1177). By contrast, the nongovernmental "think-tank," RAND Corporation, concluded that the ban could be successfully reversed. Its report found that sexual orientation is not germane to military performance and rejected the military rationale concerning unit cohesion. Further, a draft report prepared for the Personnel Security Research and Education Center of the Defense Department suggested that the military consider ending its policy of excluding homosexuals from service. However, the Defense Department rejected that draft on the basis that it exceeded its mandate.

The result of this firestorm was a compromise: the 1994 "Don't ask, Don't tell, Don't pursue" policy. It says in effect that gay and lesbian service members may serve if they don't say or do anything that might bring to the attention of peers or superiors the fact of their sexual orientation. It says further that no inquiry is to be made about sexual orientation during the enlistment process. However, once a person's sexual orientation becomes known, there is the presumption that he or she has the propensity to engage in forbidden sexual conduct. A service member can be discharged if he or she "has engaged in, attempted to engage in, or solicited another to engage in a homosexual act or acts, stated that he or she is a homosexual or bisexual, or has married or attempted to marry a person known to be of the same biological sex" (United States Code 10, s. 654).

Although conduct, not status, is ostensibly the ground for separation from military service, conduct can include "a statement by the Service member that demonstrates a propensity or intent to engage in homosexual acts" (Department of Defense Dir. 1332.14, encl. 2, par. G). Statements about homosexual orientation create a rebuttable presumption that the service member engages in homosexual acts or has a propensity or intent to do so. "Propensity" indicates a likelihood.

Legal cases brought under the final years of the old policy remain topical. In one, a female captain in the Army Reserve was discharged after a 1983 newspaper reported an interview in which she discussed her homosexual lifestyle including two marriage ceremonies with women. A federal appeals court held that the Army had to demonstrate a rational basis for its policy that was not founded upon the prejudice of others (a "rational basis with teeth" test, a more demanding justification than usually required of the military). The case was remanded to trial on an equal protection argument. However, the case was then settled without an additional court ruling on the constitutionality of the Army regulation (*Pruitt v. Cheney*, 1991).

In a case that commenced in 1987, a Naval Academy cadet was forced to resign after stating that he was gay. He fought in the courts for 7 years. After a seesaw battle, his resignation was declared final in 1995 after the full District of Columbia Court of Appeals voted 7-3 to reverse a court panel (*Steffan v. Aspin*, 1993) that had ruled in the cadet's favor. To the full court, the statement that one is homosexual is a rational expectation by the military that one will engage in forbidden conduct (*Steffan v. Perry*, 1994).

But, in another case, a federal trial and appellate court ruled in the service member's favor, holding that while the regulation banning homosexual activity is constitutional, banning *classification on status as a homosexual* is not (*Meinhold v. Department of Defense*, 1993, 1994). No assumption can be made that status will become behavior. Although heterosexuals can be discharged for practicing adultery, bigamy, sodomy, and other sex acts, they are not discharged because of their status as heterosexuals. This is an "equal protection" violation. The appeals court reaffirmed the service member's right to reinstatement. It agreed that the statement "I am in fact gay" was not equivalent to the speaker declaring that he had engaged in or intended to engage in homosexual behavior. Although a service member could not be discharged solely for statements identifying status, the court did not hold the Navy policy unconstitutional and deferred to the Navy's judgment that the presence of persons who engage in homosexual conduct or who demonstrate a propensity based on their statements impair the accomplishment of the military mission.

In 1994, a trial court ordered reinstatement in the Washington State National Guard of a nurse who had been discharged for declaring herself a lesbian. To the court, relying on *Pruitt* and *Meinhold*, her statement was not reliable evidence of her desire or propensity to engage in homosexual conduct. Her rights to due process and equal protection were violated (*Cammermeyer v. Aspin*, 1994). In 1996 the Court of Appeals refused to hear the government's appeal of this case because the policy under which she was discharged was no longer in effect (having been displaced by the "Don't Ask, Don't Tell, Don't Pursue" policy) (*Cammermeyer v. Perry*, 1996).

The new "Don't Ask, Don't Tell, Don't Pursue" policy is currently under challenge as an equal protection violation in cases climbing the appellate ladder. In 1995, one federal court issued an injunction against it (*Able v. United States*, 1995). The policy unacceptably targets status, not conduct. Thus, it was held unconstitutional, although a ban on homosexual behavior was not. In the court's uncompromising language, "Hitler taught the world what could happen when the government began to target people not for what they had done but because of their status." On appeal, the presumption of homosexual conduct following on homosexual status was found to be constitutional. However, the case was referred to the lower court to consider whether the policy violates equal protection when it treats homosexual and heterosexual service members differently (*Able v. United States*, 1996).

In *Thorne v. US Department of Defense* (1996) a federal district court held that the new policy must survive heightened scrutiny as a content-based restriction on speech (expressing a specific viewpoint). The government must show that the restriction "substantially furthers an important governmental interest."

In April 1996, the Court of Appeals for the 4th Circuit sitting *en banc* upheld by a vote of 9-4 the new policy as a legitimate use of congressional power. The policy was characterized as "a carefully crafted national political compromise" (*Thomasson v. Perry*, 1996). The equal protection argument was judged using only the weak rational basis test — here the military interest in "preserving unit cohesion." It was deemed an appropriate exercise of military authority. Later in the same year the Court of Appeals for the 8th Circuit also ruled that the policy was constitutional and that the presumption that openly homosexual people will engage in homosexual conduct was a rational means for the military to avoid the problems it expected if service people engaged in such conduct (*Richenberg v. Perry*, 1995, 1996).

Under the former military policy, "witch hunts" were common to ferret out homosexual men and women service members. Identified gay and lesbian members were often intimidated into identifying others. That policy ostensibly has been eliminated by the Department of Defense instruction that no investigative agency "shall conduct an investigation solely to determine a service member's sexual orientation" (Department of Defense Instruction 5505.8). However, a 1997 report by the Service Members Legal Defense Network describes seizures of diaries and threats of prison against those accused unless they betrayed other homosexual men and women (Brodie, 1997).

PUBLIC OPINION

Homosexuals are a relatively small minority compared with major ethnic groups. Perhaps 4 percent of men and 2.3 percent of women are exclusively homosexual. Another 2 percent of men and 1 percent of women may be actively bisexual (Michael, Gagnon, Laumann, & Kolata, 1994).

Public acceptance of homosexuality has been increasing. A 1996 poll found that 57 percent of adults said they think gay people can be as good at parenting as straight people; 36 percent thought gay couples should have the right to adopt, compared to 29 percent in 1994. In 1996 47 percent opposed gay adoption rights, down from 65 percent in 1994 (Gay families come out, *Newsweek*, November 4, 1996). Further, a National Opinion Research Center poll found that the percent of respondents agreeing that homosexual relations are "always wrong" dropped to 61 percent in 1996, down from 76 percent in 1991 (Law and Society Notes, *Lesbian/Gay Law Notes*, December 1996, p. 175).

American homosexuals have been described as victims of "cultural heterosexism." This is the lack of legal protection from discrimination in employment, housing, and services; the ban against lesbian and gay military personnel; the absence of full legal recognition for same-sex committed relationships; and sodomy laws in nearly half the states. Additionally, there is "psychological heterosexism," the individual manifestation of cultural heterosexism. It is the feelings of revulsion and hostility toward homosexuality with homosexuals being targets of verbal or physical harassment and discrimination (Herek, 1995).

A turning point politically for American homosexuals was the Stonewall Rebellion of 1969. There, in the largely homosexual area of Greenwich Village, New York City, homosexual men in a gay bar stood up to police harassment in a show of strength. The movement "out of the closets" for homosexual men and women and public displays of "gay pride," as in marches, evolved soon after.

Progress for gay civil rights has been slow. Legal cases reflect some of this movement. For example, in 1980, a gay high school student's right to attend his senior prom dance with a male partner was upheld by a federal court under First Amendment analysis (freedom of speech and association grounds) (*Fricke v. Lynch*, 1980). Thirteen years later, Massachusetts passed a law outlawing discrimination against homosexual students in public schools. A California Court of Appeal held in 1993 that a commercial photographer unlawfully discriminated in refusing to include a male couple's picture in a high school reunion book (*Engel v. Worthington*, 1993).

In the early 1980s, Oklahoma enacted a law allowing for termination of school teachers who "engage in public homosexual conduct or activity." However, a federal appellate court found that the statute failed for "overbreadth" in its conception of "public homosexual conduct advocating, soliciting,... encouraging or promoting public or private homosexual activity." It prohibited protected speech. Further, the teacher's "due process" or "fair play" right requiring the state to prove substantial work environment disruption was not necessary for employment termination. This decision was upheld on a split 4-4 vote of the US Supreme Court (a majority being required to overrule) (*Board of Education of Oklahoma City v. National Gay Task Force*, 1984).

In recent decades, only a few of the 50 states have enacted laws forbidding discrimination based on sexual orientation. In 1995, Rhode Island became the ninth state to ban sexual orientation discrimination. Others are California, Connecticut, Hawaii, Massachusetts, Minnesota, New Jersey, Vermont, and Wisconsin. Although legislation has been introduced in Congress since 1974 for federal protection against discrimination, no bill has passed.

In a backlash against these decisions, some states have tried to rescind antidiscrimination statutes. An 1992 amendment to the Colorado state constitution passed by 53 percent of the voters would "ban the state or every one of its political subdivisions from adopting laws, rules or policies that specifically protect lesbians, gay men or bisexuals from discrimination." The amendment was enjoined by a state district court and remanded for trial. The State Supreme Court held that the statute violated fundamental rights of lesbian, gay, and bisexual Coloradans and did not meet the high threshold of "strict scrutiny" as required by the Equal Protection Clause in the U.S. Constitution. However, after reviewing expert testimony, to which I contributed evidence on the unchangeable characteristic of sexual orientation, in an attempt to give heightened protection to homosexuals as a class, the courts declined to make a finding of whether homosexuality is "immutable." After the state's highest court upheld the ruling that the amendment was unconstitutional, Colorado appealed to the U.S. Supreme Court (*Evans v. Romer*, 1994). The question considered by the court was, "Does a popularly enacted state constitutional amendment precluding special state or local legal protections for homosexuals and bisexuals violate the fundamental right of independently identifiable, yet nonsuspect, classes to seek such special protections?" In May 1996 the Supreme Court answered yes by a 6-3 vote (*Romer v. Evans*, 1996). The standard of review was not heightened scrutiny but the lowest level of review. The law "lacks a rational relationship to legitimate state interests." It relegated homosexuals to inferior status. The "state interests" were pretexts.

The city of Cincinnati passed a similar law with 62 percent of the vote. It has had a seesaw judicial history. The law read that the city may not "enact, adopt, enforce or administer any ordinance, regulation, rule or policy which provides that homosexual, lesbian or bisexual orientation, status, conduct or relationship constitutes, entitles or otherwise provides a person with the basis to have any claim of minority or protected status, quota preference or other preferential treatment." A federal trial court held that laws going beyond simple repeal of existing gay rights laws violate the First and Fourteenth Amendments to the U.S. Constitution (free speech and equal protection). The court found that in Cincinnati, homosexuals were not being given any rights beyond those of other citizens. Thus the law was overturned (*Equality Foundation of Greater Cincinnati Inc. v. City of Cincinnati*, 1994). However, the Court of Appeals reversed. It held that the ordinance did not violate equal protection rights to participate in the legal process. Homosexuals were held not to be a "cognizable class" for equal protection analysis and had no fundamental right of participation (*Equality Foundation of Greater Cincinnati Inc. v. City of Cincinnati*, 1995). The appeal from this ruling was also filed with the U.S. Supreme Court. Its fate should hinge on the decision of the Supreme Court in the Colorado case.

Oregon narrowly defeated an anti-gay rights referendum in 1995 by 51.4 to 48.6 percent. A Utah proposition was also defeated by about 2 percent. Maine rejected a constitutional amendment that would have barred political subdivisions from prohibiting sexual orientation discrimination by 3 percent of the vote.

Every year in this century until 1994 the city of Boston, which has a large population of Irish descent, held a St. Patrick's Day parade. Then a federal court held that the Irish-American Gay, Lesbian and Bisexual Group of Boston must be allowed to march along with more traditional celebrants. However, the U.S. Supreme Court later overturned that ruling (but not in time to "save" the 1994 parade) (*Hurley v. Irish-American Gay, Lesbian and Bisexual Group of Boston*, 1995). By 9-0 it upheld the ban with the reasoning that to include gays and lesbians would alter the content of speech that the parade sponsors, a non-state association, wanted to convey. Homosexuals, said the court, could have their own parade. In New York City, after a similar ruling, they did just that.

Individual cases reflect slow change in the public integration of homosexual persons. One concerned four men who danced together in a Chicago sports bar and were arrested. Taking their case to the County Commission on Human Rights (which prohibits sexual orientation discrimination in public accommodation), they prevailed. The bar was fined and required to post a notice of compliance with the human rights law (Settlement in same-sex dancing controversy, *Lesbian/Gay Law Notes*, September 1995, p. 123). The American Medical Association House of Delegates in 1995 adopted a report calling for nonjudgmental recognition of sexual orientation by physicians. It abandoned a 1981 policy statement supporting treatments designed to change sexual orientation.

Hate crimes are attacks based on a class characteristic of the victim. Hate crimes against homosexuals have been reported for decades. "Queer hunting" by teenagers was described in 1961 ("Queer Hunting among Teenagers," 1961). Crimes based on sexual orientation have not been routinely punished, however. Victims of sexual orientation hate crimes generally do not report them to the police. In Philadelphia the majority of gay men in a sample who had suffered criminal violence did not report it (Gross, Aurand, & Addessa, 1988). Even in San Francisco, a city with a large integrated gay population, over 80 percent did not report hate crimes (Winslow, 1982). And, on a university campus, over 4 in 5 gay and lesbian students who had been victimized did not report at least one incident to police or campus authorities (Herek, 1986). Two principal reasons for victim nonreporting are the perception that police are antihomosexual (Comstock, 1989) and the fear many victims have of public disclosure of their sexual orientation (for a general review, see Berrill & Herek, 1992).

In 1986, the U.S. Congress held hearings on anti-gay violence (Committee on the Judiciary, 1986). The resulting Hate Crimes Statistics Act of 1990 directs the federal government to collect data on hate crimes based on race, ethnicity, religion and sexual orientation.

In 1996 there were over 1,000 reported hate crimes in consequence of the victim's sexual orientation. This constituted 13 percent of recorded hate crimes (Law and Society Notes, *Lesbian/Gay Law Notes*, December 1996, p. 175).

Some states have enacted laws providing for increased penalties against perpetrators of hate crimes. The California Supreme Court upheld that state's hate crimes law forbidding "by force or threat of force, anyone [to] wilfully injure, intimidate, interfere with, oppress or threaten a person trying to exercise legal rights because of … sexual orientation." The law provides for penalty enhancement (s. 422.7, Penal Code).

The federal Crime Bill of 1994 included a mandate to promulgate guidelines for sentencing enhancement for hate crimes (P.L. 103-322, s. 28003, 28 USCA, 1994). Many criminal sentences for "gay-bashing" are now enhanced. The death penalty has been invoked in a homicide, and in one case a prison sentence was to run for over 500 years.

Homosexual panic defenses have been invoked in many cases by a heterosexual defendant when the murder victim was gay. Homosexual panic is an involuntary explosive reaction to a perceived fear of homosexual assault. The defense has generally been unsuccessful (*People v. Milner*, 1988; *People v. Rodriguez*, 1967). In a recent case, it was held that an aggressive homosexual solicitation does not warrant a murderous response (*Commonwealth v. Pierce*, 1994).

In 1996 a television program recruited participants with a secret romantic crush. Both the holder and object of the romantic feelings were then invited to appear on the program, where the identity of the secret admirer would be revealed. In this case the man holding the crush was interested in another male. The object of those feelings was led to believe, before appearing on the program, that the person holding the crush was a former girlfriend. Three days after the identity of his secret admirer was revealed to him, he shot his admirer to death. He was convicted of second degree murder and sentenced to 25–50 years imprisonment.

Examples of gay/lesbian acceptance or at least accommodation are evident in large cities. Businesses catering to a homosexual clientele can be found in areas with major gay and lesbian populations. Thousands of entries appear in "gay guides," including travel agencies arranging holiday tours. In West Hollywood, California, a large billboard advertises vacation trips for a gay clientele. Gay pride marches are held annually in major cities with a large gay and lesbian population. Fringe newspapers containing personal or classified advertisements for persons seeking companionship have dedicated sections for men seeking men or, less often, women seeking women.

Several metropolitan areas have neighborhoods largely inhabited or frequented by homosexual men and women. Well-known ones are the Castro district of San Francisco, Greenwich Village in New York, and the city of West Hollywood in Los Angeles County. These areas are stocked with bars, clubs, and restaurants catering to gay and, less often, lesbian customers. Gay bath houses were common in large cities with substantial gay populations prior to the AIDS epidemic. Many have been closed by public health authorities, and others have withered as patrons became more cautious in seeking anonymous sexual encounters. Movie houses showing explicit male–male(s) sex continue in gay areas of large cities. More commonly, gay videos are available for rental, although police harassment of adult bookstores where erotic books and videos are purchased, or where patrons may rent a "private" booth for video viewing, continues.

Legal action groups working on behalf of homosexual litigants or defendants have carried many landmark cases forward. Principal organizations are the Lambda Legal and Educational Foundation and the American Civil Liberties Union, particularly chapters in New York and Los Angeles. Additionally, the Lesbian Mother Defense Fund has assisted in family law cases.

However, assuming 4 percent of men are homosexual and 2 percent of women are homosexual in the United States, these groups are vastly underrepresented in major public office. There have been only four openly gay Congressmen (Barney Frank, Gerry Studds, Steven Gunderson, and Jim Kolbe) serving in the House of Representatives. No member of the Senate has been openly homosexual, nor have any members of the president's cabinet, a president or vice president, or a member of the Supreme Court. Long-term mayor of New York City (Ed Koch) was frequently said to be homosexual, but he never acknowledged it.

Conclusion

A slow, uneven increase in social accommodation and legal protection of homosexual men and women characterizes the American scene.

Centuries-old state laws criminalizing same-sex genital contact have fallen one by one in half the states; enforcement is less vigorous in those remaining. Decades-old restrictions on admitting homosexual aliens into the country have been repealed.

Efforts by homosexual men and women to enjoy the civil rights of heterosexuals continue, exemplified by the fight to join the military and to marry. For the first time, the military is being seriously challenged on its policy of excluding homosexual men and women. For the first time, a state is considering seriously the right of two same-sex persons to marry.

Hesitantly, courts are acknowledging the capacity of homosexuals to be effective parents who do not compromise the best interests of children. The definition of "family" is evolving. Same-sex partners with children have become more visible and increasingly recognized by the law.

Inroads are being made to guarantee openly homosexual men and women equal opportunity both in securing employment and in working in an environment free from harassment. Homosexual men and women are more open to colleagues and relatives about their sexuality. Public opinion, especially among younger persons, is more accepting of gays and lesbians, although discrepancies exist between regions of the country. To an extent, these differences are powered by the influence of traditional religions or reflect sociopolitical differences of large urban versus rural areas.

Countering this heightened acceptance has been a recent backlash brought by those claiming to be protectors of "traditional family values." Although court decisions protecting homosexuals may not alter adverse public opinion, they are applying the brakes against enforcement of new discriminatory laws. And, although some individuals continue to beat and kill in consequence of the victim's sexual orientation, the law has taken a firm stand against these crimes of hate.

The HIV epidemic, blighting hundreds of thousands, although devastating, has bonded the gay community. Further, it has not yielded the feared isolation, scapegoating, and branding of homosexuals as the new lepers. This too reflects an evolution of the social and legal status of homosexuals in America.

Cited Cases

Able v United States, 880 F. Supp 968 EDNY (1995); 88 F3d 1280, 2nd Cir. (1996).

Baehr v Lewin, 852 P2d 44, Hi (1993); now *Baehr v Miike* (1996).

Baker v Wade, 553 F Supp 1121, ND Tex (1983); 743 F2d 236, 5th Cir. (1984); *aff'd on reh. en banc*, 769 F2d 289, 5th Cir. (1985); *cert denied* 106 S Ct 3337 (1986).

Baker v Nelson, 191 NW2d 185 (1971); *dismissed for want of a federal question* 409 US 810 (1972).

Bezio v Patenaude, 410 NE2d 1207, 1216, Mass (1980).

Birdsall v Birdsall, 197 Cal App 3d 1024 (1988).

Board of Education of Oklahoma City v National Gay Task Force, 729 F2d 1270, 10th Cir. (1984); 470 US 903 (1985).

Borquez v Ozer, 69 Fair Employment Practice Cases (BNA) 1415 (1995).

Bottoms v Bottoms, 444 SE2d 276 Va (1994); 457 SE2d 102 (1995).

Boutilier v Immigration and Naturalization Service, 363 F2d 488, 491, 2nd Cir. (1966).

Bowers v Hardwick, 478 US 186, 190–192, 196, 203, 206 (1986).

Braschi v Stahl Associates, 74 NY2d 201, 543 NE2d 49 (1989).

Cammermeyer v Aspin, 850 F Supp 910, WD Wash (1994).

Cammermeyer v Perry, 97 F. 3d 1235 9th Cir. (1996).

Campbell v Sundquist, 926 S.W. 2d 250, Tenn. (1996).

City of Dallas v England, 846 SW2d 957, Tex. App (1993).

Christensen v State, 266 Ga. 494, 468 SE2d 188 (1996).

Commonwealth v Bonadio, 415 A2d 47, Pa (1980).

Commonwealth v Pierce, 642 NE 2d 579, Mass (1994).

Commonwealth v Wasson, 842 SW 2d 487, Ky (1992).

Cox v Florida Department/Health and Rehabilitative Services, 656 So2d 902 Fla (1995).

Curiale v Reagan, 222 Cal App 3d 1597 (1994).

Curran v Mt. Diablo Council of the Boy Scouts of America, 23 Cal App 4th 1307 (1994); 239 Cal App 4th 192 (1994).

Custody of H.S.H.-K: Holtzman v Knott, 193 Wis.2d 649, 533 NW2d 419 (1995).

De Muth v Miller, 652 A2d 891, Pa Super (1995).

De Santis v Pacific Tel & Tel, 608 F2d 327, 9th Cir. (1979).

Dillon v Frank, 58 Employment Practice Decisions (CCH) p. 41, 332 (1992).

EEOC v H.J. Nassar Motor Co., No. 95-11993 JLT, E.D. Mass. (1995); cited in *Lesbian/Gay Law Notes* (October 1995), p. 137.

Eisenstadt v Baird, 405 US 438 (1972).

Engel v Worthington, 19 Cal App 4th 43 (1993).

Equality Foundation of Greater Cincinnati Inc. v City of Cincinnati, 860 F Supp 417, Ohio (1994); 54 F3d 261 (1995).

Evans v Romer, 882 P2d 1335 Colo (1994).

Fox v Sierra Development Co., 876 F Supp 1169, D.Nev (1995).

Fricke v Lynch, 491 F Supp 381, D.R.I. (1980).

Gay Law Student's Association v Pacific Tel & Tel, 24 Cal 3d 458 (1979).

Giddens v Shell Oil Co., 12 F3d 208, 5th Cir. (1993).

Greenwood v Taft, Stettinius and Hollister, 663 N.E. 2d 1030 Ohio (1995).

Griswold v Connecticut, 381 US 479 (1965).

Gryczan v State of Montana, No. BDV-93-1869 (1996), 96–202 (1997).

High Tech Gays v Defense Industrial Security Clearance Office, 895 F2d 563, 9th Cir. (1990).

Hurley v Irish-American Gay, Lesbian and Bisexual Group of Boston, 115 S Ct. 2338 (1995).
Jacobsen v Jacobsen, 608 SW2d 64, Ky Ct App (1980).
Jacobson v Jacobson, 314 NW 2d78, 81, ND (1981).
J.S and C. (1976), 324 A.2d 90, Super, Ct. N.J. (1974); *affd.* 362 A.2d 54 (1976).
Marriage of Martins, 645 NE2d 567, Ill. App. 2 Dist. (1995).
Matthews v Superior Court of Los Angeles County, 34 Cal App 4th 598 (1995).
Matter of Jacob, 660 NE 2d 397, NY (1995).
Matter of Dana (Anonymous); *G.M. (Anonymous)* (1995); cited in *Lesbian/Gay Law Notes* (March 1995), p. 159.
McKay v Johnson, C6-95-1629, Ct. App. Minn (1996).
Meinhold v Department of Defense, 808 F Supp 1455, CD Cal (1993); 34 F3d 1469, 9th Cir. (1994).
Meritor Savings Bank v Vinson, 106 S.Ct. 2399 (1986).
M.M.D., 662 A2d 837, DC App (1995).
M.P. v S.P., 404 A2d 1256, NJ Super (1979).
Music v Rachford, 654 So2d 1234, 1 Fla Dist Ct (1995).
Nancy S. v Michelle G., 228 Cal App 3d 831 (1991).
People v Milner, 45 Cal 3d 227 (1988).
People v Onofre, 51 NYS 2d 476 (1980); *cert denied* 451 US 987 (1981).
People v Rodriguez, 256 Cal App. 2d 663 (1967).
Petition of K.M. and D.M., 274 Ill. App. 3d 189, 653 N.E. 2d 888, Ill (1995).
Prescott v Independent Life and Accident Insurance, 878 F Supp 1545, Ala (1995).
Pruitt v Cheney, 963 F2d 1160, 9th Cir. (1992); 943 F2d 989, 9th Cir. (1991); *cert denied* 506 US 1020 (1992).
Pulliam v Smith, 476 S.E. 2d 466 N.C. (1996).
Reynolds v United States, 98 US 145 (1878).
Richenberg v Perry, 73 F3d 172, 8th Cir. (1995); 97 F. 3d 256 (1996).
Roe v Roe, 324 SE2d 691, 694, Va (1985).
Roe v Wade, 410 US 113 (1973).
Romer v Evans, 116 S.Ct. 1620 (1996).
Rowan v Scott, 665 So2d 760 (1995).
Rowland v Mad River Local School District, 730 F2d 444, 6th Cir. (1984).
S.E.G. v R.A.G., 735 SW2d 164, Mo (1987).
Shahar v Bowers, 836 F Supp 859, (1995); 70 F3d 1218, 11th Cir. (1995).
State v Baxley, 656 So2d 973 (1995).
State v Cox, 627 So2d 1210 (1993).
State v Cuiffini, 395 A2d 904, App Div. (1978).
State v Morales, 826 SW2d 201, Tex App. (1992), 869 SW2d 941 (1994).
State v Saunders, 381 A2d 333 NJ (1977).
Steffan v Aspin, 8 F3d 57 (1993).
Steffan v Perry, 41 F3d 677, DC Circuit (1994).
Stone v Stone, No. 71-2-D111, District Court, Knox County, Maine (1979).
Thomasson v Perry, 80 F3d 915, 4th Cir. (1996).
Thorne v US Department of Defense, 916 F Supp 1358, EDVa (1996).
Ton v Information Resources, 70 Fair Employment Practice Cases (BNA) 355, ND Ill (1996).

Townend v Townend, No. 74 CV 0670, Court of Common Pleas, Portage County Ohio April 4 (1975).

Van Driel v Van Driel, 525 NW2d 37 (1994).

Vandeventer v Wabash National Corp., 893 F Supp 827, ND Ind. (1995).

Ward v State, 636 So2d 68, Fla Ct. App. 5th Dist (1994).

Webster v Doe, 486 US 596 (1988).

Williams v District of Columbia, 916 F Supp 1, DCDC, (1996).

Williams v Saxbe, 413 F Supp 645, DCDC (1976).

REFERENCES

American Law Institute. (1962). *Model penal code, section 213.2* (proposed official draft).

American Psychiatric Association. (1957). *A Psychiatric Glossary*. Washington, DC: Author, p. 551.

Berrill, K. & Herek, G. (1992). *Hate crimes*. Newbury Park: Sage.

Brodie, I. (1997, February 28). US Army pursuing "witch-hunt over gays." *The Times*, p. 15.

Committee on the Judiciary. (1986). *Hearing before the Subcommittee on Criminal Justice, House of Representatives* (serial no. 132). Washington DC: U.S. Government Printing Office.

Comstock, C. (1989). Victims of anti-gay/lesbian violence. *Journal of Interpersonal Violence*, 4, 101–106.

General Accounting Office, Defense Force Management. (1992). *Document Gad NS IA8-92-98, 985*. Washington, DC: Author.

Gross, L., Aurand, S., & Addessa, R. (1988). *Violence and discrimination against lesbian and gay people in Philadelphia*. Philadelphia: Philadelphia Lesbian and Gay Task Office.

Herek, G. (1986). *The Yale sexual orientation survey*. Unpublished manuscript.

Herek, G. (1995). Psychological heterosexism in the United States. In A. D'Augelli & C. Patterson (Eds.), *Lesbian, gay and bisexual identities over the lifespan* (pp. 321–346). New York: Oxford University Press.

Interpreter Releases 56:387, 398 (1979).

Katz, J. (1976). *Gay American history*. New York: Crowell.

Lesbian/Gay Law Notes (1994, January), p. 7, Lesbian and Gay Law Association of Greater New York.

Lesbian/Gay Law Notes (1994, February), p. 29, Lesbian and Gay Law Association of Greater New York.

Lesbian/Gay Law Notes (1995, March), p. 36, Lesbian and Gay Law Association of Greater New York.

Lesbian/Gay Law Notes (1995, April), pp. 54, 55, Lesbian and Gay Law Association of Greater New York.

Lesbian/Gay Law Notes (1995, September), p. 123, Lesbian and Gay Law Association of Greater New York.

Lesbian/Gay Law Notes (1996, January), p. 7, Lesbian and Gay Law Association of Greater New York.

Lesbian/Gay Law Notes (1996, December), p. 175, Lesbian and Gay Law Association of Greater New York.

Michael, R. T., Gagnon, J. H., Laumann, E. U., & Kolata, G. (1994). *Sex in America: A definitive survey*. Boston: Little, Brown.

Newsweek, "Gay families come out." (1996, November 4, p. 56).

Oaks, R. (1980). Perceptions of homosexuality by justices of the peace in colonial America, pp. 35–42. In D. Knutson (Ed)., *Homosexuality and the law*. New York: Haworth Press.

Queer hunting among teenagers (1961, June). *Mattachine Review*.

Skorneck, C. (1993, January 5). FBI's first report on hate crimes. *San Francisco Examiner*, p. A5.

Winslow, C. (1982). *Mayor's survey of victims of violent personal crimes in San Francisco*. San Francisco: Office of the Mayor, Mayor's Criminal Justice Council.

11

Canada

ALEXANDER GREER, HOWARD BARBAREE, AND CHRISTINE BROWN

Introduction

In the conclusion to his article "Winning Rights and Freedoms in Canada," Adam (1993) writes, "Gay and lesbian networks, culture and organization … show increasing vitality in the 1990s and, after decades of struggle, are making headway in achieving rights and recognition in Canadian society" (p. 36). The headway can be measured, in part, by the annual Gay and Lesbian Pride March held in Toronto in July 1996; approximately 70,000 people marched, and another 600,000 viewed the parade, the largest in North America. For the first time, a separate lesbian parade was held on the day prior to the joint parade. The last decade, however, has not been one of unalloyed success for gay men and lesbians in the courts or legislatures of Canada. This chapter will briefly review the course of change in the sociolegal control of homosexuality in Canada through an examination of five issues that have been the object of recent court decisions or legislative action: the age of consent for anal intercourse, censorship of homosexual erotic material, pension rights for persons in same-sex relationships, a partial recognition of the legal status of same-sex couples in one province, and the inclusion of sexual orientation as a protected status under the Canadian Human Rights Act.

The number of homosexuals in Canada is unknown; no surveys have been conducted by either the private sector or the provincial or federal governments. In the most recent national census, StatsCan (the federal agency that conducts the census) included an optional question on same-sex couples as part of an in-depth census form, but no such question was included in the brief form that most citizens complete. The results will not be available until late 1997.

The impetus for change in the sociolegal control of homosexuality in Canada has its roots, to some degree, in England and the United States. For example, the decriminalization of consensual homosexual acts between adult males in England in 1967, following the Wolfenden Report (1957) led Pierre Trudeau, then Justice Minister, to introduce legislation to decriminalize consensual homosexual acts in Canada. During the 1950s, gays and lesbians were dependent for information on publications from the United States, such as the *Mattachine Review*, published by the Mattachine Society, and *The Ladder*, published by the Sisters of Bilitis (Kinsman, 1987). Gays in Canada still look to the United States for many publications focusing on homosexuals. During this time there were, however, individuals and groups within Canada that worked for equal rights for homosexuals. An early proponent of more tolerant and enlightened treatment of homosexuals was Jim Egan

ALEXANDER GREER, HOWARD BARBAREE, AND CHRISTINE BROWN • Clarke Institute of Psychiatry, and University of Toronto, Toronto, Ontario M5T 1R8, Canada.

Sociolegal Control of Homosexuality, edited by West and Green, Plenum Press, New York, 1997.

of Toronto, who wrote articles and letters to newspapers and provided information to governmental commissions (Kinsman, 1987). Homosexual associations and groups sprang up in major Canadian cities such as Toronto and Vancouver in the late 1950s; many were socially focused groups that worked sporadically toward changes in the law and in police behavior, but they tended to disband relatively quickly. It was not until the Stonewall riot in New York City that more permanent and active homosexual rights groups were formed in Canada. The Community Homophile Association in Toronto and the Gay Alliance toward Equality were founded in 1971 (Adam, 1993).

The 1970s and 1980s were marked by advances toward acceptance of homosexuals and the recognition of equality rights, but several setbacks also occurred. For example, in a "clean-up" campaign in Montreal in anticipation of the 1976 Olympics, police raided seven bath houses and one gay bar. But in 1979, the province of Quebec, of which Montreal is a part, enacted the first human rights code that included sexual orientation as a prohibited ground of discrimination. In 1981, Toronto police conducted a massive raid on the city's bath houses during a provincial election campaign. Yet in 1986 Ontario (of which Toronto is a part) added sexual orientation to its human rights code. These advances and retreats in the homosexual rights campaign reflect to a great degree changes in the provincial governments. Indeed, the inclusion of sexual orientation in Quebec's human rights code is directly attributable to the role homosexuals played in the election success of the Parti Quebécois (Adam, 1993).

Many of the changes in the sociolegal control of homosexuality in Canada described in this chapter have been the result of changes in government at the provincial and federal levels. The most significant single event for gay rights, however, was the enactment of the Charter of Rights and Freedoms. As will be shown, many of the changes have occurred as a result of appeals to the provisions of this Charter.

CRIMINAL PROHIBITIONS

Sexual practices between individuals of the same sex were decriminalized in 1969 by the Criminal Law Amendment Act (1968–69, SC 1968-69, Chap. 38, s.7). "Buggery" (anal intercourse) and "gross indecency" (usually, but not limited to, oral intercourse) committed in private between persons 21 years old and older were exempted from criminal prosecution. Since then, the age of consent for anal intercourse has been lowered to 18 [Criminal Code, s. 159(2)],[1] while the age of consent for all other forms of sexual expression (vaginal and oral intercourse) has been lowered to 14 [Criminal Code, s. 150.1(1)]. Additionally, consent is a defense for non-anal sexual activity between a person who is age 12 or 13 and a person who is less than 2 years older or who is under 16. No such defense is available for anal intercourse at these ages [Criminal Code, s. 150.1(2)]. Thus there is a disparity between the age of consent for heterosexual and lesbian activity and that for a form of sex predominantly engaged in by male homosexuals.[2]

This disparity in age of consent has been challenged in two provincial courts. A British Columbia court held that the distinction between the age of consent for anal intercourse

[1]Technically, Section 159(2), setting out the age of consent at 18, is a defense to a criminal charge of anal intercourse. It is proper to view it as defining the age of consent, as are Sections 150.1(1) and (2).
[2]Regarding sexual acts between two women, see *R. v. C.* (1981).

and that for other sexual practices did not offend the Canadian Charter of Rights and Freedoms (*R. v. Khadikin*, 1986). In Ontario (the most populous province) a court has held that the denial of the consent defense in anal intercourse prosecutions involving a person between the ages of 14 and 18 is a violation of Section 15(1), which provides that "Every individual is equal before and under the law and [is entitled to] ... equal protection and equal benefit of the law without discrimination and, in particular without discrimination based on race, national or ethnic origin, religion, sex, age or mental or physical disability." Section 1 of the Charter "guarantees the rights and freedoms set out ... only to such reasonable limits prescribed by law as can be demonstrably justified in a free and democratic society," but the court held that a reasonable limit was not breached.[3] Furthermore, the law that barred homosexuals from having anal intercourse — "a basic form of sexual expression among gay men" — until age 18, while heterosexuals were able to have sexual intercourse at 14, arbitrarily disadvantaged this "historically disadvantaged group" and thus violated Section 15(1).

CENSORSHIP OF HOMOSEXUAL EROTICA: THE LITTLE SISTERS DECISION

Officers of the Customs Service of Canada seized or detained publications imported from the United States that were bound for the Little Sisters Book and Art Emporium in Vancouver. This is one of only four bookstores in Canada that caters almost exclusively to homosexual customers, both lesbians and gay men. In addition to stocking and selling a wide variety of fiction and nonfiction of interest to homosexuals and serving as an informal community center for the gay community in Vancouver, Little Sisters also sells homosexual erotic materials — books, magazines, and films, much of it imported from the United States. Under the Customs Act [R.S.C. 1985, Chap. 1 (2nd Supp.)] customs officers are empowered to detain and review imported publications for obscene content and to prohibit the importation of those materials that in their opinion are obscene.[4] Customs officials identified materials imported by Little Sisters for heightened inspection, and many publications were delayed and some prohibited from importation. Over a period of years, Little Sisters had availed itself of the appeals processes provided by the Customs Act. Despite significant success in those appeals, the bookstore's imported publications continued to be closely scrutinized by customs officers. Little Sisters sought a declaration that the relevant customs regulations violated freedom of expression under Section 2(b) and equality rights under Section 15 of the Charter of Rights and Freedoms and were not justified under Section 1. The bookstore also sought a declaration that the customs regulations had been applied in a manner that violated Sections 2(b) and 15 of the

[3]The court also held that the statute violated Section 7 of the Charter in that it denied the defendant a defense available to others [*R. v. M.* (C.), 1992]. The court further reasoned — following *Haigh v. Canada* (1992) — that sexual orientation is "an analogous ground" to the groupings specified in Section 15(1) of the Charter and that sexual orientation should be "read into" that section. Although the decision in *R. v. M.* (C.) (1992) did not specifically overrule *R. v. Khadikin* (1986) (nor does the court have the power to do so), it is likely that the decision of the Ontario court reflects the true state of the law of consent for anal intercourse in Canada.

[4]Code 9956(a) of Schedule VII and Section 114 of the Customs Tariff [1985, R.S.C., c.41 (3rd Supp.)] and Sections 58 and 71 of the Customs Act [1985, R.S.C., c.1 (2nd Supp.)].

Charter.[5] Before considering the court's decision, it is necessary to review briefly the jurisprudence of obscenity in Canada.

Section 163 of the Criminal Code outlines the crime of "corrupting public morals" and includes the publication of obscene materials. Section 163(1)(a) provides that "[e]very one commits an offense who makes, prints, publishes, distributes, circulates, or has in his possession for the purpose of publication, distribution, or circulation any obscene written matter, picture, model, phonograph record, or other thing whatever." Subsection (8) of the statute provides a definition of obscene: "... any publication a dominant characteristic of which is the undue exploitation of sex, or of sex and any one or more of the following subjects, namely, crime, cruelty and violence shall be deemed to be obscene." In R. v. Butler (1992) the Supreme Court of Canada clarified the definition of obscene. Obscenity in Canada is determined by a two-stage test. First, the reviewing court must determine into which one of three categories the materials fall: explicit sex with violence, explicit sex without violence but that subjects people to treatment that is degrading or dehumanizing, or explicit sex without violence that is neither degrading or dehumanizing. (Violence in this context includes both actual physical violence and threats of physical violence.) When considering whether the material is obscene, the finder of fact (judge or jury) must determine what the community would tolerate others being exposed to on the basis of the degree of harm that may flow from such exposure. Harm means that it predisposes people to behave in an antisocial manner; the court gives the example that some material may predispose men to mistreat women. The stronger the inference of risk of harm, the less the likelihood of tolerance. Explicit sex with violence will almost always constitute undue exploitation of sex; explicit sex that is degrading or dehumanizing may be undue exploitation of sex if the risk of harm is substantial, and explicit sex without violence that is not degrading or dehumanizing is tolerated and will not be found obscene unless it involves children. If the material is found to unduly exploit sex, it will not be judged obscene if (part two of the test) considered as a whole the portrayal of sex is essential to wider artistic, literary, or other similar purposes.

In the Little Sisters case, the court (p. 521) first found that "the law is neutral on its face and applies to all obscenity, whether tailored to heterosexual or homosexual audiences. It does not draw a distinction between homosexual and heterosexual." However, a law may still be discriminatory in its effects if "it imposes burdens or disadvantages based on the enumerated or analogous grounds" of Section 15 of the Charter (p. 522). The plaintiffs were required to show that they suffered disadvantage because of their homosexuality. The bookstore argued that heterosexual pornography performs an entertainment function, while homosexual erotica is far more important to homosexuals; it serves "as an affirmation of their sexuality and as a socializing force, ... normalizes the sexual practices that the larger society has historically considered to be deviant and ... organizes homosexuals as a group and enhances their political power" (p. 522). The court also found that the unequal effect is compounded by the facts (produced through testimony of plaintiff's expert witnesses) "that such a large proportion of such materials is produced in the United States and that there are only four bookstores in Canada dealing exclusively in homosexual erotica" (p. 522). The combination of these circumstances has "adversely affected the ability of the plaintiffs ...

---

[5]A claim that a law as written violates the Charter is brought under Section 52(1) of the Constitution Act, a claim that the law is applied in a manner that violates the Charter is brought under Section 24(1) of the Charter.

and other homosexuals, to obtain material that has value to them, they have been correspondingly disadvantaged and the disadvantage is directly related to their homosexuality" (p. 523). Nevertheless, the court held that the distinctive treatment and disadvantage arose not from the Customs Act, but from Section 163(8) of the Criminal Code. Thus, "the disproportionate impact is not the responsibility of the impugned legislation and it cannot be said that this legislation imposes a burden on the plaintiffs that would amount to an infringement of their rights under s.15(1)" (p. 523). The court concluded, "[T]he point is that homosexual obscenity is proscribed because it is obscene (under s. 163(8) of the Criminal Code) not because it is homosexual (p. 539). There is "a body of social science evidence that would support Parliament's reasoned apprehension that obscene pornography produced for homosexual audiences causes harm to society" (p. 540).

The court rejected the bookstore's argument that, as applied to homosexual erotica, Section 163(8) of the Criminal Code violates the Charter, but it did issue a declaration that the Customs Services procedures in this case violated Section 24(1) of the Charter.

The court's decision cannot be seen as a victory for those who support the unfettered importation or sale of homosexual erotic materials. However, it can be seen as a qualified success for homosexual rights. At very least, it is a success for the Little Sisters Bookstore and Emporium and for other bookstores catering to homosexuals (such as the Glad Day bookstore in Toronto, which also had books seized by the Customs Service) in their efforts to import and sell nonobscene homosexual erotica without undue interference.

FAMILY LAW ACT: DEFINITION OF SPOUSE

The Family Law Act of Ontario (R.S.O. 1990, c. F.3) (hereafter FLA) regulates the economic aspects of marriage and the dissolution of marital relationships (both sanctioned and common law). Section 30 of the FLA states that "every spouse has an obligation to provide support for himself or herself and for the other spouse in accordance with need, to the extent that he or she is capable of doing so." At issue in *M. v H.* (1996) was the definition of spouse for the provision of support following the dissolution of a lesbian relationship.

A spouse under Section 1(1) of the FLA is "either of a man and woman who (a) are married to each other, or (b) have together entered into a marriage that is voidable or void, in good faith on the part of the person asserting a right under the Act." This definition applies to Part I (family property), Part II (matrimonial home), and Part IV (amendments to the common law) of the FLA. Section 29 provides a further definition for the purposes of Part III (support obligations): In addition to those who are married, a spouse is "either of a man or woman who are not married to each other and have cohabited (a) continuously for a period of not less than three years, or (b) in a relationship of some permanence, if they are the natural or adoptive parents of a child."

The lesbian couple, M. and H., had lived together for at least 5 years and, according to the plaintiff M., "shared their lives in every respect; business, financial, social, domestic, sexual, and recreational." The defendant, H., disputed this assertion, claiming that they never contemplated an interdependent financial relationship (*M. v. H.*, at p. 600). M. sought a spousal support order under Section 30 of the FLA. Her claim was rejected because she did not come within the definition of spouse under either Sections 1(1) or 29. She sought a determination that the definition of spouse in Section 29 of the FLA violated

Section 15 of the Charter in that it excluded same-sex relationships and, therefore, denied her the "equal protection and equal benefit of the law." H., joined by the attorney general for Ontario, argued that the definition of.spouse in Section 29 did not violate Section 15 of the Charter and if it did, it was justified under Section 1 of the Charter.

The court held that the exclusion of same-sex relationships from the FLA violates Section 15 of the Charter and is not saved by application of Section 1. The court granted M.'s request for a declaration that (1) Section 29 is of no force or effect to the extent that it excludes same-sex couples from its definition of spouse, (2) the words "a man and a woman" be severed from the definition of spouse, and (3) the words "two persons" be read into the definition of spouse. The decision in M. v. H. is being appealed to Ontario's court of appeal.

PENSION RIGHTS: EGAN V. CANADA

A badly divided Supreme Court of Canada rejected a claim that the exclusion of partners in same-sex relationships from the definition of spouse in the Old Age Security Act (R.S.C. 1985, c. O-9) was not a reasonable limit under Section 1 of the Charter. The 5-4 vote reflects a serious division in the court concerning economic issues and same-sex relationships.

Upon reaching 65 years of age, Egan became entitled to a pension under the Old Age Security Act. His same-sex partner of 47 years applied for a spouse's allowance, which the Act provides when the spouse of a retiree is between the ages of 60 and 65 and the couple's combined income falls below a predetermined level. Egan's partner's application was denied because he failed to meet the definition of spouse under the Act. Their application was dismissed at trial, and their appeal was dismissed at the federal court of appeals. They appealed to the Supreme Court.

Justice LaForest, Chief Justice Lamer, Justice Gonthier, and Justice Major (with LaForest writing) held that Egan and his partner did not suffer discrimination under Section 15(1) of the Charter. They employed a three-stage analysis to make this determination. First, they had to determine if the law at issue made a distinction between the appellant and others. There was no real controversy on that point: The law clearly distinguished between Egan and others. The second step required a determination that the distinction imposed a burden, obligation, or disadvantage on a group to which the claimant belongs that was not imposed on others or that this distinction did not provide them with a benefit that it granted to others. There was no controversy on this point: The group to which Egan and his partner belong — same-sex couples — are denied a benefit that others receive. It is the third step in the test that gives rise to the split in the court: Was this distinction based on an irrelevant personal characteristic that is either enumerated in Section 15(1) or is analogous thereto?

All of the justices agreed that sexual orientation is an analogous ground to those enumerated in Section 15(1). Justice LaForest and the justices that concurred with him found that sexual orientation is relevant to the functional values underlying the law and, therefore, a distinction drawn on that basis is not discriminatory. It was Parliament's intent, they held, to provide support to married couples for "reasons deeply rooted in our fundamental values and traditions" (p. 621). Parliament, they found, may "quite properly give special support to the institution of marriage" because of all social relationships it is unique because it is "anchored in the biological and social realities" that only heterosexual couples have the ability to procreate. That not all heterosexual couples have children was not a critical factor in this analysis. Parliament need not put into place procedures to separate childless couples from heterosexual couples with children, ruled to court, because it would impose on Parliament "the burden of devising administrative procedures that would be both unnecessarily intrusive and difficult to administer" (p. 622). Thus, in this analysis, "[N]either in purpose nor in effect does the legislation constitute an infringement of the fundamental values sought to be protected by the Charter."

Justice Sopinka held that the definition's underinclusiveness infringes Section 15(1) of the Charter, but is "saved" under Section 1. He held that the government must be given some flexibility in extending social benefits and need not be proactive in recognizing new social relationships. The issue is the kind of socioeconomic issue in which the government must mediate between competing groups and in which the courts should be reluctant to second-guess the choices Parliament has made. He wrote, "[G]iven that equality of same-sex couples with heterosexual couples is generally regarded as a novel concept, government has not, by its inaction to date, disentitled itself to rely on s.1 of the Charter" (p. 650).

In dissent, Justice L'Heureux-Dube argued that the statute's violation of Section 15(1) of the Charter is not saved by application of Section 1. She found that the statute is not rationally connected to the objective of the law—providing support for elderly couples. The statute, in addition, does not minimally impair the rights of same-sex couples in that it "has a significant discriminatory impact in terms of perpetuating prejudice, stereotyping, and marginalization of same-sex couples, and homosexuals and lesbians individually" (p. 673).

The dissent, written by Justice Cory and joined by Justices Iacobucci and McLachlin, noted that, first, the appeal did not challenge the definition of spouse provided in Section 1(1) of the Old Age Security Act, but only the definition of common law spouse in Section 2. The underinclusiveness of the definition, they found, violates Section 15(1) of the Charter because it denies equal benefit of the law by denying homosexual couples an economic benefit and denying them the right to make a choice regarding their relationship. The legislation cannot be saved by Section 1 of the Charter, since the remedy proposed— deleting the words "of the opposite sex" from the statute—would not "involve a significant intrusion into Parliament's budgetary decision making."

The loss of this appeal was certainly disappointing for homosexuals and particularly for those in same-sex relationships of some duration. However, the closeness of the vote and Justice Sopinka's unwillingness to follow the reasoning of the majority suggests that the court will not long tolerate Parliament's inaction on the issue. Indeed, Justice Sopinka's opinion can be seen as an exhortation to Parliament to act.

THE SEXUAL ORIENTATION AMENDMENT TO THE CANADIAN HUMAN RIGHTS ACT

The Canadian Human Rights Act [Revised Statutes (1993), c H-6] prohibits, under Section 2, discrimination in employment, housing, and the provision of goods and services in federally regulated businesses. The prohibited grounds of discrimination are race, national or ethnic origin, religion, age, sex, marital status, family status, disability, and conviction for which a pardon has been granted [s. 3(1)]. In May 1996 the government, through the Minister of Justice, put forward an amendment to the Act that would add "sexual orientation" to the list of prohibited grounds for discrimination. The amendment has proceeded through a third reading, not without controversy, and is expected to be proclaimed shortly.

Quebec was the first province to include sexual orientation as a prohibited ground in 1977; since then, seven other provinces have amended their human rights codes to include sexual orientation as a prohibited ground of discrimination. Since 1979 the Canadian Human Rights Commission has called on the government to amend the Human Rights Code, and since 1992 the Commission has been accepting complaints of discrimination based on sexual orientation. In its 1994 Annual Report the Canadian Human Rights Commission called the government's failure to include sexual orientation as a prohibited ground of discrimination "a fundamental abdication of our human rights responsibilities" (p. 61). In 1985 an all-party committee of the House of Commons unanimously endorsed an amendment that would have had the same effect as this bill.

Controversy concerning this amendment centered around the Reform Party's conviction that amending the Human Rights Act would "redefine the terms of marriage, family, or spouse" such that it would "provide state sanction of same-sex marriages, or the extension of spousal benefits to same sex couples."[6] Members of Parliament from the Reform Party and other parties offered amendments to the government's Amendment Bill that were, in their view, designed to limit the reach of the sexual orientation provision to the Canadian Human Rights Act. All of these amendments were defeated. They included those "affirming that including sexual orientation will not affect freedom of religion, expression, and association as guaranteed by the Charter of Rights and Freedoms."

Enactment of the amendment to the Canadian Human Rights Act will, in fact, do no more than codify the activities of the Human Rights Commission, which, as noted earlier, has accepted complaints based on discrimination on the basis of sexual orientation since 1992. Moreover, far more activities and industries are covered by the inclusion of sexual orientation as a prohibited ground for discrimination in the codes of eight provinces; the federal act covers only about 10 percent of the citizens of Canada. However, the addition of sexual orientation to the Human Rights Act may be significant because the Act also bars "hate speech" against members of protected groups. Hate speech directed against homosexuals was not barred by the unamended Act. The addition will also complement the inclusion of sexual orientation in the Charter of Human Rights and Freedoms, which addresses the acts of government, while the Human Rights Act applies to individuals.

CONCLUSION

In the past decade there has been a gradual loosening of the sociolegal controls on homosexuality in Canada. There has been recognition of sexual orientation as a prohibited ground of discrimination under the human rights codes of a majority of the provinces; soon the same will occur at the federal level. The courts, including the Supreme Court of

[6]Remarks of Mr. Preston Manning, leader of the National Reform Party, *Commons Debates* (1996, May 9), p. 2582.

Canada, are agreed that the prohibited grounds of discrimination under the Charter of Rights and Freedoms includes sexual orientation.

CITED CASES

Egan v Canada, 124 D.L.R. (4th) 609 (1995).

Haigh v Canada, 9 O.R. (3d) 495, 10 C.R.R. (2nd) 287 C.A. (1992).

M. v H., 27 O.R. (3d) 593 (Ont. Ct. Gen. Div.) (1996).

R. v Butler, 70 C.C.C. (3d) 129, 11 C.R. (4th) 137, 1 S.C.R. 452 (1992).

R. v C., 30 Nfld & PEIR 451 (Nfld. Dist. Ct.) (1981); revised 39 Nfld & PEIR 8 (Nfld. C.A.) (1982).

R. v Khadikin, 29 C.C.C. (3d) 154 (B.C.S.C.) (1986).

R. v M. (C.), 75 C.C.C. (3d) 556, 15 C.R. (4th) 368 (Ont. Ct. Gen. Div.) (1992).

Little Sisters Book and Art Emporium v Canada, 131 D.L.R. (4th) 486 (1996).

REFERENCES

Adam, B. D. (1992). Winning rights and freedoms in Canada. In A. Hendriks, R. Tielman, & E. van der Veen (Eds.), *The third pink book: A global view of lesbian and gay liberation and oppression.* Buffalo, NY: Prometheus Books.

Human Rights Commission. (1995). *Annual Report: 1994.* Ottawa: Federal Printing Office.

Kinsman, G. W. (1996). *The regulation of desire: Sexuality in Canada.* Montreal: Black Rose Books.

Wolfenden, J. (1957). *Report of the Committee on Homosexual Offences and Prostitution.* London: Her Majesty's Stationery Office.

12

European International Control

ALAN REEKIE

The Council of Europe

In many parts of the world minimal respect is paid to the United Nations International Covenant on Civil and Political Rights, but treaties between the nations of Europe have amplified the principles of the Covenant and have developed means of implementing them. The sovereign nations of Europe each have their own legal systems and social conventions. Nevertheless, the proliferation of international treaties and supranational institutions is gradually bringing about greater uniformity and, with it, a trend toward the lessening of legal discrimination against homosexuals and a tolerance of organizations promoting their interests.[1]

In the aftermath of World War II, several European countries collaborated to set up the Council of Europe. Their aim was to create a permanent international organization that would provide a forum for discussion and for the preparation of legal agreements that would prevent disputes arising between member states, or at least ensure that such disputes could be resolved peacefully. Probably the best-known of its achievements is the European Convention for the Protection of Human Rights and Fundamental Freedoms, adopted in Rome on November 4, 1950, which came into force in fifteen member states on September 3, 1953.

The Council of Europe has a Parliamentary Assembly made up of certain members of the national parliaments of its constituent states. This body elects the members of the European Court of Human Rights, one judge from each member state. The court, situated in Strasbourg, hears petitions forwarded to it by the European Commission of Human Rights. This commission, which also has one member from each of the contracting states, has responsibility for the initial examination and filtering of applications from individuals or groups who claim that their rights under the European Convention have been violated by some action taken by the authorities of a contracting state. The Commission of Human Rights considers whether there is a prima facie case and whether the applicant has exhausted all possible methods of appeal available in the home country. The majority of

---

[1]In addition to the standard works that appear in the list of references, this chapter has made use of some specialized sources, including *Homostudies* (University of Maastricht, The Netherlands); Homosexuelle Initiative (Wien/LAMBDA, Nachrichten, Austria); *EUROLETTER* (edited by Gay and Lesbian International Lobby, Denmark); and the survey of Alexandra Duda (% Schwule und Lesben Sentrum, Kartauserwall 18, D-50678 Köln, Germany). All of the aforementioned are members of International Gay and Lesbian Association. Much information, especially where no specific attributions are cited, has been received through the Internet, which is now being used extensively by gay and lesbian individuals and groups to circulate news and requests for help all over the world.

ALAN REEKIE • International Gay and Lesbian Association, Brussels B-1000, Belgium.

Sociolegal Control of Homosexuality, edited by West and Green, Plenum Press, New York, 1997.

applications are rejected at this stage. If an application is accepted, the next step is for the Commission of Human Rights to try to resolve the matter through discussion with the government and parties involved. Failing this, the complainant can appeal to the European Court of Human Rights. Their decision, usually reached after public hearings with all parties legally represented, is theoretically binding, so that if a complaint is upheld this should result in a change in law or practice in the country concerned. Including the time occupied by domestic legal proceedings, many years generally go by between the initial complaint and a ruling from the European Court of Human Rights.

When the European Convention on Human Rights first came into operation, legal discrimination against homosexuals was endemic, with an absolute ban on any physical expression of attraction between men being in force in most European countries (West, 1977). Social discrimination was also widespread against both male and female homosexuals. Although the Convention does not refer explicitly to sexual orientation, it was so framed that the European Court of Human Rights and the European Commission on Human Rights have been able, in later years, to interpret the standards set by the Convention in the light of an evolving social context and to apply them to the situation of homosexuals. For example, in an appeal concerning corporal punishment in the Isle of Man (*Tyrer v. UK*, 1978), it was held that the Convention was "a living Instrument that can adapt to, amongst other things, the moral perceptions of the time."

Despite an initial reluctance to do so, the court recognized in due course that national laws prohibiting homosexual acts performed by consenting adults in private breached Article 8 of the Convention because they went beyond the permitted purposes for which the right to respect for private life could be overridden. The Article states:

1. Everyone has the right to respect for his private and family life, his home and his correspondence.
2. There shall be no interference by a public authority with the exercise of this right except such as in accordance with the law and is necessary in a democratic society in the interests of national security, public safety or the economic well-being of the country, for the prevention of disorder or crime, for the protection of health or morals, or for the protection of the rights and freedoms of others.

Although the European Commission of Human Rights passes on petitions to the court only after individuals have exhausted the legal processes in their own countries, the prospect of an eventual condemnation by the court often provides national legislators with the incentive — or the excuse — to enact the required reforms. Making a final pronouncement is all the court can do, there being no effective enforcement mechanism. However, a useful criterion for the evaluation of the recent applications to join the Council of Europe, coming from emergent democracies in the East since German reunification in 1989, has been the extent to which the Convention's standards for the protection of individuals are embodied in their national laws (Tatchell, 1992).

European Court of Human Rights Case Law

In *Dudgeon v. UK* (1981), the European Court of Human Rights ruled that the complete ban on homosexuality in one province of the United Kingdom, namely Northern Ireland, contravened the European Convention on Human Rights by violating the right to privacy set forth in Article 8. The court found that the right to engage in consensual same-sex acts in private "concerns a most intimate aspect of private life. Accordingly there must exist particularly serious reasons before interferences on the part of public authorities can be legitimate for the purpose of Paragraph 2 of Article 8." The U.K. government complied with the Homosexual Offenses (Northern Ireland) Order of 1982, extending to that province the decriminalization of adult, consensual, private homosexual behavior already applicable elsewhere in Great Britain.

This was a landmark decision, particularly in view of an earlier case (*Handyside v. UK*, 1976) when the court declared that, on the requirements of morals, "State authorities are in principle in a better position than the international Judge to give an opinion." In *Handyside*, the court ruled that the destruction of an offending publication under the British Obscene Publications Acts (1956 and 1964) did not breach the right of freedom of expression, even though the material was freely available elsewhere in Europe. The court was exercising its so-called "margin of appreciation" and allowing the national court to decide, in the light of the case as a whole, whether the ban served a pressing need for the protection of morals.

The court's liberality in *Dudgeon* has to be set against an absence of positive support for equal treatment of males and females in the matter of minimum age limits (usually misleadingly called the "age of consent") for homosexual relationships. The issue was avoided in the *Dudgeon* decision, but in an earlier case (*X. v. Federal Republic of Germany*, 1976) the Commission had reported that in its view the existence of a special social danger in the case of masculine homosexuality, through its tendency to proselytize adolescents, justified unequal treatment of males and females. Similar reasoning was repeated in a 1982 decision, when the application of Richard Desmond, a U.K. teenager, protesting the differential age of consent, was rejected in a ruling that allowed account to be taken of the moral interests and welfare of young people (Helfer, 1990). As Pieter van Dijk remarks (1993, p. 196), regarding the age of consent, the legislatures of many of the member states are in advance of decisions by the Strasbourg Court.

The right to pursue adult homosexual relationships in private has been reasserted in two further decisions of the European Court of Human Rights. In *Norris v. Ireland* (1988) the Court urged the Republic of Ireland to repeal the laws against consenting adult male homosexual behavior that dated from the time when the country was a part of the United Kingdom, but were no longer being enforced there. The complainant had already brought the issue to the Irish High Court, where the judicial ruling on October 10, 1980, was that, in view of the Catholic and democratic nature of the Irish Republic, the law was valid (Norris, 1993), but the European Court held that the factors supposedly justifying retention of the impugned laws were no greater than in the prior case of *Dudgeon*. The plaintiff's lawyer was Mary Robinson, later President of Ireland, but the Irish government did not take immediate action, although the Council of Ministers repeatedly urged it to reform the law. When the Irish Parliament finally complied on June 24, 1993, gender-neutral language had already been adopted in the rest of Irish sex law, with the result that all legal discrimination was eliminated at a stroke (Rose, 1994).

In *Modinos v. Cyprus* (1993), the European Court of Human Rights again held to its earlier position that an absolute ban on homosexual acts is a breach of the Convention. Even though, in this instance, the law was not being enforced, it had a preventing and stigmatizing effect. Mr. Modinos was paid compensation, but there was no reason to believe that repeal of the relevant law (ss. 171–173, Cypriot Criminal Code) was imminnent until just before this book went to press ("Human rights group backs gay rights bill," *Cyprus Mail*, 14 May 1997).

THE EUROPEAN UNION

Closer integration among the countries of Europe is being further promoted by another great international grouping, the European Union (EU), formerly known as the European Economic Community. In accordance with the European Treaties, three international institutions are mainly responsible for defining the specific actions needed to achieve closer integration: the European Parliament, the Council of Ministers, and the European Commission. Any new EU legislation proposed by the Commission does not take effect until it has been approved by both the Parliament and the Council of Ministers (who must also agree on any amendments). For full legal effect, the decisions of the European Parliament, whose members are directly elected by the citizens of all member-states, must be adopted by an absolute majority. They tend to have less influence than the Council of Ministers, which cannot adopt any proposal unless supported by at least a "qualified majority" (i.e., a broad consensus) of the members, who are representatives of the governments of the member-states. On the most sensitive issues its decisions must be unanimous. The European Commission (not to be confused with the Human Rights Commission) is the EU's "civil service," headed by commissioners appointed by the member-states for fixed terms. In its role as "Guardian of the Treaties," it is responsible for drafting proposals to amend the patchwork of national laws among the member-states where this is needed to create a "level playing-field" by eliminating barriers to the free circulation of goods, services, capital, and people within the EU's single, internal market. Although much progress has been achieved, the prospect of enlarging the Union to include new member-states with very diverse social and economic situations has stimulated debate on what amendments to the Treaties would be appropriate.

The European Court of Justice (ECJ) in Luxembourg (not to be confused with the aforementioned European Court of Human Rights in Strasbourg) is the highest court for the interpretation of European Union law. If a question of EU law arises in any court in a member state, that court can refer the question to the ECJ for determination. In this capacity the ECJ, over the years, has greatly widened the scope of the Treaty of Rome and other EU law.

Although initially concerned primarily with economic, industrial, and employment issues, the Union now has a wider remit and encourages member-states that still maintain discriminatory legislation to follow the example of those who have already adopted gender-neutral criminal laws on sexual behaviors. Although the European treaties to which member states of the Union subscribe do not deal directly with matters of gay rights, the principles embodied in them lead in that direction. Thus, Title I–Common Provisions, Article F of the Treaty on European Union [signed at Maastricht on February 7, 1992, and published by the Office for Official Publications of the European Communities, L-2985 Luxemburg, 1992], which has become known as the Maastricht Treaty, states that:

1. The Union shall respect the national identities of its member-States, whose systems of government are founded on the principles of democracy.

2. The Union shall respect fundamental rights, as guaranteed by the European Convention for the protection of Human Rights and Fundamental Freedoms signed in Rome on 4 November 1950 and as they result from the constitutional traditions common to the member-States, as general principles of Community law.
3. The Union shall provide itself with the means necessary to attain its objectives and carry through its policies.

The Union's adherence to the European Convention on Human Rights includes respect for Article 14, which declares that the rights and freedoms set forth "shall be secured without discrimination on any ground such as sex, race, colour, language, religion, political or other opinion, national or social origin, association with a national minority, property, birth or other status." If not already within the meaning of "other status," it would seem that sexual orientation could be slotted into the list. Although this has not happened, the European Parliament has long recognized that discrimination on grounds of sexual orientation is incompatible with the Treaty of Rome's provisions for the "free circulation of goods, services, capital and people" within the Union. Its resolution on "Sexual Discrimination in the Workplace" was based on recommendations from a group headed by an Italian Member of the European Parliament, Vera Squarcialupi (1984). It urged upon member-states the abolition of laws against consenting sexual relations between adults of the same sex, equalization of the age of consent regardless of gender, and rejection of the classification of homosexuality as a mental illness.

The European Parliament, in a resolution on "Equal Rights for Homosexuals and Lesbians in the European Union," adopted on February 8, 1994, by a vote of 160-98, returns to these issues, calling upon member-states to end all differences in legal or administrative treatment of people on grounds of sexual orientation. Based on a report by Claudia Roth of the Committee on Civil Liberties and Internal Affairs (a Green Party Member of the European Parliament), the full text of the resolution is reproduced in the Appendix to this chapter. Although such resolutions do not compel the European Commission or the Council of Ministers to act, they do have an influence. Over the last few years, Luxembourg, Ireland, and Germany have all enacted liberalizing amendments to their sex laws so that, when Austria, Finland, and Sweden joined the EU in 1995, all 12 of the preexisting member states, save Portugal and the United Kingdom, had abolished penal laws discriminating against homosexual sex; Portugal did so shortly afterwards and Austria and Finland are expected to follow suit in due course.

Delays in achieving complete, Europe-wide integration of law and practice on controversial social issues result from the contorted and ambiguous terms of the successive treaties that regulate the Union, which reflect the anxiety of individual countries to preserve their sovereignty and national traditions. In particular, the vaguely-defined principle of "subsidiarity," according to which "decisions should be taken at the lowest level consistent with effective action within a political system" (Bainbridge & Teesdale, 1966, p. 430), restricts any proposed Union action to occasions when its aims can be achieved better by the Community than by the individual state. It remains a matter for negotiation what issues can be left to be dealt with by domestic law (Snyder, 1993).

On an issue with a bearing upon homosexuality that arose in the United Kingdom, the European Court of Justice decided, on April 30, 1996, that the dismissal by a local authority of a male-to-female transsexual from the post of college administrator because of a sex change was in breach of EU law. The court held that the dismissal contravened the 1976

Equal Treatment Directive [Council Directive 76/207/EEC of February 9, 1976 on the implementation of the principle of equal treatment of men and women as regards access to employment, vocational training, and promotion and working conditions (Official Journal of the European Communities No. L039, February 14, 1976, p. 40)], since the discriminatory action in this case was on the grounds of the individual's sex, which was protected (*Guardian*, 1 May, 1996).

DISCRIMINATORY PRACTICES

An impressionistic survey of the situation as it appeared to gay and lesbian activists a few years ago is provided in the *Third Pink Book* (Hendriks, Tielman, & Veen, 1993). It shows that male, and sometimes also female, homosexual acts remain imprisonable offenses regardless of consent in many parts of the world. In Europe, by September 1995, a total ban on homosexual relations between men still operated officially in Boznia-Herzegovinia, Cyprus, Macedonia, and Romania. Contrasting legal age limits for heterosexual and male homosexual relations remained in the countries listed in Table 1.

Criminal law provisions that prohibit "promoting" or "encouraging" homosexuality are on the statute book in Finland [Article 20 (9.2)], Liechtenstein, and the United Kingdom. These doubtfully efficacious laws are arguably in breach of the provisions for freedom of speech in the European Convention on Human Rights and have not been enforced in the last few years. Similar provisions in Austria (s. 220), and laws there prohibiting the creation of or membership in lesbian and gay organizations (s. 221), which appear to breach the Convention's provisions on freedom of association, were repealed with effect from March 1997. In Greece, male prostitution is an offense (Article 347), but there is no corresponding law against heterosexual prostitution.

In some countries, such as Bulgaria, Italy, Spain, and the United Kingdom, laws on "public indecency" and "obscenity" are used in discriminatory ways against gay men and lesbians who display affection by hugging and kissing in public places. Provisions concern-

TABLE 1. Legal Age Limits for Heterosexual
and Male Homosexual Acts

	Date total ban repealed	Minimum age for heterosexual contact	Minimum age for homosexual contact
Albania	1995	14	18
Austria	1971	14	18
Bulgaria	1968	14	18
Croatia	1977	14	18
Finland	1971	16	18
Hungary	1961	14	18
Liechtenstein	1989	14	18
England & Wales	1967	16	18
Gibraltar	1992	16	18
Isle of Man	1992	16	21
Scotland	1980	16	18

ing "public morals" are applied in some countries to the publications of gay and lesbian organizations, thereby trespassing upon the rights of freedom of speech and press. Such laws have also been used to prevent these organizations from obtaining the official registration needed for their incorporation. Meeting places of gay organizations have been raided by police, and gay activists have been intimidated by allegations of breaches of licensing conditions. For example, in September 1995, the Lambda group was prevented on similar legalistic pretexts from holding a gay and lesbian festival in Istanbul (Reuters, 1995).

Discriminatory legislation reflects views, more prevalent in past generations, that attribute homosexuality to genetic or mental disease. Claims of "cures" by means of drugs or electroshock are still made by some people who share these views. In many places social pressures provoke homosexuals into heterosexual marriages, which often result in great unhappiness. Except in those countries that have introduced legislation forbidding discrimination on grounds of sexual orientation, overtly homosexual persons are often excluded from sensitive occupations (notably diplomatic or military service), and many of them face a hostile climate in their workplace and restrictions on promotion and career development (Waaldijk & Clapham, 1993). Homosexuals who strive to retain a low profile risk arbitrary dismissal should their sexual orientation be discovered. Few openly homosexual persons are elected to public office, although some who have "come out" voluntarily during periods of mandate have retained their position and been reelected subsequently.

Even when formal discrimination has been eliminated from the criminal law, gays and lesbians who have had heterosexual relationships can face severe difficulties in maintaining custody of, or even visiting rights to, their children, should they become divorced or separated. Their rights are especially precarious if they are living with same-sex partners. In some countries (e.g., Austria, Norway, Italy, France, and the United Kingdom), means are already in place, or else under discussion, to prevent lesbians from becoming mothers through artificial insemination. In most European countries only heterosexual couples are allowed to adopt children.

RECENT ACTION BY THE COUNCIL OF EUROPE, THE EUROPEAN UNION, AND OTHER INTERNATIONAL ORGANIZATIONS

Pending before the Council of Europe's Committee on Human Rights and Legal Affairs is a proposal, supported by the International Gay and Lesbian Association (ILGA), for an additional protocol to the European Convention on Human Rights that would explicitly include sexual orientation among the grounds for which discrimination is prohibited.

The Parliamentary Assembly of the Council of Europe (Recommendation 934/81 and Motion for Recommendation 6348/90), as well as the European Parliament (Squarcialupi, 1984) have long been urging member-states to provide complete equality for homosexuals and heterosexuals in all fields of legislation and, in particular, to adopt the same age of consent for both. This has had some practical effect when countries applying for membership are investigated by the Council of Europe in regard to the human rights situation of their homosexual citizens. In February 1993 the Parliamentary Assembly of the Council adopted Written Declaration No. 227, which stressed the need to end discrimination against homosexuals in former communist countries. When Lithuania became a member in May 1993, its ban on homosexuality was lifted. Just 1 month later, Luxembourg, one of the existing member-states, introduced discriminatory age limits of homosexual and heterosexual relations in its penal code in 1972 (Article 372 bis), which remained in effect until the law of August 10, 1992 (Article 42) came into effect on December 25, 1992, setting a common age limit of 16.

When Romania was admitted as a member of the Council of Europe in September 1993, despite its antihomosexual legislation, the Parliamentary Assembly requested reform to bring the country into line with the ratified European Convention. Despite considerable political opposition in the country, a bill that would amend the Romanian Penal Code (Article 200) and decriminalize homosexual acts by adults that did not involve "public scandal" was put before the Chamber of Deputies. It was, however, ultimately rejected on November 21, 1995.

The Council of Europe is not alone in having tried to influence Romania on this matter. Amnesty International (1994, 1995) has also expressed concern about Article 200 of the Romanian code, which allows for the arrest, prosecution, and imprisonment of adults engaging in consenting homosexual acts in private. It has also complained about the maltreatment of homosexual suspects during police detention or imprisonment in Romania. The following account, taken from the testimony of one young Romanian prisoner, Ciprian Cocu (1995), illustrates the effect of a combination of social and legal hostility:

> Cocu confessed to his family that he was in a gay relationship with another young man slightly older than himself. They disapproved and reported the matter to the police. Cocu and his lover were arrested and held in prison where the lover was beaten unconscious and Cocu was repeatedly raped by fellow inmates. Their case received unfavorable publicity in a police journal. This caught the attention of human rights activists from abroad and Amnesty International took up the case. Probably as a result of this, when the case came to trial in June 1993 their prison sentences were suspended. On his release Cocu was expelled from the high school where he had been studying, being considered a danger to other students. His lover could not for a long time find any employer to hire him and when he finally got a job he was harassed so much he was forced to leave. He committed suicide in May 1995. (pp. 9–11)

The EU is under some pressure to improve gay rights. In 1991 the European Commission extended its code on sexual harassment in the workplace with provisions for the protection of gay men and lesbians. In April 1993 the European Human Rights Foundation launched a report, *Homosexuality: A European Community Issue*, which presented the findings of a study that had been largely funded by the EU. It set out the need for cross-national agreement in the context of the development of the "single market" in general and the "free movement" of people in particular (Waaldijk & Clapham, 1993). In November 1993, a pilot study (*Lesbian Visibility Project*) by ILGA, also mainly funded by the EU, was completed. It aimed to explore matters not often dealt with in other homosexual studies and produced recommendations and suggestions for further work.

In its proposals for the Intergovernmental Conference on the revision of the European Treaties in 1996 (IGC-96), the Reflection Group, chaired by Carlos Westendorp, responded to calls from the European Parliament and other representative bodies by recommending the inclusion, in the European treaties, of an explicit commitment to "such European values as equality between men and women, non-discrimination on grounds of race, religion, sexual orientation, age or disability and that it should include express condemnation of racism and xenophobia and a procedure for its enforcement." Despite the reluctance of the Conservative British Government, which had made no secret of its opposition to further European integration in general, and to any obligation to eliminate discrimination on grounds of sexual orientation in particular, the following text for a proposed new Article 6a of the European Treaty was included in the document: "The European Union Today and Tomorrow—A general outline for a draft revision of the Treaties" prepared for the European Council meeting in Dublin in December 1996 [Conf 2500/96]: Non discrimination—New Article 6a.

Within the scope of application of this Treaty and without prejudice to any special provisions contained therein, the Council, acting unanimously on a proposal from the Commission and after consulting the European Parliament, may take appropriate action to prohibit discrimination based on sex, racial, ethnic or social origin, religious belief, disability, age, or sexual orientation.

At the time of writing, just after a Labour British Government committed to respecting Human Rights was formed following the General Election on May 1, 1997, but before the European Council Meeting in Amsterdam at which the final text of the draft Treaty amendments will be determined, it remains to be seen whether these will include "sexual orientation" among the grounds on which the EU can prohibit discrimination.

Within the EU institutions themselves, personnel members have formed a gay, lesbian, and bisexual association known as Egalité, which advocates elimination of all staff regulations that discriminate against homosexuals in the context of their employment (such as tax benefits and social security arrangements for same-sex partnerships). By a decision of the Commission on July 9, 1996, in response to representations from Egalité, the partners of staff member, regardless of their sex, will have access to the same facilities as spouses. The European Citizen Action Service, an independent, nongovernment organization that monitors the impact of EU actions on the public, also supports the abolition of all EU practices that deny homosexuals equal enjoyment of the rights laid down in the European Treaties (such as freedom of movement between countries) and advocates the use of nondiscriminatory language in all future charters or agreements. The European Court of Human Rights is also being called upon to consider the issue of discrimination against the same-sex partners of employees in an appeal from the United Kingdom.

Although not directly concerned with sexual orientation, measures to combat AIDS are of special concern because of the relatively high incidence of the disease among European male homosexuals and reports of transmission through bisexual behavior. Through its Action Program "Europe against AIDS," the EU provides financial support for specific projects of research on the social aspects of AIDS control. Agreement has been reached recently (European Parliament Press Service: "Info Memo 17," January 31, 1996) on support for three 5-year EU Health Action Programs, one of which is for AIDS prevention. This effectively extends the currency of existing programs and provides a substantially increased budget of European Currency Unit 49.6 million (about $63 million). The main effort of the AIDS program is directed at increasing sex education and information, especially in schools; the coordination of studies on such topics as modes of transmission and situations of risk; promoting preventive schemes, such as making available both condoms and instruction on how to use them to avoid the sexual transmission of diseases; the exchanging of experience gained; and the promotion of studies on the psychosocial aspects of HIV/AIDS. The European Commission will undertake the management of the Action Program in close collaboration with member-states to ensure that actions taken are complementary to other Community policies. The legal basis of this activity is Article 129 of the Treaty on European Union [signed at Maastricht on February 7, 1992, and published by the Office for Official Publications of the European Communities L-2985 Luxemburg, 1992], which provides for action "directed towards the prevention of diseases," but within the Commission there have been desires expressed to include "treatment actions" such as therapy and assistance to HIV-positive persons and AIDS patients.

Other international bodies that have taken a stance on gay issues include Amnesty International, which, in 1989, following a long campaign by organizations of gays and their supporters, decided to recognize people imprisoned solely because of consensual homosexual behavior or orientation as "prisoners of conscience."

In 1992 the World Health Organization, an agency of the United Nations, published a revision of its *International Classification of Mental and Behavioural Disorders* (ICD 10) in which it stated, under the heading "Disorders associated with sexual development and orientation" (F66), that sexual orientation alone is not to be regarded as a disorder. Remarkably, this decision came nearly two decades after the American Psychiatric Association had opted for a similar position in its *Diagnostic and Statistical Manual*.

In March 1993 the United Nations was prepared, for the first time, to grant Roster Non-Governmental Organization status at the Council of Economic and Social Affairs to an organization advocating homosexual equality, the ILGA. However, at the instigation of the United States, following a Congressional Resolution sponsored by Senator Jesse Helms, this status was suspended until the ILGA was able to satisfy the committee that neither it nor any of its member groups supported, condoned or sought the legislation of pedophilia. Despite ILGA's clear resolutions on the subject and its exclusion of three member groups that refused to give the required assurances, the ban was upheld, owing to the variety of views about legal ages of consent and the problem of trying to prove a negative (*ILGA Bulletin*, March 1993; January 1994; February 1994). A different outcome emerged from the first meeting of the Organization for Security and Cooperation in Europe (OSCE), held in Ottawa in 1995, when it adopted what is known as the Ottawa Declaration. This calls upon member-states to ensure that all persons belonging to different segments of their population be accorded equal respect and consideration in their constitutions, legislation, and administration and that there be no subordination, explicit or implied, on the basis of ethnicity, race, color, language, religion, sex, sexual orientation, national or social origin, or minority status. The reference to sexual orientation was inserted at the initiative of Danish parliamentarians in response to repeated requests from ILGA. Unlike other OSCE bodies, the Assembly does not require unanimous agreement when making its decisions.

For gay activists, it is of concern that until relatively recently the rulings from the European Court of Human Rights have been based on breaches of privacy rather than on the more fundamental issues of discrimination (e.g., absence of equality, equal protection and benefit under the law). However, European countries that have ratified the United Nations International Covenant on Political and Civil Rights (adopted by the General Assembly December 1966 and coming into force March 1976) are affected by decisions of the United Nations Human Rights Committee. In *Toonen v. Australia* (1994) the Human Rights Committee decided that the criminalization of homosexuality in the Australian state of Tasmania not only violated the right to privacy (Article 17) but also violated the nondiscriminatory clauses of the International Covenant (Articles 2 and 26) as it involved discrimination based on sex. Following sustained pressure, the Tasmanian law was ultimately repealed by the State legislature on May 1, 1997, so that the minimum age limit for both homosexual and heterosexual acts there is now 17 years ("Reformer weeps as Tasmania dumps its gay laws," *Sydney Morning Herald*, 2 May 1997).

Developments in Individual European Countries

The liberalizing changes that have occurred in different jurisdictions in the last few years (some described briefly in the following paragraphs) reflect the trend toward closer integration between European countries. Despite this, the social aspects of homosexuality remain very much national issues. As the descriptions of developments in particular countries show, formal adherence to nondiscrimination does not necessarily eradicate the varying concerns and levels of tolerance belonging to the disparate cultural and political traditions of European states.

In 1991 a total ban on homosexuality was abolished in the Ukraine. In 1990 and 1992 Estonia and Latvia, respectively, abolished laws penalizing homosexual behavior. In August 1994 the total ban on homosexual relations, repealed in Lithuania the year before, was repealed also in Serbia, including Kosovo, and a common age of consent was established. On January 20, 1995 the Albanian Parliament legalized homosexual relations, finally abolishing Article 137 of the penal code, which had been promulgated under the communist dictatorship and specified up to 10 years imprisonment for simply "being homosexual." The new code provides sanctions only for sex relations involving minors or the use of violence. In January 1995 the Cyprus Parliament introduced a bill to abolish the ban on homosexuality under Article 171 of their penal code. The repeal of the ban by the Irish Parliament in June 1993 was in accordance with recommendations from the Report on Child Abuse by the Law Reform Commission of Ireland (1990) and followed a long campaign by gay rights organizations. The reform left a minimum age of 17 for penetrative sexual acts, both heterosexual and homosexual (Rose, 1994). Hate speech against homosexuals in Ireland was already covered by the Prohibition of Incitement to Hatred Act 1989. In October 1993 the Unfair Dismissal Act was extended to include a prohibition of discrimination on grounds of sexual orientation. The Irish Parliament is now planning to establish an Equality Commission that will monitor all forms of discrimination against homosexuals.

A legislative reform in Switzerland, enacted as federal law on June 21, 1991, effective from October 1, 1992 (RO 1992, 1670-78, FF II 1985 II 1021), eliminated all discrimination against homosexuality from the penal code that had been contained in Articles 187–212. This was largely in accordance with recommendations by an official committee chaired by Professor B. Schultz and approved by 73 percent of voters in a national referendum held on May 17, 1992. One of the more controversial aspects of the new legislation in Switzerland was the replacement of an absolute prohibition on sexual activity by or with persons under 16 by the provision in Article 187(2) that consensual sexual acts by or with persons below that age limit are not offenses as long as the participants' ages do not differ by more than 3 years.

Various regulations to prevent discrimination have been enacted in Norway (1981),

France (1985), Denmark (1987), Sweden (1987), and Ireland (1989). In Finland, the provisions of Chapter 11, Article 9 of the penal code came into force on September 1, 1995, making it a criminal offense to discriminate on grounds of race, faith, gender, nationality, age, or sexual orientation.

In 1986 Denmark equated married and homosexual couples in regard to inheritance rights. In May 1989 the Danish Parliament passed a "law on registered partnership" that gave homosexual couples the same rights as heterosexual partnerships, save for the right, as a couple, to adopt children. In the spring of 1993 the Norwegian Parliament adopted legislation for the registration of same-sex partnerships, closely following the law in Denmark, where 3000 partnerships had already been registered. On June 7, 1994, by a vote of 171-141, the Parliament of Sweden adopted a partnership law based on the Norwegian and Danish precedents. In the summer of 1995 the governments of Denmark, Norway, and Sweden agreed formally that the administrations in each country would recognize civil partnerships registered in either of the other two countries. On March 8, 1995, in response to a test case submitted by the homosexual rights group Homeros Lambda, the Hungarian Constitutional Court ruled that the legal position of two persons of the same sex living together as a de facto couple should be the same as for unmarried heterosexuals living together in what are sometimes called common-law marriages. The necessary statutory changes had to be enacted before March 1, 1996. Following a favorable vote in the Dutch Parliament in April 1996, the possibility of legal marriage between same-sex partners is presently being considered.

In autumn 1993 the French government adopted a law directing insurance companies to accept joint insurance coverage for unmarried couples. On July 25, 1995, for the first time in France, a homosexual couple received legal recognition in France when the Belfast Tribunal Correctional ordered an insurance company to pay damages of FF732,121 (about $150,000) to a 49-year-old woman whose female partner had been killed by one of their policyholders in a road accident. The insurance company withdrew its appeal after the "Centre gai et lesbien" had pointed out that the homosexual community might be expected to react if the plaintiff were to lose (*Liberation*, September 14, 1995).

On February 15, 1996, the Italian Parliament passed a law on sexual violence (*Norme contro la violenza sessuale*). Nearly all sexual offenses, except public obscenity and pornography, were transferred from the chapter covering offenses against public morals to the chapter covering offenses against the person, thereby directing the criminal law to the more limited target of protection of self-determination. The changes effectively reduced the age of consent for "innocent" adolescents (a concept very occasionally used to discriminate against homosexual relations) from 16 and fixed it in all cases at 14 (Article 609 quater). It also provided that consensual relations with 13-year-olds should not be punishable if the partner concerned is not older than 16.

CONCLUSIONS

The elimination of discrimination against homosexuals typically occurs in stages approximately corresponding to an evolution of public attitudes from ignorance, fear, and loathing, through tolerance, to understanding and acceptance (Waaldijk, 1992). Although as yet incomplete, the process must be fairly advanced in Western Europe since, in most countries, enforcement of discriminatory laws became exceptional before the provisions themselves were repealed. In a democratic society, lesbians and gay men, being in a minority, must convince the majority to accord them equality through rational argument and everyday experience, as they cannot rely on weight of numbers.

Obviously, these stages in the evolution of public opinion do not appear smoothly or simultaneously in all countries, given the diversity of social, political, and cultural traditions. Gay activists are well aware that premature legislation can prove counterproductive. For example, antidiscrimination laws pushed through a hostile parliament are liable to be hedged with reservations and restrictions that would be unacceptable to a parliament meeting in a different and more tolerant climate. Reversions to discriminatory legislation have occasionally occurred, usually enacted rapidly in response to media reports, such as that recently engendered by what is called "sex tourism." Even when legal equality is attained formally, continuing vigilance is needed to ensure the elimination of bias in enforcement policy.

The influence of the mass media in "demystifying" homosexuality has been an important factor in the evolution of opinion in many European countries. This is not just through documentary reports of the effect of discrimination on the individuals concerned, but also in the manner in which newsworthy events are covered, such as proposed legislative changes or the annual Gay and Lesbian Pride parades, as well as through the inclusion of sympathetic gay and lesbian characters in popular television drama. Although this seldom occurs in American escapist productions, which are broadcast all over the world, the European tradition of realistic program making has led public service broadcasters to depict homosexual people in everyday settings — in films like *Priest* and also in adaptations of American gay classics such as Armistead Maupin's *Tales of the City*.

The main impetus for change, however, has come from homosexuals themselves, generally through the local, regional, and national groups that are members of the IGLA. This active organization was launched through an initiative by the British Campaign for Homosexual Equality in 1978. In representing some 400 member organizations from more than 45 countries worldwide, ILGA's first priority has been to work toward the abolition of all legal, social, cultural, and economic discrimination against homosexuals. Its experience in promoting the changes described is now being applied all over the world, including many territories where the prejudices and prohibitions, first introduced in colonial times, have been retained after independence and after they have been eliminated in the colonial powers' homelands.

Experience has demonstrated the importance and value of ensuring that all human beings, regardless of their sexual orientation, are able to enjoy full human rights. The achievement of this goal should contribute to mutual understanding and peaceful coexistence throughout the new Europe.

APPENDIX: EUROPEAN PARLIAMENT RESOLUTION ON EQUAL RIGHTS FOR HOMOSEXUALS AND LESBIANS IN THE EUROPEAN COMMUNITY (A3-0028/94)

The European Parliament,

- having regard to the motions for resolutions by:
    (a) Mr. Blak and Mrs. Jensen, on discrimination in relation to freedom of movement (B3-0884/92),
    (b) Mr. Bettini and others, on recognition of civil unions for couples consisting of persons of the same sex (B3-1079/92),
    (c) Mr. Lomas, on civil rights for homosexuals and lesbians (B3-1186/93),

- having regard to its resolution of 13 March 1984 on sex discrimination at work,
- having regard to its resolution of 13 March 1991 on a plan of action in the context of the 1991–1992 "Europe against AIDS" programme,
- having regard to its recommendations on sexual harassment at work and the corresponding provisions on protection for lesbians and homosexuals,
- having regard to the Commission report, "Homosexuality, a Community Issue," on the impact on lesbians and homosexuals of the completion of the European internal market,
- having regard to its resolution of 8 July 1992 on a European A Charter of children's rights,
- having regard to the legal discrimination against lesbians and homosexuals which still exists in a number of Member States,
- having regard to the draft directive on combating discrimination on the basis of sexual orientation at work and in other legal areas, drawn up by the German Gay Union (SVD),
- having regard to the law on registered partnerships in Denmark and other anti-discrimination laws for homosexual people,
- having regard to Clause 28 of the Local Government Bill in the United Kingdom,
- having regard to Rule 45 of its Rules of procedure,
- having regard to the report of the Committee on Civil Liberties and Internal Affairs (A3-0028/94),

A. having regard to its action in support of equal treatment for all citizens, irrespective of their sexual orientation,

B. having regard to the greater public visibility of lesbians and homosexuals and the growing pluralization of lifestyles,

C. whereas lesbians and homosexuals are still exposed nonetheless, to ridicule, intimidation, discrimination and violent attacks in many social spheres, often from their earliest youth,

D. whereas social change in many Member States calls for a corresponding adjustment of the civil, penal and administrative provisions in force, to end discrimination on the basis of sexual orientation, and whereas such adjustments have already been made in a number of member States,

E. whereas the application of discriminatory provisions by Member States in a number of fields covered by EC legislation amounts to a violation of the fundamental principles of the EC Treaties and the Single European Act, particularly where freedom of movement, pursuant to Article 3 of the EEC Treaty, is concerned,

F. having regard to the European Community's special responsibility to ensure equal treatment for all citizens, irrespective of their sexual orientation, within the framework of its activities and areas of responsibility,

General Considerations

1. Affirms its conviction that all citizens must be treated equally, irrespective of their sexual orientation;

2. Considers that the European Community is under the obligation to apply the fundamental principle of equal treatment, irrespective of each individual's sexual orientation, in all legal provisions already adopted or which may be adopted in future;

3. Believes, furthermore, that the EC Treaties must make stronger provision for the defence of human rights, and therefore calls in the Community institutions to make preparations, in the context of the institutional reform scheduled for 1996, for setting up a European institution able to ensure equal treatment, without reference to nationality, religious faith, colour, sex, sexual orientation or other differences;

4. Calls on the Commission and Council to accede to the European Convention on Human Rights, provided for in the Community's 1990 programme, as a first step towards more vigorous protection for human rights;

To the Member States

5. Calls on the Member States to abolish all legal provisions which criminalize and discriminate against sexual activities between persons of the same sex;

6. Calls for the same age of consent to apply to homosexual and heterosexual activities alike;

7. Calls for an end to the unequal treatment of persons with a homosexual orientation under the legal and administrative provisions of the social security system and where social benefits, adoption law, laws on inheritance and housing and criminal law and all related legal provisions are concerned;

8. Calls on the United Kingdom to abolish its discriminatory provisions to stem the supposed propagation of homosexuality and thus to restore freedom of opinion, the press, information, science and art for homosexual citizens and in relation to the subject of homosexuality and calls upon all Member States to respect such rights to freedom of opinion in the future;

9. Calls on the Member States, together with the national lesbian and homosexual organizations, to take measures and initiate campaigns against the increasing acts of violence perpetrated against homosexuals and to ensure prosecution of the perpetrators of these acts of violence;

10. Calls upon the Member States, together with the national lesbian and homosexual organizations, to take measures and initiate campaigns to combat all forms of social discrimination against homosexuals;

11. Recommends that Member States take steps to ensure that homosexual women's and men's social and cultural organizations have access to national funds on the same basis as other social and cultural organizations, that applications are judged according to the same criteria as applications from other organizations and that they are not disadvantaged by the fact that they are organizations for homosexual women or men;

To the Commission of the European Community

12. Calls on the Commission to present a draft Recommendation on equal rights for lesbians and homosexuals;

13. Considers that the basis of the Recommendation should be equal treatment for all Community citizens regardless of their sexual orientation and the ending of all forms of legal discrimination on the grounds of sexual orientation, calls on the Commission to submit a report to parliament at five-yearly intervals on the situation of homosexual men and women in the Community;

14. Believes that the Recommendation should as a minimum seek to end:
- different and discriminatory ages of consent for homosexual and heterosexual acts
- prosecution of homosexuality as a public nuisance or gross indecency,
- all forms of discrimination in labour and public serviced law and discrimination in criminal, civil, contract and commercial law,
- the electronic storage of data concerning the sexual orientation of an individual without her or his knowledge and consent, or the unauthorised disclosure or improper use of this data,
- the barring of lesbians and homosexual couples from marriage or from an equivalent legal framework, and should guarantee the full rights and benefits of marriage, allowing the registration of partnerships,
- any restriction on the right of lesbians and homosexuals to be parents or to adopt or foster children.

15. Calls on the Commission, in line with the Parliament's opinion of 19 November 1993 on the proposal for a regulation amending the Staff Regulations of Officials and the Conditions of Employment of Other Servants of the European Communities in respect of equal treatment of men and women to undertake to combat any discrimination on the basis of sexual orientation in its own staffing policy;

16.   Instructs its President to forward this resolution to the Council, the Commission and the governments and parliaments of the Member States and the states which have applied for membership.

CITED CASES

Dudgeon v U.K., 45 EC Series A, (1981, October 22).
Handyside v U.K., 24 EC Series A, (1976).
Modinos v Cyprus, 259 EC Series A (1993, April 22).
Norris v Ireland, 142 EC Series A (1988, October 26).
Toonen v Australia, Community No. 488/1992, 50th Session, United Nations Human Rights Commission CCPR /C/50/D/488/1992 (1994, March 31).
Tyrer v UK, 26 EC Series A (1978).
X v Federal Republic of Germany, Yearbook of the European Convention on Human Rights, XIX, 276 (1976).

REFERENCES

Amnesty International USA. (1994). *Breaking the silence: Human rights violations based on sexual orientation.* New York: Author.
Amnesty International. (1995). *Romania: Broken commitments to human rights.* London: Author.
Bainbridge, T., & Teesdale, A. (1966). *Penguin companion to the European Union.* London: Penguin.
Cucu, C. (1995). *International Tribunal on Human Rights Violations against Sexual Minorities.* San Francisco: International Gay and Lesbian Human Rights Commission.
Dijk, P. van (1993). The treatment of homosexuals under the European Convention on Human Rights. In K. Waaldijk & A. Clapham (Eds.), *Homosexuality: A European Community issue* (pp. 179–206). Dordrecht, The Netherlands: Martinus Nijhoff.
European Community Reflection Group. (1995). *Laying the foundations of Europe of the future* (doc. SN 400/95, Section 4, Annexe 14). Office for Official Publications of the European Communities, L-2895 Luxemburg, 1995.
European Parliament. (1994). *Resolution on equal rights for homosexuals and lesbians in the European Community* (A3-0028/94). Office for Official Publications of the European Communities, L-2985 Luxemburg, 1995.
Hendriks, A., Tielman, R., & Veen, E. van der. (Eds.). (1993). *The third pink book: A global view of gay and lesbian liberation and oppression.* Buffalo, NY: Prometheus Books.
Helfer, L.P. (1990). Finding a consensus on equality: The homosexual age of consent and the European Convention on Human Rights. *New York University Law Review, 65,* 1044–1100.
Law Reform Commission of Ireland. (1990). *Report on child sex abuse.* (no. 32, s. 4.29). Dublin: Author.
Norris, D. (1993). The development of the gay movement in Ireland. In A. Hendriks, R. Tielman, & E. van der Veen (Eds.), *The third pink book: A global view of gay and lesbian liberation and oppression* (pp. 149–164). Buffalo, NY: Prometheus Books.
Official Journal of the European Communities. No. L 039, February 14, 1976, p. 4.
Reuters news report 1557-3 OVR 108 (1995, September 1).
Rose, K. (1994). *Diverse communities: The evolution of lesbian and gay politics in Ireland.* Cork, Ireland: Cork University Press.
Snyder, F. (1993). Subsidiarity: An aspect of European Community law and its relevance to lesbians and gay men. In K. Waaldijk & A. Clapham (Eds.), *Homosexuality: A European Community issue* (pp. 221–246). Dordrecht, The Netherlands: Martinus Nijhoff.

Squarcialupi, V. (1984). Sexual Discrimination in the Workplace. *Official Journal*, C[104 16(4)], 46–48.

Tatchell, P. (1992). *Europe in the pink*. London: Gay Men's Press.

Waaldijk, K. (1992). Standard sequences in the legal recognition of homosexuality: Europe past, present and future. *Australian Gay and Lesbian Law Journal*, 4, 50–72.

Waaldijk, K., & Clapham, A. (Eds.). (1993). *Homosexuality: A European Community issue*. Dordrecht, The Netherlands: Martinus Nijhoff.

West, D. J. (1977). *Homosexuality re-examined*. London: Duckworth.

13

ENGLAND

DONALD J. WEST AND ANDREA WÖELKE

THE CRIMINAL LAW

The English System

As there are two different legal systems in Britain, one for England and Wales (and a similar one for Northern Ireland) and one for Scotland, we will concentrate on English law for our discussion. In the absence of a written constitution such as that operating in the United States and because the government has only recently proposed to incorporate the European Convention on Human Rights into U.K. law, British citizens had little formal protection against discrimination on grounds of sexual orientation. Since English law is based on the common law system, it includes many rules and principles that are not written down in statutes and only appear in the judgments of higher courts, which then set binding precedent for future similar cases. In the criminal law relating to sexual offenses one finds different rules for heterosexual and homosexual conduct while some ostensibly nonsexual offenses are applied disproportionately against homosexuals. Although civil law does not target homosexuality as overtly as does the criminal law, it nevertheless produces discriminatory effects.

A Punitive Tradition

English criminal law differs from that of many other European countries in having had a long tradition of criminalizing both partners in any form of sexual behavior between males. When "buggery," (i.e., anal intercourse) first became a matter for the secular courts in 1553 (25 Henry VIII c. 6) the penalty was death, and so it remained until the Offences against the Person Act 1861, which lowered the punishment for the "Abominable Crime of Buggery with either mankind or any animal" to penal servitude for life or for any period not less than 10 years. Life imprisonment remained the maximum penalty until 1967.

Acts of "gross indecency between men" (Sexual Offences Act 1956, s. 13) usually refer to fellatio or mutual masturbation, but can even include behavior where the participants do not actually touch each other. These were first made crimes by the Criminal Law Amendment Act 1885. This act, criticized from its inception as "a blackmailer's charter," was used to imprison the writer Oscar Wilde in 1895. On the centenary of this event a plaque commemorating Wilde was installed in Poets' Corner in Westminster Abbey.

In 1953 and 1954, coincidentally in time with the McCarthy purges of male homosex-

DONALD J. WEST • Institute of Criminology, University of Cambridge, Cambridge CB3 9DT, England, United Kingdom.   ANDREA WÖELKE • Solicitor, Anthony, Gold, Lerman and Muirhead, London, SE1, England, United Kingdom.

Sociolegal Control of Homosexuality, edited by West and Green, Plenum Press, New York, 1997.

uals in the United States, some sensational trials reminiscent of the Wilde scandal took place in England. A number of prominent people, including a Peer of the Realm, were convicted of homosexual behavior in private on the evidence of young men who had been their party guests. The young men escaped punishment for their own participation by appearing as prosecution witnesses and agreeing that they had been seduced into immoral acts by the lavish hospitality they had received from their social superiors (Wildeblood, 1955). In one case the forbidden relationships came to light through letters unexpectedly discovered by police searching through servicemen's kit bags for stolen property. The arbitrary way people could be selected for prosecution for their private sexual habits began to arouse public concern, and the government set up the Wolfenden Committee to consider the role of the law. Their report (Home Office, 1957) concluded that there was a realm of private morality that was "not the law's business" and recommended the decriminalization of consensual homosexual acts between adult men in private. In the decade that followed there were numerous and vitriolic debates in Parliament as repeated attempts were made to introduce the proposed reform. It was finally enacted, with various exceptions, in the Sexual Offences Act 1967 (Grey, 1992).

The State of the Law Today

For male homosexual behavior to be allowed under the terms of the 1967 Act the men had to be over 21, fully consenting, and in complete privacy. Section 1(2) specifies that, where there are more than two persons present (including a female) the behavior is not "in private" and that a lavatory accessible to the public is not a private place. Consensual homosexual behavior between members of the armed forces or between members of the crew of U.K. merchant ships remained criminal. Furthermore, a man who "procures" another male for "an act of buggery" [s. 4(1)] or for gross indecency with a third party [Sexual Offences Act 1956, s. 13; cf. Sexual Offences Act 1967, s. 4(3)] commits a crime, even though the acts in question may be between consenting adults and not in themselves offenses. This puts at risk a man (but not a woman) who introduces two homosexual male friends to each other. The law has had an inhibiting effect on social or counseling groups for homosexuals, especially if men under 21 are included. In contrast, the "procuring" of women for sex is illegal under the Sexual Offences Act 1956 only if prostitution [s. 22(1)], deception [s. 3(1)], or threats [s. 2(1)] are involved or the woman is mentally incapacitated [s. 9(1)]. In Scotland the act did not apply and male homosexual conduct remained totally illegal until the passing of the Criminal Justice (Scotland) Act 1980, although in practice prosecutions for private behavior between consenting adults had long since ceased. Following a judgment by the European Court of Human Rights (*Dudgeon v. UK*, 1981) the provisions were extended to Northern Ireland in 1982, to the Channel Islands in 1990, and to the Isle of Man in 1992.

Some of the stipulations in the 1967 act have been relaxed by the Criminal Justice and Public Order Act 1994. The privacy conditions have remained unchanged, but the age prohibition on male homosexual contact was lowered to 18 (s. 145) and homosexual behavior in the armed forces or on merchant ships was decriminalized, although it remained grounds for dismissal. In addition, the definition of rape [in the Sexual Offences (Amendment) Act 1976, s. 1], an offense carrying the possibility of life imprisonment, was extended to include nonconsensual anal penetration of a person of either sex. The present law fixes 16 as the minimum age for sexual contact (other than anal sex) with the opposite sex or with the same sex in the case of women, but 18 for sex between males and then only under defined circumstances. For anal sex with man or woman the permitted age is now 18. Age limits below which the conduct is deemed criminal are commonly called "ages of consent," but the law uses various other age limits to define the maximum penalties that can be applied to either or both partners in a sexual offense.

The revisions introduced in the Criminal Justice and Public Order Act 1994 leave very severe maximum penalties for penetrative sex with underage males, even when they are clearly (but not legally) consenting. Buggery with a boy under 16, whether or not he is a cooperating participant, carries a maximum penalty of life imprisonment, the same as for rape. In other cases the maximum penalties for buggery and gross indecency are the same, that is, 5 years regardless of consent if the accused is over 21 and his partner is under 18, otherwise 2 years, save where a consenting couple, both of them over 18. are behaving in private, in which case no offense is committed.

Nonconsensual acts of a nonpenetrative kind are governed by the offense of "indecent assault" (Sexual Offenses Act 1956) "on a male" (s. 15) or "on a female" (s. 14). The maximum penalty for either is now 10 years, that for indecent assault on a female having been increased [Sexual Offences Act 1985, s. 3(3)]. Since no one under 16 can give valid consent to indecent assault, it follows that women can be so charged for sexual acts with a girl under 16. This would appear to be the only situation in which lesbians are affected by the criminal law.

Sexual indecency with a child under 14 that need not involve actual physical interference, defined as "gross indecency with or towards a child" by a person of either sex, carries a maximum penalty of 2 years imprisonment (Indecency with Children Act 1960, s. 10). This offense includes masturbating in front of a child or inducing a child to touch the offender indecently.

Vaginal intercourse with a consenting girl under 16 is "unlawful sexual intercourse" under the Sexual Offences Act 1956 [s. 6(I)]. Only the male partner can be prosecuted for this heterosexual offence (R v. Tyrell, 1894), whereas, if two men have sexual contact and at least one of them is under 18, both are guilty of either buggery or gross indecency. It is a legal anomaly that any indecent but nonpenetrative act with a girl under 16 carries a maximum penalty of 10 years, whereas for actual sexual intercourse it is only 2 years unless the girl is under 13, when it becomes life (Sexual Offences Act 1956, s. 5).

Coercive sexual behavior or harassment are rightfully punished more severely when they are directed against the very young. It seems disproportionate, however, that all forms of sexual contact between people under 16, regardless of gender or willingness to partici-pate, should render them guilty of crime and that, until they are 18, young males can be held criminally responsible for sexual contacts with each other. The U.K. law, unlike that of many other European states, makes no distinction between unwanted, aggressive assaults causing physical or psychological damage and romantic or playful behavior between or involving young people. This has the effect of leaving a great deal to the discretion of law enforcement authorities on matters about which opinions differ and also discourages education and counseling of teenagers on contraception and safer sex. Additionally, arbitrary age criteria can produce odd results. For consensual intercourse with a girl on her 13th birthday a man incurs a maximum penalty of 2 years compared with life imprisonment had it been a day earlier.

Offenses Ancillary to Sex

It is an offense, carrying a maximum penalty of 2 years imprisonment, "for a man persistently to solicit or importune in a public place for immoral purposes" (Sexual Offences Act 1956, s. 32). Although the question is really one of fact and for the jury to decide, the courts still regard homosexuality as "immoral," even when it is not illegal and does not involve prostitution. When first introduced (Vagrancy Act 1898, s. 1), the importuning law was apparently intended to control males touting for female prostitutes, but it has hardly been used except to prosecute men approaching other men. Solicitation by men of female prostitutes first became a defined offense under Section 1 of the Sexual Offences Act 1985, which introduced the offenses of "kerb crawling," that is, soliciting for prostitution from a car, or persistent soliciting in the street. The penalty is a fine up to £1,000.

Heterosexual prostitution by women is regulated by the Street Offences Act 1959 whereby "it is an offence for a common prostitute to loiter or solicit in a public place for purposes of prostitution." A woman is not charged unless she has been previously formally cautioned by the police on at least two occasions. This does not apply to men, so rent boys cannot be dealt with as common prostitutes (*DPP v. Bull*, 1994). Unlike male importuning, female soliciting for prostitution is no longer an imprisonable offense (Criminal Justice Act 1982, s.1), although many prostitutes end up in prison for nonpayment of fines.

It is an offense, with a maximum penalty of 7 years imprisonment, "for a man knowingly to live wholly or in part on the earnings of [female] prostitution" (Sexual Offences Act 1956, s. 30). The statute has been interpreted strictly by the courts to include any form of profit, so that even cab drivers who carry call girls to hotel customers can be so charged. Women prostitutes complain that their husbands or boyfriends are under constant threat of prosecution. Although a man can also be charged with benefiting from the prostitution of another man (by an analogous offense under the Sexual Offences Act 1956, s. 5), rent boys do not usually turn over any of their earnings and so do not put other men in this vulnerable position. However, organizers of male prostitution through escort agencies, massage parlors or brothels are at risk. To "keep a brothel" or to let premises to be used for prostitution are specific offenses (Sexual Offences Act 1956, ss. 33–36) whether the prostitution is homosexual or heterosexual (Sexual Offences Act 1956, s. 6).

Advertising for sexual contact or for prostitution can be illegal if it is done by more than one person. This oddity arises out of the unwritten common law offenses of Conspiracy to Corrupt Public Morals or to Outrage Public Decency, which are based on judicial precedent and not on any statute. In the House of Lords, the highest court in the country, lesbianism, fornication, or adultery have been given as examples of this offense (*Shaw v. DPP*, 1962). This charge was used to prosecute the publishers of a magazine for printing gay contact advertisements (*Knuller v. DPP*, 1972). These cases provoked much comment, and no recent similar prosecutions have been reported. To advertise for sex or prostitution by fixing a notice visible from the street is not an offense (*Burge v. DPP*, 1962), but it might be if two or more offenders "conspire." The common practice of sticking adverts for prostitution in public telephone booths can be dealt with under local bylaws.

Unlike the behavior involved in boxing and other sports, sexual acts that involve any kind of physical injury are prohibited, since the consent of the victim is no defense to a charge of "assault causing actual bodily harm" (i.e., any harm that is any more than transient or trifling, such as a scratch). Exceptions to this are made for, among other things, surgery and sporting contests such as boxing, but not when the purpose is to obtain sexual pleasure. The question was first dealt with by the Court of Criminal Appeal in *R v. Donovan* (1934), which concerned the caning of a young woman who had been persuaded to agree to it for the sexual gratification of the man involved. It was held that causing actual bodily harm in these circumstances was a crime. The decision was reasserted more forcibly by a House of Lords decision (*R v. Brown*, 1993) that rejected by a 3-2 majority the appeal of a group of men who had been imprisoned for homosexual behavior in private that had included consensual sadomasochistic acts. Nobody had complained, but the matter had come to notice through a videorecording of the activity that was sent anonymously to the police. Unaware that they had broken any law, some of the participants made self-incriminating statements when questioned. No permanent injuries resulted and no medical intervention was required, but since their injuries were more than "transient and trifling" the men were held to have been properly convicted of causing actual bodily harm and wounding contrary to Sections 47 and 20 of the Offences Against the Person Act 1861. The judgment found that it was not in the public interest that people should try to cause, or should cause, actual bodily harm for no good reason and that satisfying sadomasochistic libido did not come within the category of good reason. Although this would appear to apply equally to heterosexuals, the wording of some of the judges' remarks emphasized the homosexual context. Lord Jauncey referred to the "real danger" of "the possibility of proselytisation and corruption of young men" and Lord Lowry referred to "homosexual sado-masochism." Some of the sentences were reduced on appeal, but even so some were more severe than what might have been imposed for ordinary assaults committed in anger (Thompson, 1995). Three of the defendants appealed to the European Court of Human Rights. The decision, in February 1997, agreed that privacy had been breached, but pronounced that this was allowable under the principle of "margin of appreciation." This permits individual states to apply differing standards should they find it necessary for the protection of health or morals. Reinforcing the impression of a different standard being applied to heterosexuals, in an Appeal Court decision on February 29, 1996, the conviction of Alan Wilson, who had branded his initials on his consenting wife's buttocks with a hot knife blade, was overturned (*Times*, 1 Mar. 1996). The matter had been reported to the police by the woman's doctor. At Doncaster Crown Court, where the man had been convicted, the judge had said that he was unhappy about it but felt bound by the House of Lords decision in *Brown*; on appeal, however, the decision was reversed and Lord Justice Russell was reported as saying "Sexual activity between husband and wife in the privacy of the home is not a matter for criminal investigation, let alone criminal prosecution" [*R v. Wilson* (1996) 26.All.R241]. It was suggested that the defendant might apply for costs against the Crown Prosecution Service.

It is uncertain what effect the rejection of the *Brown* application by the European Court of Human Rights may have. It is unlikely that the prosecution of sadomasochistic practices in private, especially when heterosexual, will have much priority. In March 1996 Martin Church, who ran a club where sadomasochistic sex beatings and whippings admittedly took place, was found not guilty at Southwark Crown Court of a charge of keeping a disorderly house (Disorderly House Act, 1751). Moreover, the Law Commission (1995) has issued a consultation paper discussing at length issues of consent in the criminal law in a variety of contexts, such as circumcision, ear piercing, euthanasia, medical treatment, and hazardous sports. They review arguments against the criminalization of sadomasochistic activity These echo the arguments heard years earlier in relation to homosexual activity in general. The participants are engaging in playful, consensual activity that does no harm to others and no permanent damage to themselves; they are made to feel shame and are forced into secrecy, they fear harassment by police and others about which they dare not complain in case they are themselves prosecuted; they are hampered in making safe contacts or in joining groups with similar interests or in obtaining information about safe techniques; and finally, they are discouraged from cooperating with police when investigations of serious sex-related crimes are under way. The Law Commission cites evidence that the practices are widespread. Even though participants in sadomasochistic activity may be relatively common in the male homosexual community, they are undoubtedly outnumbered by heterosexuals, including the numerous heterosexual clients of "dominatrix" female prostitutes. In their provisional recommendations the Law Commission suggested that consent for sexual purposes should be a defense to a charge of assault except where "serious disabling injury" is inflicted. They define "serious" by such criteria as "permanent bodily injury or functional impairment or serious disfigurement" (p. 41), taken from proposals originally put forward by a Cambridge academic, Professor Glanville Williams.

Legal Targeting of Offenses

Normally, punishment is supposed to be commensurate with the seriousness of the current offense, but exceptions were introduced in the Criminal Justice Act 1991. In offenses of sex or violence, where only a custodial sentence is adequate to protect the public from "serious harm," it may be imposed even if otherwise inappropriate [s. 1(2)(b)]. Further, under Section 2(2)(b), a custodial sentence on a violent or sexual offender may be for such longer period, not exceeding the statutory maximum, as is necessary to protect the public from serious harm (i.e., serious personal injury, physical or psychological). Section 44 further empowers courts to direct that the period of supervision following the release of a sex offender on parole should be extended from the usual three quarters point to the end of the sentence. The offenses covered by the term "sexual" [s. 31(I)] include male importuning and the consensual offense of indecency between men, despite protests by gay rights organizations that these are not acts liable to cause "serious harm" to the general public (Leng & Manchester, 1991).

The new Crime (Sentences) Act 1997, part of a tougher policy on the punishment of crime, has been much criticized by members of the judiciary. It provides for the abolition of the customary one-third remission of time spent in prison in the absence of disciplinary offenses. The act introduces mandatory minimum sentences for certain offenses. Sex offenders are especially targeted. A person convicted for a second time of "a serious sexual offence" would be given a life sentence. Sex offenders sentenced to fixed terms of imprisonment would be subject to extended periods of compulsory supervision and control following release. These provisions might well increase greatly the numbers of sex offenders, including homosexual offenders, held in custody or under supervisory control. In addition, the government has legislated (Sex Offenders Act, 1997) for the introduction of a register of pedophile offenders. Heterosexual acts with children up to 16 are included; the age goes up to 18 for homosexual acts.

Some laws, although not specifically directed at sex, can be used to control homosexuality. For instance, "disorderly behaviour" or "insulting words or behaviour" that is "within the hearing of a person likely to be caused harassment, alarm or distress" are prohibited by the Public Order Act 1986. Homosexual talk or displays of affection that might provoke "queer-bashing" could be held to come under such provisions. In addition to the national criminal law, local regulations and bylaws intended for the control of nuisances in parks, railway stations, and streets can be used in place of charges of importuning or indecency between males. For example, until recently London rent boys were often charged with "highway obstruction," a minor offense that can be successfully prosecuted without proving sexual intent (West & De Villiers, 1992). Defendants may be pleased to avoid being categorized as sex offenders, but the use of these devices mean that the criminal statistics fail to reflect the true extent of sex-related offenses.

On occasion charges are brought against homosexuals in circumstances in which heterosexuals would be unlikely to be prosecuted. In 1986, two men lost an appeal against conviction for insulting behavior whereby a breach of the peace may be occasioned contrary to Section 54 (13) of the Metropolitan Police Act 1839. They had been kissing and embracing at a bus stop in London in the small hours of the morning when police arrived and arrested them. According to police testimony, they were apparently unaware of two couples passing by. One of the men had remonstrated with them for their "filthy" behavior "in front of the girls." In the appeal judgment it was suggested that the presumption that an observer would not find their behavior offensive amounted in itself to insult (*Masterson and Cooper v Holden*, 1986). Wintemute (1994) cites the case of a heterosexual couple receiving no more than a small fine for copulating in a crowded railway carriage, much less than the likely punishment for similar behavior by homosexuals.

Other instances of unusual applications of the law in homosexual situations include a revival of blasphemous libel, an offense that had not been used for 50 years. The moral campaigner Mary Whitehouse instigated a private prosecution of the editor of *Gay News* for publishing a poem describing a Roman centurion's homosexual fantasies about Christ on the cross. The conviction was confirmed on appeal by the House of Lords (*Whitehouse v Gay News Ltd and Lemon*, 1979). That the author, Professor James Kirkup, was an established poet and that blasphemy was not intended was held to be immaterial.

Legal prohibitions on the sale, distribution, possession, importation, and public display of sexually explicit materials are generally more restrictive in England than in most of Western Europe. This area of law is governed by the Obscene Publications Act 1959, which makes it an offense (ss. 1, 2) to publish anything the effect of which is such as to tend to deprave and corrupt persons who are likely to read, see, or hear it. There is a defense of justification of being for the public good on the grounds that it is in the interests of science, literature, art, or learning or of other objects of general concern (s. 4). Since the jury or the magistrates will have to decide on both tests, the likelihood of any item falling within the act is unpredictable. Thus the homosexually explicit picture books *Tom of Finland*, which are readily available in shops all over the country, have been found obscene by a provincial magistrate (*The Pink Paper*, 4 Nov. 1994). Juries have shown greater tolerance in recent years, but it is still the case that homosexual material is more likely to be affected than its heterosexual equivalents. Book shops and mail order businesses supplying material of interest to homosexuals are at risk of police raids and prosecutions. An example that attracted much publicity was the seizure in 1986 of a large amount of stock from a gay book shop in London, followed by charges of importing obscene books, charges for which no defense of public good exists (Customs Consolidation Act 1876, s. 42; cf. *R v. Bow Street Magistrate*). The seizure included many standard works freely available elsewhere. In this instance the charges were eventually dropped, so it was never tested in court whether the police were correct in regarding the material as obscene (Jeffery-Poulter, 1991).

Need for Reform

This brief review shows that when the English criminal law addresses matters of morality, as opposed to clear-cut sexual violence, it is intricate and confusing, based on common law offenses and overlapping acts drafted at different times and using inconsistent, arcane, and ill-defined terminology. The absence of clear statutory definitions of offenses makes the law far from user-friendly. The scope for arbitrary and variable decisions by courts is increased through lack of clarity as to which crime or mode of prosecution fits a particular item of behavior. Attempts to clarify the law have been mooted but not carried forward. The Criminal Law Revision Committee (1984), in its fifteenth report, discussed more precise definitions of "indecent assault" and the Law Commission (1989) later produced a draft criminal code intended "to make the criminal law more accessible, comprehensible, consistent and certain," (preface) but the government shows no sign of enacting it.

PROSECUTION AND PUNISHMENT

Although the distinction between behavior involving persons of the same or different sex is marked by extreme differences in some maximum penalties, sentencing in practice can be rather more realistic about the supposed gravity of offenses; nevertheless, considerable inequalities remain. Maximum penalties fixed by statute, which are meant to apply only to the very worst cases, allow the courts wide discretion. Although the law makes no distinction as to whether a young person under 16 was or was not a willing participant, the courts do take consent very much into account when sentencing (Walmsley & White, 1979). Sentencing "tariffs" are established by Appeal Court decisions on cases referred to them. They determine a band within which a sentence is supposed to fall in all ordinary circumstances. The tariffs suggest a tendency to award higher sentences for certain same-sex offenses than for analogous different-sex ones. For example, for consensual heterosexual intercourse with girls between 13 and 16 the tariff is a fine or a conditional discharge or imprisonment up to 1 year for older offenders. In practice, the male partner is usually given a caution or, if prosecuted at all, no more than a fine. For consensual sexual activity by a man with a boy of corresponding age, however, the tariff, which in this instance the courts tend to follow, is 3–5 years imprisonment. Thus, in *R v. Roe* (1988), for indecent acts by a man "of previous good character" with boys around 14 years of age, where there was no suggestion of coercion and where the boys received small sums in payment, the Appeal Court found 2½ years imprisonment appropriate. Because of the defendant's showing of remorse and his guilty plea, this sentence has to be regarded to be at the bottom end of the tariff. Where the young person is older, the length of the sentence decreases. In *R v.*

Harper (1993) the Appeal Court made only a modest reduction, from 2 years to 18 months imprisonment, for a man of 61 who had consenting anal intercourse with a youth of 18 who had visited him at home. There were no aggressive features and no "corruption," but the offender had a history of prior same-sex sexual offenses. Interestingly, with the lower age of consent, such behavior would not be a crime today. In contrast, sexual intercourse with a girl between 13 and 16 is often not prosecuted at all. In 1993, 1443 such offenses were recorded by the police, 553 cautions were issued, and 187 men were prosecuted. Of those prosecuted for this offense in 1992, only 22 percent were sentenced to immediate custody.

In contrast to the many prosecutions for consensual anal intercourse with young men, prosecutions of this offense with young women (until November 1994 subject to a maximum of life imprisonment) are unusual, despite evidence that the practice is far from rare among heterosexuals (see Wellings, Field, Johnson, & Wadsworth, 1994, Table 4.6).

Where sexual acts are forced or involve young children the penalties are much greater. Some of the longest-serving prisoners in England are pedophiles convicted of buggery with young boys, which is prosecuted as a serious crime even if the boys are apparently willing participants. Men who have had a close, ongoing relationships with a boy and have had ample opportunity for repeated anal intercourse may well be persuaded to confess to having done so to avoid courtroom confrontations with the boy. Such offenders are liable to heavier sentences than others against whom there is available proof of no more than indecent assault. On this point the reasoning of the Appeal Court in *R v. Willis* (1975) is still influential. In his judgment for the court, Lord Justice Lawton held that, since maximum sentences for other forms of homosexual behavior had been reduced, but not the life sentence for buggery with a boy under 16, it followed that "judges should always regard buggery with boys under the age of 16 as a serious offence — and the younger the boy the more serious the offence" (at 622j). Long imprisonment is customary for repeated buggery with young boys. For example, in *R v. Sheridan* (1986) an appellant with prior convictions for offenses with children who had committed buggery and other sex acts with three boys between ages 11 and 14, paying them for doing so, had a sentence of ten years imprisonment confirmed.

Disgust at the idea of men letting themselves be "used" like women was probably one of the reasons underlying traditionally heavy punishment for buggery. The advent of HIV and AIDS and awareness of the risks of infection from anal intercourse has provided a more plausible justification. In contrast, nonpenetrative indecencies with even young boys may receive somewhat less harsh sentences. For example, in *R v. Eames* (1992), 21 months imprisonment was deemed appropriate for a scoutmaster who had squeezed the penises of boys ages 10 and 11 during swimming lessons.

Victimless offenses between adults (when the circumstances are not strictly "in private") rarely lead to prison sentences, despite the maximum penalty for gross indecency between men being 2 years imprisonment. Even when buggery is involved, imprisonment is unusual for consenting acts between adults. In *R v. Bedbornugh* (1984) a 24-month suspended sentence of imprisonment was reduced to a conditional discharge for a man of 38 who had committed buggery with a man of 31 in a lavatory cubicle. They had been observed by police who peered under the door. The court noted that the men had effectively been in private and that the defendant had sterling qualities in other departments of life and had lost his job as a schoolteacher in a blaze of publicity.

Although soliciting by a male is an imprisonable offense, it almost never results in immediate imprisonment. In 1993, of 124 males sentenced for the offense, 119 were given fines or a conditional discharge, and none was sent to prison. The inappropriateness of imprisonment had been recognized in R v. Gray (1981), where a fine of £100 was substituted by the Appeal Court for a suspended sentence of 9 months imprisonment. The man importuned was a plainclothes police officer.

Heterosexual acts in public situations, if they are prosecuted at all, attract lesser penalties. If charged under Section 28 of the Town Police Clauses Act 1847, for instance, the maximum penalty is £1000 fine or up to 14 days imprisonment.

POLICING

Recorded offenses of rape and indecent assault on females have greatly increased over the last 10 years, partly as a result of women being encouraged to report incidents and of police being required to take every complaint seriously. In contrast, the offense of gross indecency between men has shown only a temporary increase (from 1,127 in 1987 to 2,022 in 1989), after which it fell to around 700, less than it had been in the early 1980s. It may be that the publicity surrounding the introduction in 1988 of legislation against the "promotion" of homosexuality (in the controversial Section 28 to be discussed later) gave temporary encouragement to the police to get tough on homosexual behavior in public places. A similar increase occurred in the late 1960s and early 1970s, coinciding with much public discussion of decriminalization proposals. When finally enacted in 1967, the dispensation specifically excluded behavior in public lavatories. A Home Office researcher (Walmsley, 1978) concluded that increased confidence among the police that the policy of making arrests in lavatories had support was the most likely explanation for the apparent increase in these offenses.

The chances of being arrested for minor homosexual offenses vary remarkably over time and according to the police area concerned. Some police forces appear to be proactive in tackling public indecency. Stories abound in the gay press of the use of so-called "pretty police," that is, young, provocatively dressed decoys who hang about lavatories and cruising areas waiting to arrest men attempting to importune them or seen behaving indecently. In the case of R v. Gray (1981), already mentioned, the defendant had smiled at a plainclothes policeman, who was loitering outside a gay bar, and had invited the officer home for a whiskey. In 1993 there were hardly any convictions for indecency between males in some police areas (a total of 12 from the 6 areas of Bedfordshire, Gloucestershire, Cumbria, Cleveland, Cheshire, and Leicestershire, compared with 68 from Hampshire alone and 126 from the Metropolitan Police District, which covers London). Such stark contrasts, far greater than any differences in population size, are more plausibly accounted for by differences in police activity than by variations in public behavior. Some police forces go to great lengths to detect sexual activity in men's lavatories. In Norwich they installed fiber-optic cameras no bigger than the tip of a pen (The Pink Paper, 4 November 1994), while in Suffolk they abseiled from the rafters of a public lavatory. In these cases the courts have to rely on the word of the police, which it is said may sometimes be false or exaggerated (GALOP, 1988/9), an allegation supported by a gay sergeant from Thames Valley Police (Burke, 1993).

The Civil Law

Partnership

Marriage between same-sex couples is not permitted, nor is there any other form of partnership law. So the legal protections afforded by marriage do not apply to homosexuals living together. Divorce law aims to give both partners of a broken marriage a fair distribution of the couple's joint assets, but the American concept of palimony, applicable to same-sex associations, does not exist. If a person who dies without having made a will is survived by his or her spouse, the spouse automatically inherits the bulk of the estate. When someone is killed through the fault of a third party, the spouse, as next of kin, can sue for compensation. None of these provisions apply to same-sex partners. If property is willed to a gay partner this usually ensures that the deceased's wishes are carried out. However, under the Inheritance (Provision for Family and Dependents) Act 1975, spouses, ex-spouses, children, and opposite-sex cohabitees can bring claims against a deceased's estate if they have not been provided for or have been insufficiently provided for in a will or by the intestacy rules. The court is left a wide discretion in these situations. Other dependents, which would include same-sex partners, may only claim under this act if they have been *maintained* by the deceased immediately before his or her death.

If a married couple have been inhabiting public housing, the survivor would normally be entitled to continue the tenancy. This privilege has been extended to unmarried heterosexual partners by the Housing Act 1985 [see ss. 30, 50(3)], but an appeal decision in *Harrogate Borough Council v. Simpson* (1986) denies this as a right to same-sex cohabitees: the government is now encouraging local authorities to grant joint tenancies to same-sex partners, however, so that a surviving partner has an automatic right to stay on (Wintour, 1996).

It is usual for firms to grant some shared rights in pension schemes to the legal spouse of an employee, but not to a same-sex partner. Such discrimination has been challenged recently by Lisa Grant, a railway worker, who appealed (on May 1, 1996) to an Industrial Tribunal in Southampton against her employer's decision not to grant the concessionary travel pass normally provided for the partner of a heterosexual employee. The tribunal decided to refer the case to the European Court of Justice in Luxembourg, which has the task of interpreting the treaties of the European Union. The court has been asked if "discrimination based on sex" includes discrimination based on sexual orientation.

Other repercussions follow from the fact that a long-term partner, unlike a spouse, is not defined as next of kin. A hospital patient can nominate as acting next of kin someone who is not a relative, but in the event that they are too incapacitated to do so the partner may be refused information or access. In the event of a mental illness necessitating compulsory hospitalization the individual to be informed and to have some rights of appeal, referred to as the "nearest relative," has to be selected on criteria set out in the Mental Health Act 1983 (s.26). Only if an unrelated person has been living with the patient for not less than 5 years does he or she take precedence over actual relatives, and never over a spouse. Application can be made to the Court of Protection for a power of attorney to take over an incapacitated partner's finances, but the partner's relatives have to be notified and can challenge the arrangement (Enduring Powers of Attorney Act, 1985).

As far as residence of children of divorced couples is concerned, the parent living in a same-sex relationship has generally lesser chances of convincing the court that an order should be made in his or her favor (Gooding, 1992; Wintemute, 1994). The special sense of grievance and betrayal on the part of a heterosexual parent whose spouse has left to live with a same-sex partner means that a battle over custody of, or access to, their children is likely. All such cases have to be decided on their particular facts and thus do not count as binding precedent. Legally, the interests of the child are supposed to be paramount. Lord Justice Glidewell stated in the Appeal Court that he regarded it as axiomatic that the ideal environment for the upbringing of a child is the home of loving, caring, and sensible parents, the father and mother: "In cases where the marriage has broken down the court's task is to choose the alternative which comes closest to that ideal" (C v. C, 1991). In most cases this would be a heterosexual family. Although the mother's relationship with a woman did not in itself determine the matter, a first instance decision in this case that had given "care and control" (now called *residence*) of the 7-year-old daughter to the mother was quashed. At the rehearing Justice Booth gave care and control back to the mother relying on expert evidence that the mother's sexual relationship with a woman would not involve the daughter nor influence her sexual identity (cf. Golombok & Fivusch, 1994; Green, 1978). Still, the order was not made *regardless* of, but *despite*, the mother's lesbian relationship, which it was acknowledged might lead to stigmatization of the child by her peers (cf. Beresford, 1994; B v. B, 1991, where the expert contested this assumption). This means that courts can justify discriminatory decisions on the grounds of public intolerance.

From the recent case law two assertions can be put forth. First, the majority of the judiciary seems to be ill at ease with permitting children to live with homosexuals. In B v. B (1991) Judge Callman stressed that it weighed in the mother's favor that she was not a militant lesbian but kept her sexuality in private. Second, the unease of most judges is also reflected in the fact that they are keen to rely on expert evidence, which normally supports the view that it is not seriously detrimental to a child to live with a homosexual parent. Most cases that go in favor of lesbian mothers are decided by the outweighing bond between mother and child, which does not apply in the same way to fathers. Cases have occurred where gay fathers have been entirely deprived of any link with the child through compulsory adoption by the mother's new husband (D, Re, 1977).

Only married couples or single people individually are permitted to adopt children [Adoption Act 1976, s. 14(1), 15(1)]. Adoption authorities have discretion, which they often use, to count homosexual orientation as an unfavorable factor when assessing the suitability of an unmarried person, living alone or with a same-sex partner, to be allowed to adopt a child. A member of a gay male household is most unlikely to be considered suitable. However, in Re H (1993), a lesbian couple who had been "given" a baby by a married mother who did not want it were granted an interim residence order that was later made permanent (*The Pink Paper*, 1 November 1992, cf. Wintemute, 1994). Because it is not necessarily permanent, fostering by gay couples is not unheard of, especially in cases of gay teenagers (cf. Re W, 1992). In the end the question depends on the attitudes of each local authority.

Apart from these special cases of fostering, gay men are in practice most unlikely to be allowed to raise a child they have not fathered. If a lesbian woman, on the other hand, wants to raise a child, she might do so by conceiving in any way. If, however, such a mother claims income support, she will later on face reductions if she fails to disclose the identity of the father, provided she knows it (Child Support Act 1991, ss. 6, 46). Alternatively, she can apply to National Health Service fertility clinics where the anonymous donor's sperm will be checked for diseases, but, in deciding whether to treat a woman, clinics must have regard to the welfare of any child that might be born, including the child's need for a father [Human Fertilisation and Embryology Act 1990 (HFEA), s. 13(5)]. Hence, a lesbian woman may be refused treatment on these grounds. In cases of married or unmarried opposite-sex couples the husband or boyfriend will be able to be legally regarded as the father of the child, but no such parental status exists for same-sex partners (HFEA, s. 528). Gender, as certified at birth, is legally unalterable in Britain, so even a sex change operation will not override this rule, although the issue is to be considered by the European Court of Human Rights. It is possible, however, where one of the partners has a child, either from a previous opposite-sex relationship (as in *Re C*), by donor insemination, or otherwise, for same-sex partners to be awarded a joint residence, which amounts to near full parental status.

Employment

There is no specific legal protection against discrimination in recruitment or dismissal from employment on grounds of sexual orientation as there is for discrimination on grounds of race in the Race Relations Act 1976 or of gender in the Sex Discrimination Act 1975. Where sexual orientation discrimination results in indirect gender discrimination it can be challenged under the latter act. In 1987 the Equal Opportunities Commission found unlawful a ban on the employment of men as cabin staff by an airline. It had been argued that male applicants were likely to be homosexual and therefore an AIDS risk in the event of an accident (Harris & Haigh, 1990). Generally, the Employment Protection (Consolidation) Act 1978 (s. 67) allows employees who have been in a job for at least 2 years to appeal against unfair dismissal to an industrial tribunal. At the hearing the employer has to show the reason for the dismissal, and the tribunal has then to decide whether or not it was fair [s. 57(3)]. The test is whether "the reasonable employer" would have dismissed, not whether injustice has been done to the employee. So a prejudicial but honest and genuine belief on the part of the employer (e.g., about the perceived risk to children imposed by a gay teacher) can be "reasonable," even in the light of expert evidence to the contrary (*Nottinghamshire County Council v. Bowl*, 1978). Reasons given in cases of dismissal of gay or lesbian employees in connection with their sexuality usually fall either under the category of "conduct" in Section 57(2)(b) — for example, an indecency conviction (*Wiseman v. Salford City Council*, 1981) — or under the catch-all category of "some other substantial reason" in Section 57(1)(b), which could be for just being gay (*Saunders v. Scottish National Camps Association Ltd*, 1980) What is more, pressure by fellow employees to have a gay or lesbian employee dismissed can be declared a fair reason. It is often asserted that none of the decisions establishes legal precedent as each depends on its special circumstances, but recently some employees who were dismissed when their homosexuality became known have been awarded compensation by the Employment tribunals (Palmer, 1995).

By now equal opportunities policies that include sexual orientation have been introduced by many companies and firms and by many professional bodies, including the Bar Council, the Law Society, and government departments, as well as by some police forces (Burke, 1993). In 1994 the Lord Chancellor's Department introduced a similar policy for judges. Although these policies might help in an internal disciplinary procedure, it is unlikely that a court will find that they constitute part of the contract of employment, so they are not legally enforceable. The only way they could come into play in an unfair dismissal hearing is where the tribunal might not believe, in the light of an equal opportunities policy, that "homosexuality" as an employer's reason for dismissal was "honest and genuine." However, an employer's obligation to show that dismissal was "reasonable" could be helped by showing that all has been done for the requirement of fairness, including the introduction of an equal opportunity policy. All the employer then has to convince the tribunal of is that the belief was honest and genuine. Thus, a local council with an equal opportunity policy including sexual orientation could still succeed before an industrial tribunal in arguing that it was reasonable to dismiss a gay teacher, since in this particular occupation the employee comes into close contact with minors, and therefore his sexual orientation could be seen by the reasonable employer to impose a threat. Moreover, equal opportunity policies as such do not give homosexual partners the benefits and perks of a married couple, nor give a surviving partner interest in a work pension after the death of a former employee.

Although homosexual behavior by military personnel has now been decriminalized, homosexuals are still banned from service in the armed forces since, on existing Ministry of Defence policies, a homosexual orientation is incompatible with military service. Over the period from January 1990 to May 1994, 260 servicemen and servicewomen were dismissed or administratively discharged on these grounds. The policy has brought the Ministry of Defence into conflict with Australian authorities who have refused to accede to a request to screen out gays sent for attachment to British units. Service personnel who have confessed or been "outed" complain of being subjected to intrusive interrogations by the Military Police Special Investigation Branch about the identities of their homosexual friends (Hall, 1995).

On June 7, 1995, the High Court, in deciding on an application for judicial review by four former members of the armed forces, found that the Ministry of Defence had not been unreasonable (i.e., so unreasonable as outrageously to defy logic or accepted moral standards) in dismissing the four on the grounds that their presence would disrupt the morale and discipline of the forces. It was not contended that the prior military record of any of the four had been other than exemplary, and Lord Justice Simon Brown was of the opinion that the policy violated the applicants' rights under the European Convention on Human Rights. He regretted that he could not found his decision on this, as the convention is not yet part of domestic law (Smith, 1995). Should the government lose on a (now pending) appeal before the European Court of Human Rights, those affected might be able to claim compensation. In the meantime, in March 1996 the Ministry of Defence published the outcome of an internal review that reported considerable hostility among service personnel toward gays and strong support for the ban against having them in the forces.

Immigration

For same-sex partners, where one member is not a British or European Union citizen, problems with immigration arise because they do not have the same right as married couples under the immigration laws, which allow foreign spouses to stay in the country. Consequently, the gay press features numerous advertisements for marriages of convenience, thinly disguised as "mutually beneficial arrangements." The laws do not mention unmarried opposite-sex couples, but the Home Office often used to treat them as if married and allow the partner to stay. In February 1996, however, following calls for similar discretion to be applied to same-sex couples, the minister for immigration announced that the policy of treating unmarried and married couples alike for immigration purposes had ceased.

Gay men or lesbians seeking leave to stay in Britain as refugees because homosexuality is persecuted in their home country have so far been denied the qualifying status of constituting a "social group," despite contrary decisions in other jurisdictions [cf. Article IA(2) of the Geneva Refugee Convention]. In 1995, however, a tribunal accepted the legal argument, but refused a gay Romanian leave to stay because they did not believe that he was gay. Counsel for the Home Office had demanded an anal examination to test the applicant's sexuality.

Section 28

An example of official discouragement of equality for gays and lesbians occurs in Section 28 of the Local Government Act 1988, which prohibits local authorities from intentionally promoting homosexuality, publishing material with the intention of promoting homosexuality, or promoting the teaching in state schools of "the acceptability of homosexuality as a pretended [sic] family relationship." This law was introduced following a political controversy in which local authorities controlled by the opposition Labour Party had been accused of squandering public money on support for voluntary organizations that provided services for gays and lesbians. It was also alleged that school libraries were stocking a book describing childrearing by homosexuals in a favorable light.

As a badly drafted law with unclear scope, Section 28 has limited practical significance, and no action has been taken against local authorities by the government under it. However, Section 28 has symbolic significance as a declaration that homosexual and heterosexual relationships are not of equal worth. As such it is a constant irritant to gay activists (Colvin & Hawksley, 1989). Furthermore, individuals antagonistic to homosexuals can use it to try to prevent public money from going to charities dealing with gays and lesbians or to theaters showing gay plays. For example, when the act was first passed, a promise of funding to Streetwise Youth, an organization befriending and helping young male street prostitutes, was withdrawn because it might be thought contrary to Section 28. Usually, however, authorities can plead financial stringency as a less controversial reason for reducing funding. Restrictions openly based on Section 28 have been successfully challenged on a number of occasions. In November 1994 a gay youth group funded by Shropshire County Council was closed while an investigation was launched into whether its activities were contrary to Section 28, but following protests supported by Liberty (The National Council for Civil Liberties) the County Council decided to continue its support. Liberty has also been successful in challenging the decisions of some public libraries to use Section 28 to ban or weed out publications dealing with homosexuality. (*The Pink Paper*, 14 April 1995). Arguably, Section 28 has had its most "chilling effect" in limiting discussion of homosexual issues in schools and making teachers wary of reference to homosexuality in children's sex education classes (Wintemute, 1994, p. 510). Due to the lack of clarity of Section 28's scope, it has also had an inhibitory effect on safer-sex education. However, the government has now asserted that safer-sex education is vital and does not contravene Section 28.

PUBLIC DISAPPROVAL AND ITS EFFECTS

The Effects of Publicity

The reactions of the public toward homosexual men and women and the opportunities they have for meeting each other are more relevant to their everyday lives than the letter of the law. Before 1950, when homosexuality was practiced secretly and attracted little publicity, the prohibition of homosexual behavior in private was not rigorously enforced. Only a small minority of gay men and hardly any lesbians had contact with the criminal justice system because of their sexual behavior. Police were not expected to raid houses or hotels looking for men sleeping together. Prosecutions generally arose from the involvement of children (choir boys and boy scouts were popularly believed to be at risk), complaints by disapproving third parties (such as landladies), publicly visible behavior (as in men's lavatories), or moral crusades by local police forces (as in the previously mentioned Wildeblood affair). The gay liberation movement existed only in specialist literature mainly read by sexual minorities, and the gay subculture was confined to a few discreetly run bars, private clubs, and steambaths without their real function ever being publicly advertised.

Radical changes in recent decades include the removal of the declaratory influence of a law that made homosexuals criminals and the emergence of the gay rights movement in the late 1960s as a significant political force. Far from remaining hidden, homosexual topics now feature frequently in newspapers, on television, and in the theater. Business enterprises such as magazines, bars discos, clubs, travel agencies, and clothes shops now openly advertise services for gays and lesbians. There is even a gay directory, the *Gay to Z*, set up like the yellow pages of telephone books, with about 80 pages of such listings. Nevertheless, things have not gone so far that same-sex couples are likely to be seen holding hands or kissing in public as heterosexuals might. Moreover, church authorities, bound by scriptural condemnations, continue their oppositional pronouncements. The fact that in the West anal intercourse practiced by male homosexuals has made a major contribution to the spread of AIDS allows those who disapprove on moral grounds to contend that the "plague" is a punishment for "sin." The dubious assumptions that homosexuals are more likely than heterosexuals to prey upon the young and that young people, especially boys, are easily "seduced" into becoming gay remain widespread, reinforced by an extraordinary rise in public concern about sexual abuse of children, either within the family home or in encounters elsewhere.

For homosexuals today it could be said to be "the best of times and the worst of times." Everyone has become aware of the issues, and attitudes tend to be polarized. Opinion polls show that a majority of the population remain intolerant. In a recent national survey 70 percent of men and 58 percent of women endorsed the view that sex between two men is always or mostly wrong (see Wellings et al., 1994, Table 6.5). Subsamples of this national survey were questioned in more detail in a follow-up study (Snape, Thompson, & Chetwynd, 1995). Of those who declared themselves to be heterosexual, one-half still maintained that lesbian or male homosexual relationships were always or mostly wrong and a substantial minority supported discrimination in employment. For example, being a primary school teacher was thought "never or hardly ever acceptable" for gay men by 46 percent of respondents and for lesbians by 34 percent. Similarly, for employment as hospital doctors, 35 percent of respondents found gays unacceptable and 32 percent found lesbians unacceptable, and 30 percent found either gays or lesbians unacceptable as police officers. Substantial majorities said that if they were renting out a room they would be less likely to let it to a gay or lesbian couple than to a heterosexual couple (61 and 58 percent, respectively). Nevertheless, 67 percent of heterosexuals agreed with the proposition that there should be laws to protect homosexuals from discrimination and only a minority were in favor of making homosexual relations a criminal offense. Thus, only 18 percent thought "two men aged twenty-one having sex at home" should be guilty of an offense, but 40 percent thought a 22-year-old man having sex in his own home with a 19-year-old man should be guilty of an offense. It seems that the public tolerance of homosexuality is subject to stringent age barriers.

For a significant minority of the population homosexuality arouses deep revulsion, and many who are tolerant at an intellectual level experience great unease when a member of their family becomes involved. Some older homosexuals look back on a golden age when, if they enjoyed the relative anonymity of living in a big city and knew where to go, they could compartmentalize their sex life and indulge in secret without adverse comment from family or public. Today, it may be politically incorrect in educated circles to deride the homosexual minority, but the popular tabloid newspapers still use anything from snide commentary and pejorative slang to forthright obloquy in their references to homosexuality. Occasional condemnation by the Press Complaints Commission for breach of the rule against prejudicial or pejorative reference to a person's sexuality does little to deter them. Words like "beast" and "degenerate," not customarily applied to other criminals, are commonly used for homosexual "seducers" of youths.

The strength of public disapproval is felt particularly strongly by those bold enough to have taken up what are regarded as sensitive positions as school teachers, politicians, diplomats, servicemen, policemen, or clergy. They strive to avoid drawing their employers' attention to their homosexual orientation, since exposure can mean, if not actual dismissal, then reduced chances of career advancement or risk of being shunted off to unattractive posts. Efforts to maintain an appearance of conformity can lead to the cultivation of doomed relationships with a partner of the opposite sex and disastrous marriages. Fear of condemnation by parents, siblings, or other family members often leads to semiestrangement as efforts to conceal gay relationships necessitate moving far away. Extrusion of adolescents from their homes by parents hostile to their sexual orientation is not uncommon. Since it is very difficult in England for young people under 18 who are not living with parents or enrolled in youth training schemes to obtain money through state benefits, such rejections make a significant contribution to youth crime, homelessness, and male homosexual prostitution (West & De Villiers. 1992). Juvenile peer groups can be very cruel toward anyone who fails to conform to accepted gender roles. Some young homosexuals feel great sadness and shame about their sexual orientation; the incidence of attempted suicide among them is high (Trenchard & Warren, 1984) and is recognized by the Department of Health (1993) as a significant risk.

Continuing Grievances

A survey of a sample of self-identified gay men, mostly well-educated middle-class, and resident in London (Thompson, West, & Woodhouse, 1985), revealed that only about one-third had been open about their homosexuality with friends, relatives, and coworkers and over one-fourth reported having experienced unpleasant remarks from coworkers. Interference with work careers because of homosexuality was a particularly common complaint, and it was noticeable that the men's occupations tended to be below what might have been expected from their educational backgrounds. Similar results were obtained in the more recent survey by Snape et al. (1995). Since the homosexual sample in this survey was drawn from a population study rather than from among self-selected volunteers or gay activists their experiences are of special interest. Over half reported having encountered some concrete form of discrimination because of their sexuality, 43 percent had "insults shouted in a public place," 25 percent had been "physically threatened or harassed," 8 percent had been refused promotion, and 4 percent had been dismissed from jobs.

The grievances of homosexuals treated unfairly as employees or users of services, both public and private, are occasionally heard in the courts, but far more often the grounds for discrimination are not openly acknowledged and the means are too subtle for legal challenge, even if the affected person were prepared to face the attendant publicity. The belief that homosexuals are the dysfunctional products of dysfunctional families is no longer predominant in medical opinion, but it is still supported by some religious groups, such as the Courage Trust, which has an ideological commitment to "treatment" to convert homosexuals into God-fearing Christian heterosexuals (*Guardian*, 24 Aug. 1995). An officially unacknowledged bias against homosexuals undoubtedly exists among the medical profession. Some years ago, a survey of doctors' attitudes (Bhugra, 1989) revealed that one-third of general practitioners felt uncomfortable dealing with male homosexuals, considering them a danger to children. A more recent survey revealed that some doctors found it difficult to cope with AIDS patients and that gay doctors were afraid to be open about their sexual orientation for fear it might damage their career prospects. McColl (1994), commenting on bias in the mental health services, cited the finding that one-half of medical students questioned believed that homosexuality could not form part of an acceptable lifestyle. Because of its theoretical interpretation of homosexual orientation as a developmental abnormality, the British psychoanalytic establishment can hardly be imagined to welcome gay doctors to their ranks. Recently, the Association for Psychoanalytic Psychotherapy arranged a lecture to be given by a visiting American psychoanalyst, Dr. Charles Socarides, a high-profile exponent of the concept of homosexuality as a serious disease (and this despite his having a son who is a prominent and publicly gay civil rights lawyer). The invitation provoked so much protest from gay activists that the talk was canceled at the last minute (Bunting, 1995; Rayner, 1995).

The police are reputedly fairly hostile toward gays and lesbians. According to Burke (1993), some officers wear surgical gloves whenever they deal with gay men. Few of England's regionalized police forces have equal opportunity policies that include sexual orientation. The majority of gay and lesbian police officers still conceal their sexuality from colleagues and superiors. Those who have been open about it have faced reactions ranging from tolerance or indifference to intimate interrogation and forced resignation. It is difficult for gay and lesbian officers serving in macho forces to reconcile the demands of their working culture with the feelings of the gay community, who think them hostile and oppressive. Many leave the force to escape this tension (Burke, 1993). Attitudes are changing, however. A few years ago the then chief constable of Greater Manchester was fulminating against homosexuals in public speeches; now the Manchester police are advertising for recruits in the gay press. Some forces, including the Metropolitan Police, hold regular meetings with representatives of the gay community and appoint officers to liaise with them. At these meetings, superior ranking officers deny "pretty police" or other techniques of entrapment are in use, but the behavior of police on patrol may not always conform to official policy.

In the Thompson survey (1985), a surprising proportion (nearly one-half of a sub-sample who were interviewed individually) reported having been physically assaulted at some time in connection with their homosexuality. Many of these assaults were of the queer-bashing variety, that is, attacks in public places by young men incited by behavior, appearance, or situation — such as emerging from a gay bar — that betrays homosexuality. The gay press continually reports such incidents, but there are few arrests and there has been little systematic research into the problem in England. Surveys in America, however, show that both lesbians and gay men, but particularly the latter, experience many times more physical assaults than do heterosexuals of similar social and ethnic backgrounds (Comstock, 1991). In a survey of a large sample of gay males in England (Hickson et al., 1994), over one-fourth reported having been sexually assaulted, most commonly by anal penetration. The majority of incidents were of childhood molestation by older family members or associates or occasions of coerced submission to the demands of current or former sexual partners. A significant number, however, were intentionally punitive. One example was the anal rape of a man by six of his work colleagues after they found out he was gay. The victim was subsequently dismissed from his job.

It is often alleged that some police forces do little to combat queer-bashing and that people reporting these incidents face indifference, even hostility, and are subjected to insensitive interrogation about their private lives. The situation is changing, however, and several forces, including London's Metropolitan Police, now do some monitoring of queer-bashing offenses. Furthermore, the introduction of the crime of male rape may afford male victims the same anonymity and counseling services as are available to women.

Much has been written about male rape in prisons and youth custody establishments in America, and a similar phenomenon is described in the chapter on Russia in this volume. Unaggressive types, once overpowered, are labelled "queer" or "punk" and are subjected to continued victimization (Lockwood, 1980). This may also occur to some extent in Britain, although it has not received publicity. Homosexuals in male prisons in England are liable to suffer additional restrictions and humiliations, some staff and inmates considering them a corrupting influence on other prisoners (Preece, 1993). Intolerance is not universal, however, for it appears that most staff and inmates would favor condoms being made available to prisoners and presumably some facility for privacy also, this despite anxieties about misuse (e.g., for secreting drugs) or fears of adverse reactions toward prisoners known to be using them (Greenaway, 1994). The Home Office, however, maintains that to provide condoms would be to condone crime, since it regards neither the cells nor any other part of a prison as "private places."

The depth of feeling against homosexuality reveals itself on occasion when a man's homosexuality is exposed for the first time when he is found to have AIDS. Indignant relatives may descend upon the dying man, try to expel the live-in lover, take hostile charge of affairs when the sufferer is at his most vulnerable, and, ignoring his wishes or welfare, direct their energies to concealing the situation from their friends and preventing his lover from benefiting financially at his death. Embarrassments occur at funerals of AIDS patients when relatives who have been unaware of the deceased's lifestyle are horrified at being brought into contact with the deceased's gay friends (personal communication with a priest and an AIDS worker in West London).

The fact that male homosexuals are a high-risk group for HIV creates difficulties in obtaining life or health insurance including that linked to endowment mortgages. Tests for HIV are often insisted upon, but this is becoming frequent for many other reasons.

Blackmail was an obvious danger for male homosexuals in the days when denunciation could mean imprisonment. Susceptibility to blackmail was often cited as justification for excluding suspected homosexuals from government posts involving access to official secrets, since foreign agents might force them into spying by threats of what is now called "outing" (Vassall, 1975). Although the Foreign and Commonwealth Office now includes sexual orientation in its equal opportunity policy, it recommends discretion on the part of persons posted to "sensitive" countries where homosexuality is criminal. Members of the armed forces, for whom exposure means dismissal, are also vulnerable, as are people in some other jobs. Burke (1993) quotes an ex-police officer who paid about £8500 to a colleague who blackmailed him. Of the men interviewed in the survey by Thompson et al. (1985), 15 percent reported blackmail, but usually for quite small sums, most often demanded by youths or younger men with whom they had been sexually involved. For public figures, fear of exposure can have dire consequences, the forced resignation and subsequent unsuccessful prosecution of the one-time leader of Britain's Liberal party being one example. He was alleged to have used extreme methods to combat harassment by a former lover (Penrose & Freeman, 1996). As recently as December 1995, a conservative member of Parliament, accused in a newspaper report of having a homosexual affair, felt this was so damaging that he spent hundreds of thousands of pounds on contesting it in an unsuccessful libel action (Linton, 1995).

The belief that many gay men are seducers or molesters of children is encouraged by lurid press stories about young boys, especially vulnerable runaways, being preyed upon by "rings" of pedophiles, passed on from one to another, and finally tortured and murdered. In reality, it is a small minority of pedophiles who are violent and there is little evidence that they are more prevalent among homosexuals than heterosexuals. Moreover, tests of erectile responsiveness, using the penile plethysmograph, have shown that being sexually aroused by children is not a feature of homosexuals any more than of heterosexuals. The proportion of males among molested children may be higher than the proportion of homosexuals in the male population, but there are various reasons for this. Tender age is more important to some pedophiles than the child's gender, and boys can be picked up more easily, being less shielded from contact with older males than are girls. Homosexual involvement with postadolescent boys attracts disproportionate publicity, if only because heterosexual involvements with teenage girls are too common to be newsworthy.

Men suspected of homosexuality are unlikely these days to be selected for jobs in residential care of children. Teachers and youth workers who are homosexual have to be particularly discreet if they are to keep their jobs. One of the homosexual men interviewed in the Thompson et al. (1985) survey said that when he was working at a hostel and had occasion to reprimand some young residents they retaliated by threatening him with accusations of sexual advances. Teaching unions have become concerned about a notable increase in accusations of sexual misconduct from disaffected pupils which, regardless of failure to substantiate, cause immediate suspension and damaged reputation. Englishmen's fear of being exposed as homosexual has been used for publicity purposes by the gay activist group OutRage!. In November 1994 they named publicly 10 bishops of the Church of England who were said to be homosexual, none of whom denied the charge. A little later, after receiving a letter from OutRage! and fearing he too might be outed, the Bishop of London created a sensation by announcing that although he was leading a celibate life his sexuality was "a grey area." While two members of Parliament have publicly acknowledged their homosexual orientation, the OutRage! campaign continued with letters sent to 20 members of Parliament whom they believed to be homosexual, stating that hiding one's homosexuality reinforces the idea that to be gay is shameful, whereas being open is "ethically right" and denies the press scope for scandal-mongering (Tatchell, 1995). Such tactics, denounced by other gay rights organizations such as Stonewall, were arguably justified on the grounds that clerics and politicians who are themselves in secret homosexual relationships should not preach against homosexual acts or vote for discriminatory laws.

Present Trends

Years of lobbying by gay and lesbian activists have not eliminated popular prejudices, but they have achieved a considerable shift in official establishment pronouncements, which are nowadays inclined to respectful acceptance. Soon after the attacks on bishops by OutRage! the Archbishop of Canterbury preached against intolerance of homosexuals and the Bishop of London was promoted to become Archbishop of York. There was, however, no change in the rule that homosexual clerics must remain celibate, although laymen living in "sinful" same-sex relationships can remain members of the Church. Application of the policy depends on each diocesan bishop and many operate a characteristically British "don't-ask-don't-tell" system, which allows some priests to have live-in lovers in the vicarage as long as there is no public scandal (personal communication from such a vicar). The conflict within the Church of England has reached such a pitch that such "gentlemen's agreements" may be impossible to operate much longer. In November 1996, a ceremony in Southwark Cathedral to celebrate the twentieth anniversary of the Lesbian and Gay Christian Movement met with vociferous protests from placard-carrying Evangelicals.

Far from "the love that dare not speak its name," issues of gay rights are forced into public prominence by incessant references in the press, in documentary television programs, and in popular drama. Gay and lesbian organizations challenge members of Parliament about their views on gay issues and hold demonstrations outside the House of Commons. Notwithstanding furious antagonism from some individuals and from some religious and political groups, English gays and lesbians are free to pursue their lives in their own way with varying degrees of openness and without overt harassment from authorities. The notorious public lavatories, cinemas, and steambaths once known as places for male sex contacts have been closed down in the wake of public exposure, but facilities for making private sexual contacts have become plentiful. Glossy gay and lesbian magazines, such as *Gay Times* and *Diva*, are available at larger newsagents. Free advertising papers (of which the most respectable is *The Pink Paper*) are distributed in gay bars. These provide, at least as openly as do corresponding heterosexual publications, numerous contact advertisements for lesbians and male homosexuals. Some of them carry notices inserted by male prostitutes, thinly disguised as masseur or escorts services, often accompanied by a nude or seminude picture of the person on offer. The illegality of group sex and sadomasochism does not prevent these adverts mentioning the availability of "duos," "SM," "CP," "bondage," or "dungeon" or the announcement of meetings of S & M Gays and other groups with specialized homosexual interests. The gay press also informs readers about the many commercial enterprises, restaurants, entertainments, clothes shops, travel agencies, solicitors, flat finders, and others, that target a gay clientele. In London and Manchester there are streets given over to a conglomeration of gay bars, clothiers, sex shops, and similar businesses (Whittle, 1994). Scattered around the capital are gay bars with heavily blacked-out windows behind which happenings such as sex shows, underwear parties, and other uninhibited activities continue largely unmolested. For the less sex-obsessed, there are in most large towns other attractions, such as social and discussion groups, outdoor activity clubs, HIV counseling centers, and information centers.

Homosexuals may feel insecure, knowing they cannot expect acceptance everywhere outside the gay ghetto communities, but a silent majority of the homosexual population, by not announcing their status in mannerisms, clothes, or badges, are able to avoid violent confrontations, unwanted attention from the police, or overt conflicts with employers. They may feel the lack of an opposite-sex partner as a social disadvantage at office parties and the like, but such pressures are not necessarily signs of active hostility; rather, they reflect social customs geared to the majority heterosexual lifestyle. The extent of the legal and personal freedom now enjoyed by English gays and lesbians owes much to men and women of the past who have come out of the closet and taken part in public protest, sometimes paying a heavy personal price for doing so. The trend toward social acceptance may not continue. To the increasing numbers of Muslim and Christian fundamentalists homosexuality is an anathema. Trends in the United States are usually precursors of what happens in the United Kingdom. Pat Buchanan, a virulently anti-gay campaigner, was a candidate for president of the United States and is influential in the Republican party. Berlin in the 1930s, before the Nazis took over, was a city renowned for its permissiveness, but that did not prevent gay men and women from being later rounded up and put into concentration camps along with Jews and other despised minorities (Rector, 1981).

CITED CASES

B v B (Minors) (Custody Care and Control) 1 FLR 402 FD (1991).
Burge v DPP, 1 All ER 666n (1962).
C v C (A minor) (Custody Appeal) 1 FLR 223 at 228 F-G) (1991).
C, Re Guardian, 2 July (1994).
D, Re AC 602 HL (1977).
DPP v Bull, 4 All ER 411 QBD (1994).
Dudgeon v UK, 4 EHRR 149 (1981).
H, Re (A Minor) (Section 37 discretion) 2 FLR 541 (1993).
Harrogate Borough Council v Simpson, 2 FLR 91 CA (1986).

Knuller v DPP, 2 All ER 898 HL (1972).
Masterson and Cooper v Holden, 3 All ER 39 (1986).
Nottinghamshire County Council v. Bowl, 1 IRLR 252 EAT (1978).
R v Bedborough, 6 Cr. App. R. (S) 98 (1984).
R v Bow Street Magistrate, Exp. Noncyp Ltd., 3 WLR 287 (1988).
R v Brown, 2 All ER 75 (1993).
R v Donovan, 2 KB 498 (1934).
R v Eames, 14 Cr App R (S) 205 (1992).
R v Gray, 3 Cr App R (S) 363 (1981).
R v Harper, 14 Cr App R (S) 678 (1993).
R v Roe, Cr App R (S) 435 (1988).
R v Sheridan, 8 Cr App R (S) 10 (1986).
R v Tyrell, 1 QB 710 (1894).
R v Willis, 1 All ER 620 (1975).
Saunders v Scottish National Camps Association Ltd, IRLR 174 EAT (1981) IRLR 277 (Court of Session) (1980).
Shaw v DPP, AC 220 (1962).
Smith, New Law Journal, 887, HC (1995).
W, Re (Wardship Publication of Information), 1 FLR 99, CA (1991).
Whitehouse v Gay New and Lemon, AC 617 (1979).
Wiseman v. Salford City Council, IRLR 202 EAT (1981).

REFERENCES

Beresford, S. (1994, November). Lesbians in residence and parental responsibility cases. *Family Law, 24*, 643.
Bhugra, G. (1989). Doctors' attitudes to male homosexuality: A survey. *Psychiatric Bulletin, 13*, 426–428.
Bunting, M. (1995). C of E's anti-gay therapy attacked. *Guardian*, August 24, p. 3.
Burke, M. E. (1993). *Coming out of the blue*. London: Cassell.
Colvin, M. & Hawksley, J. (1989). *Section 28: A practical guide to the law and its implications*. London: Liberty.
Comstock, G. D. (1991). *Violence against lesbians and gay men*. New York: Columbia University Press.
Criminal Law Revision Committee. (1984). *Sexual offences* (15th Report: Command 9213). London: Her Majesty's Stationery Office (H.M.S.O.).
Department of Health. (1993). *Mental illness: Sometimes I don't think I can go on any more*. London: Author.
GALOP (Gay London Policing Group). (1988/9). *Fifth Annual Report*. London: GALOP.
Golombok, S., Spencer, A., & Rutter, M. (1983). Children of lesbian and single-parent households. *Journal of Child Psychology and Psychiatry, 24*, 551–572.
Golombok, S., & Fivusch, R. (1994). *Gender development*. Cambridge, England: Cambridge University Press.
Gooding, C. (1992). *Trouble with the law*. London: Gay Men's Press.
Green, R. (1978). Sexual identity of 37 children raised by homosexual and transsexual parents. *American Journal of Psychiatry, 135*, 692–697.
Greenaway, D. (1994). Safer sex in prisons. *Prison Service Journal*, 37–40.
Grey, A. (1992). *Quest for justice: Towards homosexual emancipation*. London: Sinclair Stevenson.
Hall, E. (1995). *We can't even march straight: Homosexuality in the British armed services*. London: Vintage.
Harris, D., & Haigh, R. (Eds.). (1990). *AIDS: A guide to the law*. London: Routledge.
Hickson, F. C. L., Davies, P. M., Hunt, A. J., Weatherburn, P., McMannus, T. J., & Coxon, A. P. M. (1994). Gay men as victims of nonconsensual sex. *Archives of Sexual Behavior, 23*, 281–294.
Home Office. (1957). *Report of the Committee on Homosexual Offences and Prostitution* (Command 247). London: H.M.S.O.
Home Office. (1994). *Criminal statistics England and Wales 1993*. London: H.M.S.O.

Jeffery-Poulter, S. (1991). *Peers, queers and commons: The struggle for gay law reform from 1950 to the present.* London: Routledge.

Law Commission. (1989). *A Criminal Code for England and Wales.* London: H.M.S.O.

Law Commission. (1995). *Consent in the Criminal Law* (Consultation Paper 139). London: H.M.S.O.

Leng, R., & Manchester, C. (1991). *A guide to the Criminal Justice Act.* London: Fourmat.

Liberty. (1995). *Sexuality and the state.* London: National Council for Civil Liberties.

Linton, M. (1995). £400,000 bill for MP. *Guardian*, December 20, p. 1.

Lockwood, D. (1980). *Prison sexual violence.* New York: Elsevier.

McColl, P. (1994, February 26). Homosexuality and mental health services. *British Medical Journal*, 308, 550–551.

Palmer, A. (1995). Industrial tribunals support gay employment rights. *Gay Times*, (201) June, p. 40.

Penrose, B., & Freeman, S. (1996). *Rinkagate, the rise and fall of Jeremy Thorpe.* London: Bloomsbury.

Pink Paper, The. (1992, November; 1994, November; 1995, April). 72 Holloway Road, London N7 8NZ, England.

Preece, A. (1993). Being gay in prison. *Probation Journal*, 40, 85–87.

Rayner, J. (1995). Shrink resistant. *Guardian*, April 25, p. 2.

Rector, F. (1981). *The Nazi extermination of homosexuals.* New York: Stein and Day.

Snape, D., Thompson, K., & Chetwynd, M. (1995). *Discrimination against gay men and lesbians.* London: Social and Community Planning Research.

Tatchell, P. (1995). Tatchell is derided for his closet gay election stance. *Guardian*, March 22, p. 2.

Thompson, B. (1995). *Sadomasochism: Painful perversion or pleasurable pain.* New York: Cassell.

Thompson, N. L., West, D. J., & Woodhouse, T. P. (1985). Socio-legal problems of male homosexuals in Britain. In D. J. West (Ed.), *Sexual Victimisation* (pp. 95–159). Aldershot, England: Gower.

Trenchard, L., & Warren, H. (1984). *Something to tell you.* London: Gay Teenage Group.

Vassall, J. (1975). *Vassall: The autobiography of a spy.* London: Sidgwick and Jackson.

Walmsley, R. (1978, July). Indecency between men and the Sexual Offences Act 1967. *Criminal Law Review*, 400.

Walmsley, R., & White, K. (1979). *Sexual offences, consent and sentencing* (Home Office Research Study 54). London: H.M.S.O.

Wellings, K., Field, J., Johnson, A. M., & Wadsworth, J. (1994). *Sexual behaviour in Britain. The national survey of sexual attitudes and lifestyles.* London: Penguin.

West, D. J., & De Villiers, B. (1992). *Male prostitution.* London: Duckworth.

Whittle, S. (1994). *The margins of the city: Gay men's urban lives.* Aldershot, England: Arena, Ashgate.

Wildeblood, P. (1955). *Against the law.* London: Weidenfeld and Nicolson.

Wintemute, R. (1994). Sexual orientation discrimination. In C. McCrudden & G. Chambers (Eds.), *Individual rights and the law in Britain* (pp. 491–533). Oxford: Clarendon Press.

Wintour, P. (1996). Gays get joint rights. *Guardian*, April 27, p. 10.

14

RUSSIA

IGOR S. KON

HISTORICAL PRELUDE

Same-sex love has a long history in Russia (Burgin, 1994; Engelstein, 1992, 1995; Healey, 1991; Karlinsky, 1976, 1989; Kon, 1995; Levin, 1989). The Russian Orthodox Church, like other Christian denominations, defined it as a mortal sin, but the concept of sodomy in Ancient Russ was vague and included both homosexual relations and heterosexual anal intercourse, as well as any deviations from "normal" gender roles and partners, such as intercourse in the "woman-on-top" position. The most serious deviation was *muzhebludie* [male lechery] or *muzhelozhstvo* [male fornication] wherein coitus with the "wrong" gender partner was compounded with the "wrong" sexual position, that is, anal penetration. The punishment depended on the sinner's age, marital status, how often he had indulged, and the extent of his own active involvement. The penalties for juveniles and young men were more lenient than those for married men. If no anal penetration took place, reference was no longer made to *muzhelozhstvo*, but to masturbation. Lesbianism was usually categorized as a form of masturbation. The Orthodox church was very concerned about homosexuality spreading in the monasteries but were fairly tolerant of its practice among laymen (Levin, 1989).

Inconsistencies were inevitable, as the process of Christianization of Russia, which lasted over centuries—all the while involving new territories and peoples—was in many ways incomplete and superficial. Christian norms not only coexisted with pagan norms, but also frequently incorporated them. During the 15th through 17th centuries travelers and diplomats in Russia frequently remarked on the widespread occurrence of homosexuality in all milieux and the surprisingly tolerant—by European standards—public attitudes toward it (Karlinsky, 1976). This probably came less from a conscious tolerance than from a primitive acceptance of the "realities of life." A similar situation existed in Western Europe in the early Middle Ages; it was only much later that the bonfires and persecutions of the Inquisition flared up. Be this as it may, homosexuality was neither mentioned nor punished in any Russian secular legislation until the time of Peter the Great (Nabokov, 1902; Piatnitsky, 1910; Popov, 1904).

It was not until 1706 that punishment for "unnatural lechery" first appeared in Peter the Great's military code, which was based on the Swedish model. Yet 10 years later Peter, himself not averse to bisexual relations, in Chapter 20 of the broadened military code (*O sodomskom grekhe, o nasilii i blude*) watered down the punishment for sodomy. Burning at the stake was replaced by corporal punishment, but by the death penalty or hard labor for

IGOR S. KON • Institute of Ethnology and Anthropology, Russian Academy of Sciences, Moscow 117334, Russia.

Sociolegal Control of Homosexuality, edited by West and Green, Plenum Press, New York, 1997.

life if rape or other use of violence was proven. However, these regulations applied only to military personnel, not to the civilian population.

By the close of the 18th century, with the growth of civilization and closer contacts with Europe, genteel society began to feel uneasy about homosexuality. Among the common people it was mainly associated with the religious sects of Skoptsy and Khlysty. Among the aristocracy homosexuality tended to cause scandal mostly by the nepotism and corruption it fostered, notably in various government ministries, when powerful men repaid their young protégés by appointing them to high positions that in no way corresponded to their abilities. Otherwise such matters were spoken of scornfully, but at the same time rather humorously.

As one finds everywhere, homosexuality was most rife in closed educational institutions, such as the high ranking Page Corps, Cadet Corps, the Junker colleges, and the School of Jurisprudence. Since it was so commonplace, boys were quite phlegmatic, even lighthearted, about it, reserving for it a host of bawdy, jesting verses. Attempts by the administrators of these institutions to put a stop to such "indecent conduct" came to nothing (Karlinsky, 1976; Poznansky, 1988, 1991).

There were also strong unconscious homoerotic undertones in Russian classic art and literature. According to Billington (1970)

> there is, in general, little room for women in the egocentric world of Russian romanticism. Lonely brooding was relieved primarily by exclusively masculine companionship in the Masonic lodges. From Skovoroda to Bakunin there are strong hints of homosexuality, though apparently of the sublimated, Platonic variety. Homoeroticism appears closer to the surface in Ivanov's predilection for painting naked boys, and finds philosophical expression in the fashionable belief that spiritual perfection required androgyny, or a return to the original union of male and female characteristics. (p. 349)

In 1835, during the reign of Nicolas I, a new criminal code was introduced, based on the German (Würtemberg) model. In 1845 another version of it was accepted. *Muzhelozhstvo* [man lying with man], which had been interpreted exclusively as anal penetration, was now criminalized for all social strata as a "vice contrary to nature." According to Article 995 of the 1845 code, a man convicted for *muzhelozhstvo* was punished by deprivation of all rights and resettlement in Siberia for 4–5 years. If the *muzhelozhstvo* was aggravated by rape or by seduction of a minor or a mentally ill man (Article 996), it was punished by 10–20 years hard labor in Siberia.

In 1903, a new, more lenient, code was adopted. According to Article 516 of this code, *muzhelozhstvo* was punished by imprisonment for not less than 3 months or, in aggravating circumstances such as rape or seduction of a minor, by 3–8 years imprisonment (*Ugolovnoe ulozhenie*, 1903).

When the draft was in preparation, eminent lawyers, including Vladimir D. Nabokov (1902), father of the famed writer, proposed decriminalizing homosexuality altogether, but this was rejected. The punitive legislation was rarely enforced, however. Russian doctors, like their European counterparts, considered homosexuality "a perversion of the sexual feelings" and debated the possibility of treating it, but many ordinary people simply turned a blind eye to it. Some members of the royal family, like Nikolai II's uncle Grand Duke Sergei Alexandrovich, led a blatantly homosexual lifestyle. Intellectuals were also able to avoid prosecution for homosexuality. The legend of Tchaikovsky's suicide following the sentence of a court of honor made up of his former classmates is thus patently absurd (Poznansky, 1988). Thus,

> While it is true that few men were ever prosecuted in tsarist courts for the crime of consenting (homosexual) sodomy, it is not the case that imperial legislation, or even the dominant opinion among progressive legal scholars and lawmakers, exempted sodomy from repression. The tsarist regime was notorious both for ignoring the law ... and for its laxity in implementing the laws it did endorse. The relative neglect of sodomy in the courts may say more about the inefficiency of the legal system than about active tolerance for sexual diversity. (Engelstein, 1995, p. 158)

SOVIET HOMOPHOBIA

The Soviet and post-Soviet policies toward homosexuals[1] may be divided into five key periods:

1. 1917–1933: decriminalization of homosexuality, relative tolerance, homosexuality officially labelled a disease
2. 1934–1986: homosexuality recriminalized and severely dealt with by prosecution, discrimination and silence
3. 1987–1990: beginning of open public discussions of the status of homosexuality from a scientific and humanitarian point of view by professionals and journalists
4. 1990–May 1993: gay men and lesbians themselves take up the cause, putting human rights in the forefront, resulting exacerbation of conflict and sharp politicization of the issue
5. June 1993: decriminalization of homosexuality; the homosexual underground begins to develop into a gay and lesbian subculture, with its own organizations, publications, and centers; continued social discrimination and defamation of same-sex love and relationships

The initiative for revocation of antihomosexual legislation, following the Revolution of February 1917, had come, not from the Bolsheviks but from the Cadets (Constitutional Democrats) and the anarchists (Karlinsky, 1989). Nevertheless, once the old criminal code had been repealed after the October Revolution, the antihomosexual article also ceased to be valid. The Russian Federation criminal codes for 1922 and 1926 did not mention homosexuality, although the corresponding laws remained in force in places where homosexuality was most prevalent — in the Islamic republics of Azerbaijan, Turkmenia, and Uzbekistan, as well as in Christian Georgia.

Soviet medical and legal experts were very proud of the progressive nature of their legislation. In 1930, the medical expert Sereisky (1930) wrote in the *Great Soviet Encyclopedia*: "Soviet legislation does not recognize so-called crimes against morality. Our laws proceed from the principle of protection of society and therefore countenance punishment only in those instances when juveniles and minors are the objects of homosexual interest" (p. 593).

---

[1]The most important collection of documents and texts on Soviet homosexuality is Kozlovsky (1986).

As Engelstein (1995) justly mentions, the formal decriminalization of sodomy did not mean that such conduct was invulnerable to prosecution. The absence of formal statutes against anal intercourse or lesbianism did not stop the prosecution of homosexual behavior as a form of disorderly conduct. After the 1922 Penal Code was published there were in that same year at least two known trials for homosexual practices. The eminent psychiatrist Vladimir Bekhterev testified that "public demonstration of such impulses ... is socially harmful and cannot be permitted" (Engelstein, 1995, p. 167). The official stance of Soviet medicine and law in the 1920s, as reflected by Sereisky's encyclopedia article, was that homosexuality was a disease that was difficult, perhaps even impossible, to cure. So "while recognizing the incorrectness of homosexual development ... our society combines prophylactic and other therapeutic measures with all the necessary conditions for making the conflicts that afflict homosexuals as painless as possible and for resolving their typical estrangement from society within the collective" (Sereisky, 1930, p. 593).

Although, during the 1920s, a few homosexual intellectuals still played important roles in Soviet culture, the opportunity for an open, philosophical, and artistic discussion of the topic, which had been opened up at the start of the century, was gradually whittled away. By the decree of December 17, 1933, and by the law of March 7, 1934, *muzhelozhstvo* once again became a criminal offense. The exact reasons for this abrupt change are still unknown, but it was clearly part of the "sexual Termidor" and of a general repressive trend. Criminalizing clauses were inserted into the codes of all the Soviet republics. According to Article 121 of the Russian Federation criminal code, *muzhelozhstvo* was punishable by deprivation of freedom of up to 5 years and, by Article 121.2, in cases of physical force or threat thereof, or exploitation of the victim's dependent status or involvement of a minor, a term of up to 8 years.

In January 1936, Nikolai Krylenko, People's Commissar for Justice, announced that homosexuality was a product of the decadence of the exploiting classes who knew no better, but that in a democratic society founded on healthy principles there was no place for such people (Kozlovsky, 1986). Homosexuality was thus tied to counterrevolution. Later, Soviet medical authorities and lawyers described homosexuality as a manifestation of "moral decadence of the bourgeoisie," reiterating verbatim the arguments of German fascists. Typical of this stance was an anonymous article on *gomoseksualizm* in the *Great Soviet Encyclopedia* in 1952. References to possible biological causes of homosexuality, which had hitherto been used for humanistic purposes as reasons for decriminalizing homosexuality, were now rejected:

> The origin of H[omosexualism] is linked to everyday social conditions; for the overwhelming majority of people indulging in H[omosexualism], these perversions stop as soon as the person finds himself in a favorable social environment.... In Soviet society with its healthy mores, H[omosexualism] as a sexual perversion is considered shameful and criminal. Soviet criminal legislation regards H[omosexualism] as punishable with the exception of those instances where H[omosexualism] is a manifestation of marked psychic disorder. (Gomoseksualizm, 1952, p. 35)

The precise number of persons prosecuted under Article 121 is unknown (the first official information was released only in 1988), but it is believed to be about 1000 a year. Since the late 1980s, according to official data, the number of men convicted under Article 121 has been steadily decreasing. In 1987, 831 men were sentenced (this figure refers to the entire Soviet Union); in 1989, 539; in 1990, 497; in 1991, 462; and for the first 6 months of 1992, 227, among whom all but 10 were sentenced under Article 121.2 (figures are for Russia only) (Gessen, 1994). According to Russian lawyers, most convictions have indeed been under Article 121.2, 80 percent of cases being related to the involvement of minors up to 18 years of age (Ignatov, 1974). In an analysis of 130 convictions under Article 121 between 1985 and 1992, it was found that 74 percent of the accused were convicted under 121.2, of whom 20 percent were for rape using physical force, 8 percent for using threats, 52 percent for having sexual contact with minors and 2 and 18 percent, respectively, for exploiting the victim's dependent or vulnerable status (Dyachenko, 1995). These statistics should be viewed skeptically, however, bearing in mind that many of these and other accusations may have been fabricated or falsified and that many confessions have been "beaten out" of accused persons and witnesses.

Article 121 was not aimed just at homosexuals. The authorities frequently exploited it for dealing with dissidents and for augmenting labor camp sentences. Sometimes the KGB was clearly involved in the prosecution, as, for example, in the case of the well-known Leningrad archaeologist Lev Klein: His trial was orchestrated from start to finish by the local KGB in gross violation of all procedural norms (Samoilov, 1993). Typically, the purpose of such actions was to scare the intelligentsia. Application of the law was selective. If eminent cultural figures took care not to offend the authorities, they enjoyed a kind of immunity and a blind eye was turned to their homosexual proclivities, but they had only to fall foul of an influential bigwig for the law to go into high gear. This was the scenario that destroyed the life of the great Armenian filmmaker Sergei Paradzhanov. As late as the latter part of the 1980s, the chief director of the Leningrad Yuny Zritel Theater, Zinovy Korogodsky, was arraigned before a court, fired from his post, and deprived of all his honorary titles. Examples of this kind were legion.

The antihomosexual campaign in the press in the early 1930s was short-lived. By the middle of the decade utter silence on the subject had descended. Homosexuality had become unmentionable in the full sense of the term. The conspiracy of silence even embraced such academic subjects as phallic cults and ancient Greek pederasty. Its gloomy silence further intensified the tragedy of Soviet homosexuals, who not only feared prosecution and blackmail, but who also could not even develop adequate self-awareness and self-identity. Apart from legal prosecution, widespread and unlimited illegal discrimination and persecution of all kinds have been aimed not only at male homosexuals, but equally at lesbians.

Lesbian relations did not fall under the rubric of any criminal code, and close relations between women have been less visible and less liable to harassment. Public attitudes about lesbians have been just as obdurate as those about gay men. Lesbians have been exposed to ridicule, persecution, expulsion from university, termination of employment, and threats to take custody of their children away from them.

A typical scenario, recounted by more than a dozen young Russian lesbians ages 15–19 who were interviewed from 1991 to 1993 by Masha Gessen (1994),

> involves a parent or other guardian (such as a teacher at a residential school) finding out about a lesbian relationship and committing one or both of the — usually — very young women. A diagnosis and a relatively brief hospitalization — two to three months — and forced treatment with mind-altering medication followed. After her release from the

psychiatric hospital, the patient was to remain registered with a local psychiatric ambulatory clinic. (pp. 17–18)

Soviet punitive psychiatry was one of the main weapons of both legal and illegal repression. Sexologically ignorant psychiatrists were always ready to find some serious diagnosis that enabled persons so stigmatized to be put under lifelong medical and police observation or detained in a psychiatric hospital under conditions often much worse than prison. Even after the emergence in the late 1970s of a more tolerant and better-informed "sexopathology" (the Russian term for a medical sexology suggesting that all sexual problems are pathological), medicine offered little help. In all Soviet books on sexopathology, homosexuality was described as a pernicious "sexual perversion," a disease that must be treated (Vasilchenko, 1977, 1983).

In the early 1980s, an antihomosexual campaign was launched in educational publications. In the first, and at the time the nation's only, teachers' manual on sex education (1 million copies of which were published and immediately sold out), homosexuality was defined as a dangerous pathology and was said to be "a violation of normal principles of sexual relationships.... Homosexuality challenges both normal heterosexual relationships and society's cultural, moral attainments. It therefore merits condemnation both as a social phenomenon and as a specific person's behavior and mental attitude" (Khripkova & Kolesov, 1982, pp. 96–100). Thus, teachers as well as police and doctors were being warned against homosexuality.

Still today, with rare exceptions, Russian sexopathologists and psychiatrists, even those who supported the decriminalization of homosexuality, regard it as a disease and reproduce in their writings the many absurdities and negative stereotypes prevalent in the mass consciousness. The latest medical reference book on sexopathology, published in 1990, defines homosexuality as a "pathological drive." It states that, in addition to biological causes, "a strong pathogenic factor encouraging the formation of homosexual attraction can be the inculcation by parents and teachers of a hostile attitude towards the opposite sex" (Vasilchenko, 1990, p. 429–430).

In a doctoral dissertation in psychiatry in 1994, prepared under the guidance of Professor A. Tkachenko, not only is homosexual behavior described as "anomalous," but most of the 117 gay men studied by the author are diagnosed as having "psychic, psychophysical and disharmonic infantilism," "signs of organic defects of the central nervous system," and "overvaluation of the sexual sphere" (Vvedensky, 1994, p. 8).

The AIDS epidemic worsened the position of gays still further. In 1986 Professor Nikolai Burgasov, then Deputy Minister for Health and Chief Hygiene Doctor for the USSR, publicly announced: "We have no conditions in our country conducive to the spread of the disease; homosexuality is prosecuted by law as a grave sexual perversion (Russian Criminal Code Article 121) and we are constantly warning people of the dangers of drug abuse" (Burgasov, 1986, p. 15). When AIDS did appear in the Soviet Union, the heads of the state epidemiological program, the president of the USSR (now Russian) Academy of Medical Sciences, Professor Valentin I. Pokrovsky, and his son, Dr. Vadim V. Pokrovsky, once again blamed homosexuals, accusing them in public of being carriers of HIV infection and of displaying every kind of vice.

In the USSR the only nonjudgmental sexological and psychological books on homosexuality were written by the present author (Isayev, Kagan, & Kon, 1986; Kon, 1988, 1989,

1991). It was extremely difficult to get these books published. *Introduction to Sexology* was banned in the USSR for 10 years, even though the book had either completely avoided or merely hinted at the most important legal, social, and human rights issues.

STRUGGLE FOR DECRIMINALIZATION

After 1987, the question of what exactly homosexuality was — whether to regard the "blues" (the Russian word for homosexuals) as sick, as criminals, or as victims of fate — began to be discussed in the popular press, especially the youth press, on radio, and television. Although these venues were extremely diverse in approach and level of sophistication, it was of huge significance. For the first time, ordinary Soviet people began to learn, from journalistic articles and through letters from gays, lesbians, and their parents, about the crippling of human lives, arbitrary police behavior, legal repression, and the tragic and inevitable loneliness of people doomed to live in constant fear, unable to meet others like themselves. Every article produced a stream of contradictory reactions, which editors had no idea how to handle.

The key issue was decriminalization of homosexuality, which had long been a matter for debate in professional circles. In 1973, a textbook of criminal law had discussed the illogicality of Article 121:

> In Soviet literature of jurisprudence, never has an attempt been made to articulate a sound scientific basis for the existence of criminal penalties for voluntary *muzhelo-zhestvo* [sex between men]. The only reason that is usually given — that the individual is morally depraved and has violated the rules of socialist morality — cannot be considered substantive, since negative personal traits cannot serve as grounds for criminal penalties and the amoral nature of an act is insufficient for declaring it criminal.... Serious doubts exist regarding the expediency of retaining criminal penalties for the unqualified act of *muzheloshestvo*. (Shargorodsky & Osipov, 1973, p. 656)

This professional opinion was completely ignored. Back in 1979, Professor Alexei N. Ignatov, a leading legal expert on so-called sex crimes, had raised the question with those in charge of the USSR Ministry of Internal Affairs. The present author tried unsuccessfully to publish an article on the topic in the legal journal *Sovetskoye gosudarstvo i pravo* in 1982. Although it was strongly supported by the medical experts, professors G. S. Vasilchenko and D. N. Isayev, the editorial board decided against publication of the paper.

Arguments for the decriminalization of homosexuality were advanced from a variety of points of view:

1. Legal: Soviet legislation on the subject is not in accord with the standards and principles of international law; it lacks internal logic, since only males are punished under Article 121 and criminalization of homosexuality invites abuse and corruption on the part of law enforcement agencies.
2. Humanitarian: If an individual's sexual orientation is a matter of biology, not personal choice, he should not be punished for pursuing it.
3. Scientific: Criminalization goes against current sexological opinion.

4. Medical and hygienic: Criminalization makes it more difficult to combat the spread of AIDS and other sexually transmitted diseases.[2]
5. Social: Criminalization is damaging because it alienates homosexuals from the rest of society, forcing them into a squalid underworld.

Although these arguments never made their way into the press, the draft of the revised Russian Criminal Code, prepared by a commission of lawyers in the mid-1980s, excluded Article 121. However, as discussion and adoption of the new code was delayed, disputes about Article 121 finally spilled out into the popular press and onto television. Three major lines of thought emerged:

1. Article 121 should be fully revoked; there should be no mention of sexual orientation in the Criminal Code, since children and adolescents, as well as victims of rape and sexual coercion, irrespective of gender, are protected by other laws.
2. Criminal prosecution for same-sex contacts between consenting adult males (Article 121.1) should be revoked, but Article 121.2, covering aggravating circumstances, should be retained. This was the opinion of the Ministry of Internal Affairs.
3. Article 121 should remain unchanged. This was the demand of the nationalists and religious organizations.

During the initial years of *glasnost*, experts were alone in discussing the problems of sexual minorities, which they mentioned in sympathetic, but distanced, tones. Gradually, gays and lesbians themselves broke through to the press, gaining courage to fight for themselves. In this emerging self-awareness, they received considerable support from international gay and lesbian organizations and publications. An international conference devoted to the status of sexual minorities and to changing attitudes toward homosexuality took place in Tallinn in May 1990 on the premises of the History Institute of the Estonian Academy of Sciences.

In late 1989, the first Association of Sexual Minorities (ASM) was established in Moscow. Its declared aim was to be "primarily a human rights organization with the main purpose of obtaining complete equality of persons of different sexual orientations." It saw its prime objective as being campaigning for the revocation of Article 121, changing the public's prejudicial attitudes, pressing for the social rehabilitation of AIDS sufferers and employing for these purposes all the opportunities presented by the official mass media. The group began to publish a newspaper, *Tema* [*The Theme*]. The *SPID-info* newspaper (no. 12, 1990) published the Association's appeal to the USSR's president and Supreme

---

[2]According to statistics from Ukranian and Belorussian venereological centers, male homosexuals comprised over 30 percent of all syphilis sufferers in the 1980s, while in Latvia they made up over half. Fearful of exposure, homosexuals have typically avoided doctors or have gone to them too late. In Moscow, 84 percent of cases of late hospitalization of syphilis sufferers were homosexuals. It was hard to locate the source of their infection. According to Moscow Venereologist Professor Konstantin Borisenko, the source of syphilitic infection among male homosexuals was identified in no more than 7.5 to 10 percent of cases, compared with 50 to 70 percent in the rest of the syphilitic population (Borisenko, 1990). This is why he advocated the decriminalization of homosexuality, realizing that otherwise the epidemiological situation would not improve.

Soviets of the USSR and Union Republics. Signed pseudonymously by V. Ortanov, K. Yevgeniev, and A. Zubov (1990), the appeal requested removal of discriminatory statutes from the Penal Code and an amnesty for those convicted under them. At the same time the authors declared their "resolute condemnation of any attempts to seduce minors or to use violence, in any form or against persons of any age and regardless of who actually makes such attempts." They went on to say, "We do not desire to convert anyone to our beliefs, but we are what nature made us. Help us to stop being afraid. We are part of your life and your spirituality, whether you or we like it or not" (pp. 58–62).

Unfortunately, the political climate of Soviet society and the impossibility of having a constructive dialogue with the authorities created a situation in which all democratic movements quickly began to splinter into factions of "radicals" and "moderates" who refused to work with one another. Gays and lesbians groups were no different (Kon, 1993, 1995). Immediately following the publication of *Tema*'s second trial issue a split emerged in the ASM and it ceased to exist and was replaced by the Moscow Union of Lesbians and Homosexuals (MULH), headed by Yevgeniya Debryanskaya and Roman Kalinin, who became the sole editor and publisher of *Tema*. The paper was officially registered by the Moscow City Council (Mossovet) in October 1990.

These developments opened up new opportunities. That a few courageous people had come out openly, demanding civil rights instead of compassion and pity, was hailed as a moral victory. MULH now decided to operate through street meetings and protest demonstrations, employing trenchant political slogans aimed more at the Western press than at Soviet citizens. It was a tactic favored by American radical gay activists. Funds collected in the United States enabled the International Tema Organization to hold international symposia on gay and lesbian rights and AIDS prevention in both Leningrad and Moscow in the summer of 1991. The organizers openly showed the first gay and lesbian films to be seen in Russia. But the characteristics of Soviet-Russian politics — extremism, lack of political experience, unwillingness to confront reality — soon began to manifest in the Kalinin group. Demands by the Libertarian Party, of which MULH was a part, to legalize prostitution and drugs as well as homosexuality — each of which was controversial enough taken separately — when lumped together without detailed argument, the press being given only the bare slogans, proved counterproductive. The stereotype of homosexuality as equivalent to drug addiction and prostitution, thus deserving of equal condemnation, was reinforced. Kalinin's clumsy statements provoked public scandal and have been used by the communist and fascist mass media to compromise and defame the gay and lesbian movement. Ongoing quarrels between their leaders also diminished their political influence so that the repeal of Article 121.1 "came as a surprise to the gay and lesbian community" (Gessen, 1994, p. 56).

THE REPEAL OF ARTICLE 121

After the dissolution of the Soviet Union, some of its republics (Ukraine, Estonia, Latvia, and Armenia) revoked their antihomosexual legislation. Under strong pressure from Western public opinion and in order to obtain a place in the Council of Europe, Russian President Boris Yeltsin also followed this line and Article 121.1 was repealed as part of a wide-ranging reform law that he signed on April 29, 1993, and published 1 month later.

Article 121.2 remained in force, but the maximum punishment was reduced from 8 to 7 years imprisonment. The changes were made quietly in a package of many small legal changes without detailed explanation in the mass media. Incorporating these changes into the new Russian Criminal Code proved a long and painful process. The first draft, prepared by the Russian Ministry of Justice and published in a special issue of the magazine *Zakon* in early 1992, omitted Article 121, but included instead a new Article 132 titled "Muzhelozhstvo or gratification of sexual passion in other perverted forms." According to this, "gratification of sexual passion [or, in another version, "sexual needs"] in other perverted forms (including lesbianism)," if carried out with the use or threat of physical force, or exploiting the vulnerable state of the victim, was punishable by deprivation of freedom of up to 3 years. The punishment had to be much more severe for repeated offenses, for actions committed by persons guilty of rape or by a group, for serious damage done to the victim, or if the victim was a minor under 14. This early draft was extremely confused. Homosexual relations between consenting adults were no longer punishable, but homosexuality was still a "perversion," and the mention of lesbianism in this context was a regressive step.

In Russian law, rape is forced sexual intercourse with a nonconsenting female other than one's own wife. Technically, it must include actual vaginal penetration by the penis, so rape of a male is by definition impossible. Having no acceptable legal terms for oral or anal penetration, jurists call them "perverted forms" of sexual gratification. Sexologically, this is nonsense; in Russia, as elsewhere, anal and especially oral sex are quite popular among both heterosexuals and homosexuals.

The principle of gender equality in sexual relations also presented difficulty. Because rape was believed to be a more serious offense than any other sexual assault, the rape of an adult woman or a young girl was punishable much more severely than any forced sexual assault or penetration inflicted upon an adult male or young boy. In this context, men and boys were "cheaper" than females, but if a man had consensual sex with a sexually mature 17-year-old male he was to be imprisoned for up to 7 years, whereas the same act with a 17-year-old female would go unpunished.

This draft was criticized also for many other shortcomings and was rejected by the Supreme Soviet. A new draft Criminal Code, prepared by a group of lawyers and presented to the Duma by the Ministry of Justice and the president's legal office in mid-1994 was much better (*Ugolovny kodeks*, 1994). It still had an Article 142 on "Forced Mutzhelozhstvo," which this time was punishable exactly the same as rape. *Muzelozhstvo*, but not lesbianism, was also mentioned in Article 144 dealing with "coercion of a person to sexual intercourse." The draft as a whole was prepared carelessly. In the table of contents, Article 143, which referred to sexual coercion other than rape, was entitled, "The satisfaction of a sexual passion in the perverted forms," whereas in the text itself it was named "Forced actions directed to the satisfaction of sexual needs." In a later version of the draft "perverted forms" has been reinstated. An earlier version, formulated by A. N. Ignatov,[3] in which

---

[3]Professor Ignatov was especially active and persistent as a member of the working group trying to convince his more conservative colleagues. After I sent my criticisms and suggestions in a letter to the Duma, I was invited for a personal discussion with the Duma's Committee on Legislation. The Deputy Chairman of the Committee, V. V. Pokhmelkin, agreed with almost all of my suggestions, but Professor I. M. Galperin was against them. To clear the matter of "perverted forms" I asked them, "Gentlemen, I imagine you have oral sex with your wives and lovers without any remorse, yet in your draft law you call it "perversion." Have we not enough hypocrisy in this country?"

sexual orientation was not mentioned at all, had mysteriously disappeared at the last moment without the working group as a whole having been told of the change.

After prolonged discussion a compromise version was accepted. The new Penal Code was accepted by the State Duma in July 1995, but it was rejected by the Council of the federation and by President Yeltsin. The newly elected (December 1995) Duma again returned to the issue, and the new version of the code was finally approved by both Houses in June 1996, was signed by the president, and has been in effect since January 1, 1997.

Chapter 18 of the Code is named "Crimes against sexual inviolability and sexual freedom of individuality," which is an improvement on the 1994 draft title, "Crimes in the sphere of sexual relations." The separate articles on "forced Muzhelozhstvo" and "perverted forms of sexual satisfaction" are deleted, but Article 132 covers "forced actions of a sexual nature":

(1) Muzhelozhstvo, lesbianism or other actions of a sexual character committed by use of force or threat thereof against the victim or against other persons, or by exploiting the victim's vulnerability are punished by deprivation of freedom from three to six years.

(2) The same actions, if they are committed:
  a) several times or by a person previously convicted of the crimes foreseen by the articles of this chapter;
  b) by a group of persons with a premeditated conspiracy or by an organized group;
  c) which resulted in a victim's infection of a venereal disease;
  d) wittingly against an underaged person;
  are punished by deprivation of freedom from four to ten years.

(3) Actions which are foreseen by the first and second parts of the present Article if they:
  a) carelessly brought about the death of a victim;
  b) carelessly inflicted heavy damage to his/her health, caused HIV infection or some other heavy consequences;
  c) are committed wittingly against a person under fourteen years old;
  are punished by deprivation of freedom from eight to fifteen years. (Ugolovny Kodeks, 1996)

Article 133 on "Coercive acts of a sexual character" states that: "Coercion of a person into sexual intercourse, *muzhelozhstvo*, lesbianism or other actions of a sexual nature by use of blackmail, threat of destruction, damage or withdrawal of property, or by exploiting the victim's material or other dependency, is punished by fines or corrective work up to two years or deprivation of freedom up to one year." No specific sexual acts, such as oral or anal penetration, are mentioned, and whether the behavior is homosexual or heterosexual makes no difference.

The law makes an important symbolic tribute to the principle of gender equality in that, with the exception of rape, which requires a female victim, all other criminal sexual actions, such as violence, compulsion, or coercion, can be directed against persons of either gender, the victims in all cases being referred to in the law as she or he. The legal age of consent for voluntary sexual relations in the 1995 draft was set at 14 without any of the differences for gender or for heterosexual or homosexual behavior, which still exist in some countries. In the final version of the code, Article 134 provides that sexual intercourse, *muzhelozhstvo*, or lesbianism wittingly committed by a person over 18 on a person under 16 is punished by limitation of freedom up to 3 years or deprivation of freedom up to 4 years.

Generally, the new law represents a compromise solution. Partly through personal conviction and partly for political reasons, the legislators refused to eliminate homosexuality altogether from the criminal code. An open defense of homosexuality could be detrimental to the electoral prospects of any political party. Paradoxically, only the arch-reactionary Vladimir Zhirinovsky, among all Russian political leaders, had the courage, before the 1993 elections, to defend publicly, in a long speech on television, the human rights and reputation of homosexuals. But since that was the only evidence of his "liberalism," his words can't be taken seriously. All other political parties, including "democrats" (who have been accused of being pro-Western and ruining the Russian economy), try to appear as conservative as possible on family matters. The defense of "traditional Russian family values" is hardly compatible with sexual liberalism.

All the same, homosexual contacts between consenting adults have finally been decriminalized. The inclusion of lesbianism for the first time in Russian legislation follows the principle of gender equality; possibly the provision will receive only lip service with no practical consequences. The fact that *muzhelozhstvo* and lesbianism are no longer defined offensively as "perverted" or "unnatural," but mentioned at the same level as sexual intercourse, is a reminder that all forms of otherwise acceptable sexual acts are illegal if nonconsenting.

CHANGING PUBLIC OPINION

The social situation of sexual minorities is everywhere affected by public attitudes, which do not change overnight. Homophobia and discrimination against gay men and lesbians are still conspicuous in present-day Russian sexual and political culture. Soviet society has been characterized by extreme intolerance of any dissident thinking or uncommon behavior, even if entirely innocent, and homosexuals are the most stigmatized of social minorities.

According to a national survey in November 1989 by VTsIOM, which used a representative sample of 2600 people from all over the Soviet Union, attitudes toward homosexuals were considerably more hostile than toward all other negatively evaluated social groups, including prostitutes and drug addicts, with whom homosexuals are frequently linked through tendentious anti-AIDS propaganda. Among responses to the question: "How are we to treat homosexuals?", 33 percent were in favor of "liquidation," 30 percent for "isolation," 10 percent for "leaving them alone," and only 6 percent for "helping them."[4] The degrees of intolerance varied with educational level (38 percent of those with incomplete secondary education favored "liquidation," compared with 22 percent of those with higher education) and also with age, the most intolerant being those over 50. Intolerance was virtually unrelated to gender. Old-age pensioners, housewives, and military personnel exhibited maximum homophobia, while small-scale entrepreneurs ("cooperators") were the least intolerant, with none for "liquidation" and 25 percent for helping. Regionally, homophobia was strongest in Uzbekistan, where 54 percent were for "liquida-

[4]Because not all VCIOM data from this and later surveys have been published, VCIOM's Director, Professor Yury Levada, generously gave me permission to quote directly from the tables. Some of the data can be found in Levada (1994, 1995) and Bocharova (1994).

tion," followed by Georgia and Armenia, with 45 percent for "liquidation." Muslims seemed to be less tolerant than Christians, but much depended on the size of the local community, Muscovites being more tolerant than villagers or residents of far-flung towns.

Another sociological survey, undertaken in July 1990 by the Youth Institute in 16 regions of Russia, with a sample of 1500, of whom 26 percent were under 30, again revealed homosexuals to be the most hated group: 62 percent of answers were sharply condemnatory, 20 percent were neutral, and only 0.6 percent were positive, with 8 percent declining to answer (Rylyova, 1991).

It used to be difficult for Russians even to discuss these issues. In analyzing the results of the VTsIOM survey, sociologists identified two extreme groups of respondents, *tolerants* and *rigid repressors*, who were opposites in virtually all their opinions, including those about homosexuality. One group favored social assistance for homosexuals; the other wanted extermination. The only point on which they agreed was that the problem of homosexual relationships should not be debated in the press (Gudkov, 1991).

In 1990, the Russian Academy of Sciences Sociology Institute and the International Center for Human Values surveyed the views of people in the European part of the USSR (a sample of 4309) on their attitudes toward various ethnic and political groups, including homosexuals. Evaluated on an 11-point scale from "I do not like at all" to "I like very much," homosexuals were shown once again to be highly unpopular, taking third place in terms of hostility after neo-Nazis and Stalinists; 68.7 percent of men and 69.4 percent of women took the extreme negative position on the scale. In terms of age, the most hostile were those in the 41–50 age range. In this sample education did not reduce homophobia; those with a secondary professional education showed maximum hostility, and those with a university education were in second place with 70.4 percent extremely negative.[5]

In 1991, a survey by the U.S. scholars James Gibson and Ray Duch, covering the entire territory of the USSR, produced similar findings: Homosexuals took second place in hostility after neo-fascists and were placed in the "don't like at all" category by 58.2 percent of men and 58.6 percent of women. Youths' responses were slightly more tolerant (by 4–6 percent) than those of older persons (Gibson & Duch, 1991).

In the June 1993 Russian survey by VTsIOM, with 1665 respondents, the question was put: "How would you evaluate, on a scale from 1 to 5, the behavior of people having homosexual contacts?" The negative pole was chosen by 69.4 percent of men and 71.6 percent of women. The positive pole (nothing bad) was taken by only 8.8 and 7.8 percent, respectively. The oldest age group (55–84) was the least tolerant, with 82.6 and 4.8 percent being at the negative and positive ends of the scale, respectively. However, the youngest age group (16–25) was less negative, with corresponding percentages of 54.3 and 18.5, respectively. Women of this age were the most tolerant, 22 percent seeing "nothing bad," compared with only 13 percent of males of similar age. The degree of polarization of opinion was less among the better educated. Whereas 16 percent of the general population endorsed the second or third points on the scale (that is neutral or only mild, conditional censure), a quarter of the more socially advanced, young, and better educated people did so, as did almost 30 percent of students. Attitudes were not so much related to political views (those supporting economic reforms were only slightly less censorious than the average for the whole sample) than upon principles of evaluation. For some who were not censorious,

[5]Quoted by kind permission of Professor Mikhail S. Matskovsky.

"normal" was not what is demanded by society, but what is good and acceptable to the participants in any interaction.

The VTsIOM survey of July 1994 (1771 respondents) asked "What is your attitude to homosexuals?" Negative expressions were endorsed by 56 percent, neutral by 30 percent, and positive by only 9 percent. To the question "Should homosexuals have equal rights with other people?" the percentages saying "yes," "uncertain," and "no" were 38, 21, and 41, respectively. Seemingly, even some who dislike homosexuality are ready to accept the principle of equal civil rights.

Despite the prevailing negative attitude toward homosexuals, there have been some positive trends in public consciousness in the last 5 years. When, in November 1994, VTsIOM replicated its 1989 survey, it appeared that Russians had become somewhat more tolerant of all stigmatized groups, including homosexuals. Those wanting to "liquidate" them dropped from 27 to 18 percent and those wishing to "isolate" them from 32 to 23 percent, while those wishing to "help" them rose from 6 to 8 percent and those opting "to leave them to themselves" rose from 12 to 29. (These figures are not for the whole of the USSR, which were quoted in the 1989 survey, but for the Russian Federation only) (Levada, 1994). In this latest survey the demographic differences were slightly changed. Gender differences were small, but women appeared a little more tolerant than men. Age differences were strong. In the youngest group (up to age 24) the percentages for "liquidation," "isolation," "helping," and "leaving to themselves" were 17.5, 14.7, 14.8, and 40.8, respectively. The corresponding figures for the oldest group (over 55) were 32.1, 28.7, 5.3, and 12.3. Educational level was another important factor. Among those with a completed or unfinished university education, 11 percent were for "liquidation" and 43.3 percent for "leaving to themselves"; the corresponding figures for those with less than secondary school education were 28.9 and 20.4, respectively. By occupation, managers and professionals were the most tolerant, pensioners the least tolerant. Place of residence and degree of urbanization were also important correlates. In Moscow and St. Petersburg only 16.6 percent were for "liquidation" compared with 21 percent in other cities and 27 percent in rural communities. Siberia and the Far East were the most intolerant areas.

The attitudes of youth have been also surveyed (Chervyakov, Kon, & Shapiro, unpublished data). In a 1995 survey of 2872 16- to 19-year-olds in Moscow, Novgorod, (a medium-sized city), and Borisoglebsk and Yeletz (two small towns in central Russia), the question was asked: "What is your attitude to homosexuals of your own sex?" The option "no attitude, never thought about this topic" was chosen by 29.5 percent of males and 37 percent of females. "I regard them with sympathy and understanding" was chosen by 2.6 percent and 9.3 percent, respectively. The neutral option, "I regard them tolerantly, don't see anything extraordinary in them" was chosen by 19.2 percent and 32.5 percent, and the negative option "I feel aversion to them" was chosen by 48.4 percent and 21.2 percent.

In a more impersonal question on social policy, 28.3 percent of males and 35.6 percent of females strongly agreed with the statement: "At present same-sex intimacy should not be condemned." The percentages responding "rather agree than disagree" were 15.2 and 22.1, while 32.3 and 21.3 expressed strong or moderate disagreement, and 24.2 and 21.1 were unsure. Young men were generally less tolerant than young women and less willing to acknowledge having experienced some same-sex contact, attraction, or even attention. This may be related to the general adolescent male machismo complex and the difficulties of male gender socialization. Nevertheless, according to opinion surveys, Russian male adolescents appear to be less intolerant than their U.S. counterparts.

In the context of Russian politics, the social groups that are ready to accept a market economy and welcome political democracy are the ones who promote ideas of tolerance. In the context of a broad international picture, the trends identified in Russian cohorts are quite similar to those found in Western countries (Inglehart, 1990). But public opinion polls need to be interpreted with caution. The VTsIOM surveys of June 1993 and July 1994 suggest that the general level of homophobia in Russia is much the same as in the United States (Laumann, Gagnon, Michael, & Michael, 1994; Smith, 1990). Considering that as recently as 1993 any homosexual behavior was a criminal offense in Russia, that for 70 years the topic had been unmentionable, that Russia had no scholars comparable to Kinsey or Freud, and that Western sexological ideas are still unknown even to professionals, the similarity of opinion trends is remarkable. Yet, despite the similarities, American and Russian mentality and behavior are different. Americans may express moral disapproval, but it is unlikely that one-third or even one-sixth of Americans would vote for the extermination of their fellow citizens. A liberal American intellectual may privately despise gays and lesbians but hesitate to express such feelings, knowing that they have become politically incorrect and open to challenge. Some people are even ashamed of their true feelings.

In contemporary Russia, antisemitism, homophobia, and xenophobia are unconcealed, even fashionable. The chauvinist mass media (e.g., *Sovetskaya Rossiya, Zavtra, Russkoye voskresenie, Nash sovremennik, Molodaya gvardia*) deliberately incite and actively propagate homophobia. The fascist press methodically and consistently lumps together Bolshevism, Zionism, democracy, and homosexuality. The newspaper *Russkoye voskresenie*, for example, ran an article under the title "Let us defend Russian orthodoxy against the Yids." "Both the Bolsheviks and democratic leaders are of foreign extraction. Both are sexual perverts. You will recall that the first decree issued by the Soviet Government was to revoke punishment for homosexuality. Now it's the democrats who are after the same thing" (Deutsch, 1991, p. 8).

There is strong opposition in Russia to the legalization or "normalization" of same-sex love and relationships. In a television interview on June 28, 1993, the former vice president, Alexander Rutskoy, said with a squeamish gesture, as if pushing something away from him, "In a civilized society there should be no sexual minorities." Valery Skurlatov, a leader of the extreme nationalistic Vozrozhdenie Party, said at a press conference in August 1993 that "70 percent of the men in Yeltsin's cabinet are homosexuals" who pose a danger to state security because of their "hostility toward healthy citizens" and "their links to foreign homosexuals." He proposed forming a parliamentary commission to investigate the sexual preferences of government officials. "Russians have never stood for homosexuality," he said. "We have decided to campaign actively to bring the truth about homosexuality in the government to the people" (Filipov, 1993, p. 1).

Reactionary politicians are supported in such views by police officers and by some representatives of the medical profession. In 1988, the eminent Russian epidemiologist, Professor Valentin Pokrovsky, expressed his utmost distaste for the views of a group of medical students who wanted the extermination of AIDS sufferers and homosexuals. Not long after, however, as a member of the Gorbachev presidential commission for combating pornography, he said that in his opinion AIDS was "a moral sickness in society" and that demands to legalize homosexuality were absurd. When the interviewer mentioned that homosexuality was a disease he replied, "That's exactly the point. There are people who are genetically predisposed to that kind of sexual contact. It is ridiculous to call that normal. It is even more so to regard as normal and healthy people who get mixed up in homosexual affairs and seduce young children in their sexual excesses. It is not a disease, it is dissipation that must be combated, particularly through the courts" (Likholitov, 1991, p. 14). Professor Pokrovsky did not explain by what criteria or by whom — doctors or police — the sick and the dissolute should be differentiated.

Dr. Mikhail Buyanov (1994), a well-known Moscow psychiatrist who had been during *perestroika* a vocal critic of the former Soviet "repressive psychiatry," published a newspaper article entitled "Pathology Should Not Take Hold of the Masses," which was full of hatred toward homosexuals and their sympathizers and advocated strong, repressive measures. He claimed that homosexuality had always been alien to Russia and that its current popularity was the result of Western, mostly American and British, ideological expansionism. A St. Petersburg doctor, B. Irzak (1993), unlike Buyanov, supports decriminalization and is against society's interference in private life, but is worried about "normalization" and "popularizing" of same-sex love: "As a biological phenomenon, homosexuality is in need of research, and as a social phenomenon it should be put under strict control" (p. 4).

AIDS is also often used as a pretext for an anti-gay stance. Dr. Vadim V. Pokrovsky (1995), head of the Russian state AIDS prevention center, several times supported the decriminalization of homosexuality. Nevertheless, in a programmatic article about AIDS prevention strategy, including work with sexual minorities, he talks about the "moral degradation of the population" that manifests in particular in the "homosexualization of the culture (p.)." Same-sex love is for him as undesirable as sexual promiscuity, drug addiction, and prostitution.

Even some liberal and prodemocratic Russian intellectuals, who reject fascism and antisemitism, talk publicly about the existence of a dangerous international homosexual conspiracy. At the meeting of leading Russian intellectuals with the presidential administration, famous Russian writer Fazil Iskander suggested introduction of a moral censorship against the "invasion on TV of the aggressive strata of sexual minorities" (Polevaya, 1996). This idea was supported by pianist Nikolai Petrov and mildly opposed only by Mstislav Rostropovich. Such statements sometimes reflect a psychological overreaction against the excessive, noisy, sensationalist, and exhibitionistic presentation of homosexuality in the mass media.

Russians are unaccustomed to such display. Especially for the strongly normative and repressive Russian psychiatry, a pluralistic attitude toward sexual orientation is also unacceptable. This intolerance may have serious practical consequences. Should the country take a radical turn towards a new authoritarian regime, gays and lesbians and their sympathizers, along with Jewish intellectuals, could be the first candidates for concentration camps and liquidation.

PROBLEMS AND PROSPECTS

The most obvious social change in Russia is the disappearance of the old conspiracy of silence and the appearance of same-sex love as a fashionable topic for newspapers, art, and salon conversation. Roman Viktyuk, the most popular theater director in Moscow, is openly gay and his theater is always full. A famous St. Petersburg choreographer, Boris Eifman, has staged a successful ballet dedicated to Tchaikovsky's life. Problems of gay and lesbian life are openly discussed on television as well as in newspapers. Classic films from the West with homosexual allusions, or even completely devoted to gay and lesbian life, are shown in the cinemas and on television. Literature about homosexuality, such as Mikhail Kuzmin's classical poetry and his famous novel *Krylya*, as well as novels by Jean Genet, James Baldwin, and Truman Capote, are now available, and a two-volume collection of the late Russian gay writer, actor, and theater director Evengii Kharitonov was published for the first time in 1993.

Changes can also be seen in everyday life. Whereas Russian gays used to have to meet each other in the streets or public toilets, which was dirty and risky, now there are a few openly gay discos and bars in Moscow and St. Petersburg; they are very expensive, however, and are practically monopolized by *nouveau riches* and foreigners on the one hand and male prostitutes on the other. Describing a gay restaurant in Moscow, a visitor commented: "The street-sex heritage, in combination with the typical male mentality — all men are sexy animals — turns many victims of passion into a commodity in this market. Here men buy others and sell themselves. It is a constant haggle, a real market where attractive but impecunious youth pay for merriment and satiety to rich, but no longer fresh, old age, using the only currency youth has — their own bodies (Paramonov, 1993, p. 60).

Gays and lesbians now have their own newspapers and journals. After 13 issues, Roman Kalinin's *Tema* ceased in 1993, having, according to him, "fulfilled its historical mission," but the magazine *Ravenstvo Iskrennost-Svoboda-Kompromis* (RISK) [*Equality/Sincerity/Freedom/Compromise*], founded by Vladislav Ortanov, of which seven issues with a print run of about 5000 have been published by 1995, continues. In 1994 Ortanov turned over his editorial position to Dimitry Kuzmin and launched a new illustrated homoerotic journal, *ARGO*. The most stable of the Russian lesbian and gay newspapers is *1/10*, edited by Dmitry Lyshov, which has a print run of about 30,000. Similar gay and lesbian newspapers are published in the provinces (e.g., *Gei-dialog, Dialog-plus*). An information bulletin of Russian organization "Genderdoc" *Zerkalo* [*The Mirror*] has been published in Moscow since January 1995.

Letters and notices appearing in such periodicals show that the lifestyles and problems of Russian gays are as multifarious as in the West. One typical personal ad reads: "Social, easy-going, intelligent young man, 22/180.58, seeks tall, sports-loving, educated gay friend with decent statistics and 22–28 cm. size penis." Many of these young men frankly are seeking rich patrons, but there are other ads searching for love and friendship.

In 1992 *RISK* (no. 2–3) opened up a debate on permanent partnerships, and one 19-year-old wrote, "In my view all this talk about constancy is just a load of rubbish.... To sleep all the time with the same person is boring: it's hardly conceivable! I'm not a monster, thank God, and can find any number of fellows I want: Different bodies, different lips, different pricks — a new thrill every time. Maybe in a score or more years, when I won't need any of this, I'll have to tie myself down with someone permanent, but for the time being you can keep it, thank you very much" (p. 5). Alongside this note was another letter from a 27-year-old:

> I don't see any problem with having a permanent partner. Simply speaking, since he walked into my life a year ago, my life has gained a purpose and fullness. I want him constantly, all the time, but that isn't the point. For some time now sex has been secondary: we haven't anywhere to live anyway, so we spend most of our time walking

the streets and drinking tea with his or my friends whom we have both known for some time. You could probably call us permanent partners, but he is no "partner" to me, he is the man I love. And that's forever" (p. 6)

Gay and lesbian organizations now operate in many big cities. St. Petersburg, for example, has the Tchaikovsky Cultural Initiative and Defense Fund and the Krylya [Wings] Homosexual Defense Association. Krylya was initially called Nevskie berega [the banks of the river Neva] and then Nevskaya Perspektiva [Neva Perspectives], but the city fathers thought these names were advocating the homosexualization of the district. Similar organizations and publications have arisen in the former Soviet republics (Ukraine, Belarus, Latvia, Estonia) and in other Russian cities (e.q., Nizhny Tagil, Barnaul, Kaluga, Murmansk, Rostov).

Separate associations for lesbians also exist in Moscow and St. Petersburg. Moskovskaye Obyedinenie Lesbijskoi Literatury i Iskusstva (MOLLI) — The Moscow Union of Lesbian Literature and Art — was founded in 1991 by Mila Ugolkova and Lyubov Zinovieva for humanitarian and cultural activities. In St. Petersburg there is a lesbian Club of Independent Women, which published six issues of a magazine *Probuzhdenie* [*Awakening*]. The anonymous editors complained bitterly about the attitude of the feminist Center of Gender Problems: "You are right, honorable ladies, we are not your sisters!" (Publication data not available). This was in reference to the feminist bulletin *All People are Sisters*.

The political clout of the lesbian and gay organizations is negligible. Although most of the groups were formed as political organizations, they have actually focused primarily on community building, social gatherings, discos, dating services, and setting up telephone hotlines (Gessen, 1994). Prominent artists and intellectuals are in no hurry to "come out" and join these organizations. This is because they are, with reason, afraid, partly because they prefer privacy to American-style publicity and partly because, like most Russians today, they feel a general aversion to politics and believe that gay politics is no better than any other.

The idea of a separate gay identity does not appeal to many Russians. The American author Andrew Solomon (1993) was told by a gay Russian friend: "Activism occurs here because Westerners put Russians up to it. My good friends know I am gay, but it's my private business. I'm not interested in telling everyone that I like to sleep with men." Another informant added: "I don't want to be part of a subculture. I know that's the fashion in the West, but though I may choose to sleep mainly with gay men that doesn't mean I want to socialize primarily with them (p. 22).

Without some sort of organizational support, however, there is nobody to defend the human rights of sexual minorities. The Russian state and all its established political parties are either openly hostile or indifferent. In August 1994 Treugolnik [Triangle] Center, a regional social lesbian, gay, and bisexual organization was established. This association is supported by the International Gay and Lesbian Human Rights Commission (IGLHRC) and is linked to the International Lesbian and Gay Association (ILGA). However, the Moscow Justice Department refused its legal registration (in a letter of July 21, 1995) on the grounds that the organization "contradicts social norms of morality" and fails to meet the requirements of the federal law on "voluntary social organizations."

Despite obvious achievements, homosexuals in Russia remain "a marginalized and maligned community" (Gessen, 1994, p. 59). They are subject both to public prejudice and to state discrimination in every field of social and private life. If the Moscow Justice Department can discriminate against the organization of homosexuals on "moral" grounds, an even worse reception may be expected in the provinces. Most Russian state officials, especially police officers, are strongly homophobic, and gay-bashing is widespread. Organized bands of hooligans, sometimes acting with the silent acquiescence of the police, blackmail, rob, assault, and even murder gay men. They portray their actions as protecting public morals, calling it *remont* [repair work] — that is, eliminating vice with their own methods. The police often blame the victims for having provoked such crimes. Since gays are afraid of reporting such incidents, they mostly go unpunished. Many common murders and robberies of gays are attributed by the police to pathological homosexual jealousy. Old police records and lists of known homosexuals are preserved and can be used for blackmail. In the absence of effective legal control, the victims have no defense. But then, practically any Russian citizen risks facing such situations.

In 1993 the IGLHRC reported numerous cases of discrimination. After the repeal of Article 121.1, legal and prison authorities have been in no hurry to release the victims of that law. When an IGLHRC delegation tried to collect information about prisoners and their possible release, many officials were unwilling to help. Sometimes it was through mere bureaucratic inertia and lack of specific instructions. One official told them: "We have a thousand inmates here. Do you want me to look through everybody's file?" In other cases, open animosity was expressed: "I don't care what has been repealed. They're still in there and they will stay in there." Or, "They chose this life for themselves, don't deny that they are this way, so why should we try to protect them?" (Gessen, 1994. pp. 28–29).

Sexual abuse is a serious problem in Russian prisons and, to a lesser extent, in the army. According to a medicopsychological investigation of 246 male convicts registered by one prison camp's administration as having had homosexual contacts, all claimed to have been raped. Half of them said it had happened for the first time during their preliminary confinement before trial, 39 percent while on their way to the penal colony and 11 percent in the camp itself (Shakirov, 1991). Most of these young men had had no previous homosexual experience, but after these incidents they became so-called *opushchennye* [degraded], required to submit to anything others demanded of them. The authorities are aware that this is a serious problem. When questioned by a police sociologist, 74 percent of police officers working in correctional institutions acknowledged that homosexual contacts were rife there (Dyachenko, 1995), yet 13 percent thought this was the result of "inborn homosexual drive," and 45 percent blamed the bad influence of older homosexuals. In their view the only means of prevention of prison rapes and homosexual contacts were stronger punitive measures. Given the present legislation and attitudes, the obvious risk of prison epidemics are not tackled. For example, one HIV-prevention agency was not allowed to give inmates free condoms. Since prisoners are supposed to have no sex life, condoms are formally forbidden.

The strong public and official homophobia means that gays and lesbians are afraid to come out to their work colleagues, friends, or even parents. Some are terribly lonely, and gay newspapers are full of sad letters. Most people understand that in the relations between men and women there is much more involved than sex, but same-sex love tends to be thought of as exclusively a matter of exotic, unusual, and dangerous sex. To combat this stereotype, I organized, within the framework of a large, government-sponsored international conference in Moscow in June 1994 (Family on the Eve of the Third Millennium), a roundtable entitled "Same-Sex Marriages: Moral and Legal Issues." The discussion was lively and interesting; as a result, the participants, and later the plenary session of the conference, recommended unanimously the inclusion of some form of state registration of same-sex couples in the Russian family code. Although several deputies belonging to the Women of Russia faction had been present and voiced no objection to the proposal, they did not inform the Duma's legislative committee about it. No Russian newspaper saw fit to cover the discussion.

Public health authorities are equally resistive. Official governmental health services, headed by Dr. Pokrovsky, openly despise and ignore lesbian and gay organizations that are actively involved with AIDS prevention. The dislike is mutual. Sexual health education is generally poor in Russia, and this is true among gay men as well. Among a sample of 290 gay men in St. Petersburg who were questioned at gay organizations, beaches, and discos in 1993 (Dmitry D. Isaev, personal communication) promiscuity was high, with 40.5 percent reporting more than 20 partners and 27.5 percent more than 50 partners. Anonymous and short-time contacts were preferred by 14 percent, and only 12 percent had had sex only with a permanent partner. Although 47 percent said they had worried about HIV infection, only 12.5 percent used condoms regularly, a third never did so, and another third thought it sufficient to use them only for casual contacts and anal sex. Unsurprisingly, 19 percent had had some sexually transmitted disease; 2 percent had one more than once.[6]

As previously mentioned, AIDS is often used as an argument against decriminalization of homosexuality. A new federal law gives the government an unchecked power to establish a list of professions and occupations whose members must pass HIV testing. In view of past experience of Soviet repressive medicine, gays have reason to fear this provision will be applied in a discriminatory manner.

Living in an atmosphere of secrecy and fear, many gays and lesbians have personal problems, but for them access to effective psychological services is difficult. They are afraid to approach official Russian state psychiatry, which always was, and still is, prejudiced, hostile, and ignorant about homosexuality. The new breed of self-educated, private psychoanalysts are even more ignorant. Even in Moscow and St. Petersburg it is difficult to find a doctor who is both well educated and sympathetic.

Finally, it has to be said that, however bad the situation may be for homosexuals in Russia today, it is much better than it was in most times past, say 2, 5, 10, 20, or 60 years ago. Some of the present difficulties should disappear in time, but some will need special measures. Russian gay organizations receive a little money from abroad, mainly for political purposes, but collaboration in comparative social research or help with the education of doctors, social workers, and other professionals dealing with individuals seems harder to obtain. Continual pressure on the Russian government by the West on matters of human rights is very welcome, but other forms of constructive help are also needed.

Acknowledgments

This chapter was prepared with the financial help of grants from the John D. and Catherine T. MacArthur Foundation and the Russian Foundation for research in Humanities. Also gratefully acknowledged is the support of the Center for Multiethnic and

[6]Preliminary data of this survey, based on a sample of 160 gay men, were published in Isayev (1993).

Transcultural Studies and the Center for Feminist Research at the University of Southern California and ONE Institute/International Gay and Lesbian Archives. Some materials in this chapter have been earlier published by the author in *The Sexual Revolution in Russia: From the Time of the Czar to Today* (James Riordan, trans.), New York, The Free Press, 1995. They are reprinted with the kind permission of the publisher.

REFERENCES

Billington, J. H. (1970). *The icon and the axe: An interpretative history of Russian culture*. New York: Vintage.

Bocharova, O. A. (1994). Seksualnaya svoboda: slova i dela. *Chelovek*, 5, 98–107.

Borisenko, K. K. (1990). *Zabolevaniya, peredavaevye polovym putyom u muzhchingomosekualistov (diagnostika, taktika vedenyia lechenie). Metodicheskie rekomendatsii*. Moscow: Ministerstvo zdravookhranenia RSFSR.

Burgasov, N. P. (1986). Vystuplenic na kruglom stole. Literaturnaya gazeta, No. 7, p. 15.

Burgin, D. L. (1994). *Sophia Parnok. The life and work of Russia's Sappho*. New York: New York University Press.

Buyanov, M. (1994, March 17) Pathology should not take hold of the masses. *Rossiiskie vesti*, p. 4.

Deutsch, M. (1991). Uzelki na 'Pamyat' *Ogonyok*, 51, p. 8.

Dyachenko, A. P. (1995). *Ugolovno-pravovaya okhrana grazhdan v sfere seksualnykh otnoshenii*. Moscow: Akademia MVD Rossii.

Engelstein, L. (1992). *The keys to happiness: Sex and the search for modernity in fin de siècle Russia*. Ithaca: Cornell University Press.

Engelstein, L. (1995). Soviet policy toward male homosexuality: Its origins and historical roots. In G. Hekma, H. Oosterhuis, & J. Steakley (Eds.), *Gay men and the sexual history of the political left* (pp. 155–178). New York: Haworth Press.

Filipov, D. (1993, August 28). From graft to gays: Nationalists alter attack. *The Moscow Times*, pp. 1–2.

Gessen, M. (1994). *The rights of lesbians and gay men in the Russian Federation*. San Francisco: International Gay and Lesbian Human Rights Commission.

Gibson, J. L., & Duch, R. M. (1991). *Post-materialism and the emerging Soviet democracy*. Paper presented at the 1991 meeting of the American Political Science Association, Washington, DC.

Gomoseksualizm. (1952). Bolshaya Sovestskaya Ensiklopedia, Second ed., Vol. 12, Moscow, 1952, p. 35.

Gudkov, L. D. (1991). Fenomen 'prostoty.' O natsionalnom samosoznanii russkikh. *Chelovek*, 1, pp. 13–23.

Healey, D. (1991). *A social history of homosexuality 1917–1934*. Unpublished master's thesis, School of Slavonic and East European Studies, University of London.

Ignatov, A. N. (1974). *Kvalifikatsia ugolovnykh prestuplenlii*. Moscow: Yurizdat.

Inglehart, R. (1990). *Culture shift in advanced industrial society*. Princeton, NJ: Princeton University Press.

Irzak, B. (1993, July 1). Zholtyi, krasnyi, goluboy — vybirai sebe lyuboi? Shto dolshno delat' bolshinstvo, kogda gomoseksualizm vkhodit v modu? *Komsomolskaya pravda*, p. 4.

Isayev, D. D. (1993, June–August). Survey of the sexual behavior of gay men in Russia. *ILGA Bulletin*, 3, 12.

Isayev, D. N., Kagan, V. Y., & Kon, I. S. (1986). Formirovanie seksualnoi orientatsii. In D. N. Isayev & V. Y. Kagan (Eds.), *Psikhogigiena pola u detei* (pp. 47–65). Leningrad: Meditsina.

Karlinsky, S. (1976). Russia's gay literature and history (11th to 20th centuries). *Gay Sunshine*, 29/30, 1–7.

Karlinsky, S. (1989). Russia's gay history and culture: The impact of the October Revolution. In M. L. Duberman, M. Vicinus, & G. Chauncey Jr. (Eds.), *Hidden from history: Reclaiming the gay and lesbian past* (pp. 347–363). New York: NAL Books.

Khripkova, A. G., & Kolesov, D. V. (1982). *Malchik-podrostok-yunosha*. Moscow: Prosveshchenie.

Kon, I. S. (1988). *Vvedenie v seksologiyu*. Moscow: Meditsina.

Kon, I. S. (1989). *Psikhologiya rannei yunosti*. Moscow: Prosveshchenie.

Kon, I. S. (1991). *Vkus zapretnovo ploda*. Moscow: Molodaya gvardia.

Kon, I. S. (1993). Sexual minorities. In I. Kon & J. Riordan (Eds.), *Sex and Russian society* (pp. 89–115). Bloomington: Indiana University Press.

Kon, I. S. (1995). *The sexual revolution in Russia: From the age of the czars to today* (Trans. James Riordan). New York: Free Press.

Kozlovsky, V. (1986). *Argo Russkoi gomoseksualnoi subcultury*. Benson, VT: Chalidze.

Laumann, E. O., Gagnon, J. H., Michael, R. T., & Michael, S. (1994). *The social organization of sexuality: Sexual practices in the United States.* Chicago: Chicago University Press.

Levada, Y. A. (1994). *Sovetskii prostoi chelovek.* Moscow: Mizoui Okean.

Levada, Y. A. (1995, January/February). 'Chelovek sovetskii' pyat' let spustya: 1989–1994 (predvaritelnye itogi ravnitelnovo issledovania). *Informatsionnyi byulleten monitoringa,* 10.

Levin, E. (1989). *Sex and society in the world of the Orthodox Slavs, 900–1700.* Ithaca, NY: Cornell University Press.

Likholitov, V. (1991, February 1). Obnazhonnaya natura—sevodnya i ezhednevno. Interviews Valentinom Pokrovskim. *Megapolis-Express,* 6, 14.

Nabokov, V. D. (1902). Plotskie prestupleniya, po proektu ugolovnovo ulozheniya. *Vestnik prava,* #9-10. Reprinted in V. D. Nabokov (1904) *Sbornik statei po ugolovnomu pravu.* St. Petersburg.

Ortanov, V., Yevgeniev, K., & Zubov, A. (1950). Obraschchenie assotsiataii seksualnykh menshinstr-SPID-info, 12, p. 10.

Paramonov, S. (1993). Noch otrazenij. *TY,* 2, pp. 58–62.

Piatnitsky, B. I. (1910). *Polovye izvrashchenia i ugolovnoe pravo.* Mogilev.

Pokrovsky, V. (1995, March 1). Lozhka myoda v bochke dyogtya. *Meditsinskaya gazeta,* p. 4.

Polevaya, T. (1996). Chevo khotyat deyateli Kultury? *Nezarisimaya gazeta.* August, 210, p. 7.

Popov, A. (1904). *Sud i nakazaniya za prestupleniya protiv very i nravstvennosti po russkomu pravu.* Kazan, Russia.

Poznansky, A. (1988). Tchaikovsky's suicide: Myth and reality. *19th Century Music,* 11, 199–220.

Poznansky, A. (1991). *Tschaikovsky: The quest for the inner man.* New York: Schirmer.

Rylyova, S. I. (1991). Plyuralizatsia tsernnostnovo soznanyia molodyozhi *Tsennosti sotsialnykh grupp i krizis obshchestva.* Moscow: Institute Filosofii.

Samoilov, L. (1993). *Perevyornutyi mir.* St. Petersburg: FARN.

Sereisky, M. (1930). Gomoseksualizm. *Bolshaya Sovetskaya Entsiklopediya* (vol. 17, pp. 593–596). Moscow: Columns.

Shakirov, M. T. (1991). *Zabolevaniya, peredavaemye polovym putyom, u mushchin-gomoseksualistov.* Avtoreferat dissertatsii na soiskanie uchenoi stepeni doctora meditsinskikh nauk. Moscow.

Shargorodsky, M., & Osipov, P. (1973). *Kurs sovetskovo ugolovnovo prava* (part 3). Leningrad: Izdatelstvo LGU.

Smith, T. W. (1990). The sexual revolution (the polls—a report). *Public Opinion Quarterly,* 54(3), 415–421.

Solomon, A. (1993, July 18). Young Russia's defiant decadence. *New York Times Magazine.*

Ugolovnoe ulhozhenie, Vysochaishe utverzhdennoe 23 marta 1903 goda (1903). St. Petersburg.

Ugolovny kodeks Rossiiskoi Federatsii (Osobennaya chast). Proekt (1994). Moscow: Ministerstro yustitsii.

Ugolovny kodeks Rossiiskoi Federatsii. (1996, June 15). Russiiskie vesti.

Vasilchenko, G. S. (Ed.). (1977). *Obshchaya seksopatologiya.* Moscow: Meditsina.

Vasilchenko, G. S. (Ed.). (1983). *Chastnaya seksopatologiya* (2 vols.). Moscow: Meditsina.

Vasilchenko, G. S. (Ed.). (1990). *Seksopatologiya. Spravochnik.* Moscow: Meditsina.

Vvedensky, G. E. (1994). *Kliniko-diagnosticheskie aspecty anomalnovo seksualnovo povedeniya.* Avtoreferat dissertatsii na soiskanie uchenoi stepeni kandidata meditsinskikh nauk. Moscow, Gosudarstrennyi nauchnyi tscentr setscialnoi indebnoi psikhiatrii imeni, V. P. Serbskovo.

15

The Czech and Slovak Republics

IVO PROCHÁZKA

Short History of the Czech and Slovak Republics

The Czech Republic consists of two very close regions with the same language, Bohemia and Moravia. The main difference between them is in their strength of religion. The Eastern part of the Czech republic, Moravia, is more religious and Catholic. Some people in Moravia consider it to be an independent nation, but the majority identify as Czechs.

The Czech territories had their own histories as independent states from the tenth to the start of the seventeenth century, with a Golden age in the fourteenth century when King Charles IV was also the German Emperor. He founded in Prague the first university in Central Europe. In the beginning of the fifteenth century a strong Protestant movement emerged in the area, influenced by the ideas of Jan Hus. The Czech territories lost their independence during the Thirty Years War when they were joined through the Habsburgs to the Austrian monarchy. This change was followed by a resurgence of Catholicism and stronger German influence in the Czech countries.

The Slovak Republic has a shorter history. This country was never independent until the twentieth century. With the exception of a short period in the early Middle Ages it was part of Hungary. The Slovak language is Slavonic and not very different from Czech. Slovaks are more religious and Catholic than the Czechs.

As a result of a Czech movement for independence and the breakup of the Austro-Hungarian Empire after World War I, a single Czecho-Slovak state was formed in 1918. Living in Czechoslovakia were a mixture of national minorities—Germans, Hungarians, Jews, Poles, Gypsies, and Ukrainians. Czechoslovakia was a democratic state until the onset of the war of 1938–1939, when Nazi armies occupied the Czech part of the country and it became a German protectorate. During the war, for the first time in its history, Slovakia attained independence, but as a religious and fascist state. The war era saw great ethnic changes in Czech and Slovak societies. Many Jews and Gypsies died in the concentration camps. The traditional coexistence of Czechs and Germans in the country was interrupted when, after the war, almost all Germans and many Hungarians, because they had strongly supported a fascist and nationalist ideology, were made to move back against their will to their respective nations of origin. Three years after the war a coup d'état enabled the Communist Party to gain total political power in Czechoslovakia. In 1968, an attempt to change the political system toward democracy was unsuccessful; its support was destroyed by the Soviet army. From then until 1989 Czechoslovakia was under occupation, still an independent state officially, but under the control and dominant influence of Soviet power. In November 1989, as Soviet control over Eastern Europe collapsed, the so-called "Velvet

IVO PROCHÁZKA • Institute of Sexology, Charles University, Prague 120 00, Czech Republic.

Sociolegal Control of Homosexuality, edited by West and Green, Plenum Press, New York, 1997.

Revolution" changed the political system to democracy. The new system permitted an open declaration of Slovak wishes for independence. Coupled with differences in the political development of the areas, this led to a peaceful split of Czechoslovakia into the Czech and Slovak Republics in January 1993.

THE SOCIAL SITUATION IN CZECH AND SLOVAK SOCIETIES

In the first part of the twentieth century Czechoslovakia was a developed country with a developed political democracy and an effective economic system. These advantages were mostly destroyed by 40 years of communism. The main political preoccupations today in the Czech Republic are with economic growth and democratic reform. The Czech Republic now has a generally homogeneous population of 10 million inhabitants, with Slovaks and Gypsies the largest national minorities, each estimated at about 300,000. The predominant religion is Catholicism, but about half the inhabitants consider themselves atheists or without religious affinities, and the role of religion is relatively small.

Slovakia is now a democratic country. The main political parties are nationalistically oriented. The role of the Catholic Church is much stronger than in the Czech Republic; the vast majority of Slovaks are Catholics. About one-tenth of inhabitants of Slovakia are Hungarians; other minorities are Gypsies, Czechs, and Ukrainians. The communist period was one of strong industrialization and economic development in Slovakia. Relations between Czechs and Slovaks are predominantly friendly.

CRIMINALIZATION AND LEGAL HISTORY OF HOMOSEXUALITY

Data about the legal situation of homosexuals and homosexual acts in the Czech and Slovak societies of the Middle Ages are unavailable. We assume that attitudes were similar to those of other Christian countries of Europe, with criminalization and punishment continuing to the end of the Middle Ages (Boswell, 1980). In the sixteenth and seventeenth centuries there was no unified criminal law in the Czech territories; each city or region had its own legal rules. Data regarding criminalization of homosexuality are scarce, but generally all sexual behavior outside marriage was criminalized at this time. Homosexual behavior was considered "sodomy" and was punished by death. Nevertheless, the chief meaning of "sodomy" was sexual acts with animals (zoophilic behavior), although some cases are recorded where even the indecent exposure of genitalia was counted as sodomy. Homosexual behavior was called "Italian sodomy", the better to distinguish it from other offenses (Malý, 1979). The extent of these criminal practices is unknown and difficult to estimate from existing records.

The first relevant criminal law applied in German-speaking countries was Constitutio Criminalis Carolina, introduced by the sixteenth-century Holy Roman Emperor Charles V. Under this law, homosexual offenders could be sentenced to death, but this law was not generally applied in Czech territories.

The first attempt to apply unified criminal law in the Czech territories was in 1708: Constitutio Criminalis Josephina, introduced by the Emperor Joseph I. The first criminal law to be applied generally under the Habsburg monarchy was Constitutio Criminalis Theresiana, from the year 1769. Published also in the Czech language, this law specified which offenders were punishable by death. Article 74, paragraph 6, in the chapter of offenses against good mores and chastity, defines "unnatural lechery" and includes not only zoophilic and homosexual behaviors, but also masturbation. The punishment for sex with animals was more severe than for homosexual behavior (zoophile offenders were sentenced to death by fire, homosexuals were incinerated only after beheading by the sword). Under extenuating circumstances, such as youth, mental impairment, or an uncompleted offense (without ejaculation), prolonged imprisonment and corporal punishment could be applied in place of execution.

After 1787, following the Law Josephina introduced by the Emperor Joseph II, homosexual acts were no longer punished by death. This law distinguishes between so-called criminal and police offenses, homosexual behavior being included among the police offenses. These were not heard by the court; instead, they were dealt with as misdemeanors by the executive administration. Death for homosexual offenses was permanently replaced by imprisonment, corporal punishment, and/or obligatory community work. Austria was probably the first European country to abandon the death penalty for homosexuality.

Yet another penal code was introduced in 1803. This amalgamated the criminal and police offenses, all of them being heard by the courts. A new criminal law, Allgemeine Bundesgesetz, was introduced in 1852 and lasted in the Czech lands for almost 100 years, until 1950. Chapter 14 of this law, covering violent fornication, rape, and other serious cases of fornication, included paragraph 129 concerning "fornication against nature" through zoophilic and homosexual behavior. The punishment was imprisonment from 1–5 years, in more serious circumstances up to 10 years, and in the case of injury up to 20 years. It was specified that not just intercourse but also mutual masturbation between persons of the same gender constituted this criminal act. The passive person who allowed homosexual behavior with his or her body also committed the crime.

With the medicalization of homosexuality that began in the beginning of the twentieth century, it was recommended that a distinction be made between constitutional and acquired homosexuality (Bondy, 1926). Constitutional homosexual orientation was considered a mental state for which more lenient punishment was recommended. The general medical view at the beginning of the century underestimated the frequency of so-called constitutional homosexuality.

The first indications of criminalization of homosexuality in Slovakia (then an eastern region of the Austrian-Hungarian Monarchy) are in Jurisprudentia Criminalis of 1751, Article 74, where anal intercourse between two men is punished by death. No other homosexual activities are mentioned. The previously cited provisions of Codex Theresianus Criminalis and Law Josephina were applied also in Slovakia. The Hungarian criminal law of 1843, paragraph 229, included homosexual behavior with bestiophilia and punished homosexual behavior with up to 3 years imprisonment. From 1852, for the next 9 years, the General Austrian Penal Code Allgemeine Bundesgesetz was also applied in the eastern part of Austria, but when Hungarians reached more autonomy, they brought back their original law. Later, an 1878 version of Hungarian criminal law decreased the level of punishment to up to 1 year imprisonment (according to par. 241) or up to 5 years if violence or threat was used (Hudec, 1926).

When the independent state of Czechoslovakia was first formed it adopted, with small changes, the criminal law of the former Austrian-Hungarian monarchy. Despite attempts at unification and codification of criminal law, small differences between Czech and Slovak areas persisted until 1950 (Bianchi, 1973). It seems the main reason for surviving differences in legal attitudes toward homosexuality was the discussion among experts about whether criminalization of homosexual behavior was sensible and justified. Čeřovský (1926) criticized the fact that in the year 1924 the Prague courts alone heard 20 cases of accusations under paragraph 129 of Allegemeine Bundesgesetz. Medical examination of the accused was generally required and, if "constitutional homosexuality" was diagnosed, this was considered an extenuating circumstance, but one that usually meant obligatory medical treatment as part of the judicial decision.

In 1922, in support of a campaign against venereal diseases, a law was introduced that imposed penalties for endangering anyone with these infections.

During World War II Czech justice lost more of its relative autonomy. After 1941 "moral offenses" including homosexuality were treated according to the German fascist law. Some people accused of homosexuality were sent to concentration camps, but no data about this were published. In May 1945 these German criminal laws were cancelled by the Decret, a law proclaimed by President Benes.

The unified Czechoslovak Penal Code was accepted by the parliament in 1950 as Law 86\1950. Homosexual behavior was still criminalized under Chapter 7, "acts against human dignity" (par. 241). The penalty was up to 1 year imprisonment, but 1–5 if the partner was younger than 18 or if there was payment for sex. An offer of homosexual activities for money was an offense punishable by imprisonment from 6 months to 3 years.

Consensual homosexual behavior between adults was decriminalized in 1961 (Law 140/1961). However, under the new Penal Code, some homosexual acts could still be punished. According to paragraph 244, if the sex was with a person of the same gender under 18 years of age (the age of consent for heterosexuals was 15), if a dependent person was exploited (e.g., as in a relationship between teacher and student or among soldiers of different rank), or if the sex was for money (with no distinction made between client and prostitute) then the punishment was 1–5 years imprisonment. The penalty for homosexual behavior provoking public nuisance was from 1–5 years imprisonment, higher than for similar heterosexual offenses. The law allowed the suspension of a sentence.

The latest legal change of the Penal Code concerning homosexual behavior came in 1990 (Law 175/1990), when homosexuality and heterosexuality were treated equally. Paragraph 244 was excluded from the Penal Code, the age of consent became 15 years for homosexual and heterosexual behavior, and homosexual prostitution was no longer regulated by the criminal law.

Under paragraph 242, there is no longer any difference in the legal protection of minors under 15 from heterosexual or homosexual abuse. Protection of adolescents in relation to sexual behavior is mentioned in paragraph 217 (disturbance of moral education of youth) and in paragraph 243 (sexual abuse of dependent adolescents under 18), but these provisions are applied without regard to the gender of victim or offender.

OTHER LEGAL ATTITUDES TOWARD HOMOSEXUALITY

There are no other Czech or Slovak laws dealing specifically with homosexuality and/or homosexual behavior, even though there have been attempts to include some gay/lesbian issues in the statutes. There are no antidiscrimination laws to protect gays and lesbians.

A constitutional list of human rights and freedom was accepted by the Czechoslovak Parliament in 1991 (Law 23/1991). Deputy Klára Samková proposed a change to Article 3 in Part 1 of this law, which read: "Basic rights and freedoms are guaranteed for all people without distinction in gender, color of skin, language, religion, political or other opinion, national or social origin, belonging to national or ethnic minorities, possessions or other status." She wanted "sexual orientation" to be added to the list, but this was not approved by the majority of Parliament.

A law concerning once-and-for all financial compensation for victims of World War II was accepted by the Czech Parliament in 1994 (Law 217/1994), but persons sentenced to confinement in fascist concentration camps because of homosexual orientation were not included. This was because the definition of wrongful imprisonment was according to Law 255 from the year 1947 when homosexuality was still criminalized; gays and lesbians were, therefore, criminals. The Czech gay and lesbian organization Sdružení Organizaeí Homo-sexualních Občanů (SOHO), Association of Organizations of Homosexual Citizens, appealed to governmental authorities, but their intervention was disregarded. No actual case of discrimination on these grounds is on record, and the only discussion of the issue has been in the newspaper *Lidové noviny*.

The Civic Code recognizes the legal status of "persons living in the common household". This can be applied to gay and lesbian couples, but it is sometimes necessary to prove that they really live together. Even if one dies intestate, the surviving partner has a right to inherit and to continue to use their apartment. Efforts by the lesbian and gay movement to assert this right are strengthened by the acceptance of registered same-sex partnerships in Denmark, Norway, and elsewhere (Bruns & Beck, 1991) and by recommendations from the Council of Europe. However, in November 1995 the Czech government discussed proposals for a new Civic and Family Law and, from three options put forward, rejected all proposals for registered partnerships.

Transsexuals can request the medical services necessary for sex reassignment. Legal change of gender is permitted under the law concerning registers of births and deaths (268/1949), which covers mistakes and changes of gender. The law covering the use and change of first names and surnames (55/1950) allows transsexuals to change both names to accord with their new gender. The first sex reassignments were done by sexologists in the 1960s; in the 1970s, sex reassignments had to be sanctioned by legal instructions from the ministeries (Brzek & Šípová, 1983). This law is applied in Slovakia also, but there is little professional acceptance of sex changes there (Molčan et al., 1989).

DISCRIMINATION AGAINST GAYS AND LESBIANS IN CZECH SOCIETY

No comprehensive survey of the experiences of gay men and lesbians with discrimination has yet been completed, but a first study of this topic began at the end of 1995. A behavioral study of 841 gay men and 35 lesbians, which focused on HIV infection and related issues, has been completed. It showed that 76 percent believed that homosexuals are discriminated against in our society; even more, 81 percent, agreed with the statement that AIDS is often misused to discriminate against homosexuals (Stehlíková, Procházka, & Hromada, 1995).

Other surveys, concerning knowledge of AIDS/HIV and related issues, repeated with a random sample of the Czech population in 1988 and 1993, found that the greatest change in attitudes over these 5 years was an increasing tolerance toward homosexuality (Dvořák et al., 1992; Tuček & Holub, 1994). In 1988 two-thirds of respondents considered suppression of homosexuality to be an important part of AIDS prevention; 5 years later this opinion was endorsed by only 17 percent of citizens. By 1993, 18 percent of respondents considered homosexuality to be a normal and respectable variant of human sexuality, and another 30 percent considered it a harmless form of deviance. The most prevalent opinion was that homosexuality is a medical disturbance (43 percent of respondents). Only 2 percent of respondents wanted homosexual behavior criminalized.

The opinion that homosexuality is today more frequent was supported by one-third of respondents, but most people stated that they did not have an opinion. In 1993, fewer respondents asked for more information about homosexuality. In 1988 the topic was just starting to be openly discussed. In 1993 twice as many respondents as in 1988, 60 percent of the total sample, supported the idea of registered partnerships for gays and lesbians. The existence of gay and lesbian clubs and social activities was accepted by 73 percent in 1993, almost three times more than in 1988, when there were no official social organizations.

Nevertheless, despite the apparently increasing tolerance of society toward homosexuality there are some contrary indicators. The same sociological study showed that the number of people who know anybody to be gay or lesbian had stayed almost the same, with nearly two-thirds of respondents claiming not to know personally any homosexual person. It is still the case that relatively few Czech gays and lesbians are willing to be open.

There are some activities and trends indicative of increasing racism and intolerance toward minorities, especially Gypsies. Racially motivated physical attacks, including murders, have occurred. The newspaper *Mladá fronta* published 3 years ago a short survey in which the vast majority of respondents claimed they did not wish to have Gypsies as neighbors; half of them rejected HIV-positive persons as neighbors, 40 percent did not want homosexual neighbors, and about 20 percent rejected Jews.

An explanation for the rapid change toward tolerance of homosexual people could be the increasing social openness about gay and lesbian issues, the prevalence of tolerant and liberal information in the media, and the inclusion of homosexual issues among the topics of sexual education. During the communist period, even though legal attitudes were relatively tolerant, people were forbidden in practice to speak openly about homosexuality. The youth journal *Mladý svet* published a liberal article by a sexologist entitled "They Live among Us" (Zemek, 1973), which rejected the identification of homosexuality with disease and moral or criminal deviance and criticized as obsolete attempts to cure homosexuality. The reaction of state and communist authorities was very negative, and there was some threat to stop publication of the journal. As it was medically oriented, *Zdravi* [*Health*] was the only popular journal allowed upon occasion to carry information about homosexuality, but always from the medical point of view (Brzek & Hubálek, 1988).

Contact advertisements for homosexuals sometimes appeared in the 1970s, but they were not explicit. They were totally forbidden by the censors in the 1980s because they were thought to be often misused for criminal purposes. This interdiction was cancelled in 1989, when the taboo about homosexuality was broken following the activities of one gay activist (Procházka, Bobřik, & Kodl, 1991).

The comparatively small power of religion is probably one important reason why social attitudes toward homosexuality have rapidly become more tolerant. It seems to be different in Slovakia, however, where the Catholic Church is much stronger and where attitudes are thought to be less tolerant.

The Slovakian gay and lesbian movement Ganymedes developed during the early 1990s and was an integral part of SOHO until 1993 when, one-half year after the separation of Slovakia, it became independent and is now attached to the umbrella organization for lesbian and gay groups in that country.

The Czech gay and lesbian movement is almost unique. It is grouped into 21 gay and lesbian organizations covered by the umbrella association SOHO. Its political strategy has been to avoid confrontation with the rest of society and to promote closer integration of gays and lesbians. This peaceful strategy can reduce the negative reactions in society that some more aggressive approaches provoke. On the other hand, the softer approach makes it more difficult for gays and lesbians to develop a group identity, contribute to the multidimensional culture of democratic society, and grow toward openness and pride.

Job Discrimination

No official instruction exists that discriminates against homosexuals. Employers do not actively investigate whether a job candidate is homosexual (Brzek & Hubalek, 1988). Some data on job discrimination, especially from the past, are available, but only from rare cases. In such situations the employer did not usually give his or her real reason for job cancellation or rejection of a qualified applicant. Teachers, soldiers, and policemen who are open about their sexual orientation can have problems.

Army Discrimination

No official instruction exists that discriminates according to sexual orientation among professional soldiers or recruits for regular obligatory military service. If a recruit for regular obligatory service claims he is a gay and has the backing of a medical (sexological) certificate, he usually is released from duty.

Housing Discrimination

In the time of communist rule housing was an important means of state control over the people. Shortage of free apartments allowed the authorities to distribute them according to state priorities. In access to the available apartments, single people were disadvantaged in comparison with families having children, who were considered to have greater need. This was probably one reason why many homosexual men and women decided to marry. Gay and lesbian couples are not considered to form a family. State regulations and lack of apartments caused many single men and women to stay in their parental homes. Now that housing is changing to the market system and private ownership of apartments is possible, there is no law in existence for the protection of gay men and lesbians from discrimination in the right to housing. A rented apartment can continue to be used by the partner of a deceased tenant if the legal status of "person living in the common household" is not open to challenge.

AIDS and Discrimination in Health Facilities

Cases of discrimination have occurred against HIV-positive gays or homosexual men who were supposedly at risk. Some homosexual men were obligatorily tested for HIV antibodies.

In 1988 one HIV-positive gay man was sentenced for causing intentional bodily harm; he knew he was infected by HIV and gonorrhea, some of his sexual partners appeared to be also HIV-positive, and transmission from him through unprotected anal sex by him was proved. Discussion about this case appeared in the media because health authorities wanted to warn other people and to use the case as a precedent. Liberal opinions criticizing this breach of medical confidentiality and doubts about the justification for the conviction were expressed (Hanušová, 1989). Another person was similarly accused at this time. AIDS and HIV infection was also included in the list of infectious diseases the spreading of which is punishable according to paragraphs 189–190 of the Penal Code by imprisonment for up to 3 years in the case of intentional spreading and up to 1 year if the spreading was unintentional. The sentenced man was freed by President Havel in 1990. Since then, no HIV-positive person has been charged for his or her behavior.

Some anecdotal reports have come from health facilities of difficulties experienced by gay men with their neighbors, or even in their nuclear families, because of the association of homosexuality with possible HIV infection, but the extent of this problem is not known.

SOHO, the organization representing the gay and lesbian movement, is now a regular member of the National Commission on AIDS and of its executive committee, which is responsible for a human rights agenda.

Since 1990, preventive medicine programs have not considered sexual orientation as in itself a risk, but stress only the importance of safe behavior. Free and anonymous HIV testing is available and recommended (Šejda, 1993). It has been reported recently that some blood donor centers recommend that homosexual people not become blood donors without prior discussion of their risk behavior. The notification form for sexually transmitted diseases was successfully criticized because promiscuous and homosexual behaviors were listed together as risk factors for acquiring infection. The form has been changed accordingly.

In 1994 the Czech and Slovak Republics accepted the new tenth revision of *Mezinárodní Klasifikace Nemocí* (*The International Classification of Diseases*), in which homosexuality is excluded and only the diagnosis "egodystonic sexual orientation" (F66) remains. Nevertheless, the latest textbook of sexology still includes homosexuality among types of sexual deviance, even though tolerant attitudes and demedicalization opinions are also described (Zvěřina, 1994).

Political Discrimination

There is little information about the misuse of knowledge of an individual's homosexual orientation for political purpose in these countries. A well-known historical example is the Redl affair of 1913. A colonel in the Austrian army in Prague, Redl is believed to have worked as a spy after being drawn into collaboration with the enemies of Austria by threat of revelation of his homosexuality (Dobai, 1990). The former minister of defense in the communist government and the son-in-law of the first communist president, Gottwald

Alexej Čepička, was said to have lost his power and position after having sex with an *agent provocateur* from the state secret police (Frolík, 1990). The last attempt at the use of homosexuality to cause political scandal appeared in summer 1993 in the newspaper *Lidové noviny*, where it was reported that the murdered young gay journalist Zdeněk Válka had been a very good friend of a former Czechoslovak vice premier at the beginning of 1990s. This attempt to stir up scandal was found objectionable and was rejected by the political authorities.

During the communist era the state secret police kept lists of homosexual persons. The information was misused for blackmail when police needed to influence homosexual men and women. These police records were officially destroyed in the early 1990s after homosexuality was removed from the Penal Code and after protests from the gay movement. Most gay venues were subjected to random surveillance by communist authorities, and persons frequenting them were identified and recorded. There were two unofficial gay bars and two cafés in Prague at this time that were suspected to be under permanent secret police surveillance. Since the political change in 1989, police surveillance of bars, clubs, cruising areas, and other gay venues has become rare, limited to the investigation of crime.

No important political figure has disclosed his or her homosexual orientation, except for two open, but unsuccessful, candidates in the parliamentary elections in 1990 and 1992. The policy of "outing" is not considered to be useful by the gay and lesbian community.

Gay-Bashing

Criminal attacks and victimization of homosexual people have occurred, but data recording frequency are not yet available. Usually the criminal attack is connected with robbery or theft, homosexuals being chosen as victims because of the perceived difficulties in securing a conviction in such circumstances. Visiting cruising areas and looking for hustlers are dangerous behaviors, but physical and verbal attacks against gay men and lesbians simply for their sexual orientation seems to be relatively uncommon. This may reflect the general lack of public openness about personal sexual orientation.

Sexology and Gay and Lesbian Issues and Movements

Czech sexology is a medical disipline that impinges on psychological, sociological, and political issues. The Institute of Sexology of Charles University was founded in 1921 under the influence of German sexology — represented especially by Magnus Hirschfeld — and was the first institute of sexology in the university field in the world. The medical and psychological care of homosexual patients has always been an important concern of sexology.

Sexologists played an active role in efforts to bring about decriminalization of homosexual behavior in the 1920s and 1930s. They supported and argued for the belief that homosexuality was predominantly biological in nature (Bondy, 1926) but declined to coordinate their activities with the intellectual gay group founded in 1924 and kept their main activity oriented toward the decriminalization of homosexuality. That same year the first Czech book about homosexuality written from a tolerant viewpoint was published by a student of medicine (Jelínek, 1924). In 1932 and 1933, six issues of the first gay journal *Hlas* [*Voice*] were published. The difficult political situation brought to an end attempts to decriminalize homosexuality and the creation of a gay movement, but it seems that there was some influence on public opinion, and a decrease was seen in the number of prosecutions under paragraph 129. Some German gay intellectuals, such as Klaus Mann, obtained political asylum in Czechoslovakia in the 1930s (Oosterhuis, n.d.), but it is not clear if their sexual orientation played any role in this.

Freund and Nedoma were the other sexologists who pressed for decriminalization of homosexuality in the early 1960s, arguing on the basis of their own scientific studies that homosexual behavior does not constitute a social danger. Moreover, they felt that decriminalization would allow homosexuals to lead a normal life and would decrease the connection of homosexuality with negative social phenomena like prostitution and criminality. They were skeptical about the prospects of treatment (Freund, 1962). Freund introduced the penile plethysmograph, a device used in the assessment of sexual orientation. It is also used in the examination of sexual delinquents, notably pedophiles, when required by the courts.

Attempts by some sexologists to treat homosexuality continued into the late 1970s, but only when the patient asked the doctor to do so. However, in the new therapeutic approach that appeared at this time, the main effort was directed not toward change in sexual orientation nor toward adoption of a heterosexual lifestyle, but toward reducing the negative effects on health of the consequences of coming out as homosexual. Another development at this time was the foundation of psychotherapeutic groups for homosexual men (Bártová, 1979; Hubálek,1988).

Psychotherapeutic groups helped people cope with their sexual orientation but did not help them avoid social isolation. The so-called Socio-therapeutic Club was started in 1988 as an informal attempt to found a gay and lesbian movement under the protection of the Institute of Sexology (Procházka, 1989). At that time it was not permitted to found any public activity without the permission of communist leaders, permission which was almost impossible to obtain. Nevertheless, in that same year another independent illegal gay group was formed and the two collaborated closely. Early in 1989, when the communist government was still in power, the first gay journal was successfully published and the officially named Socio-therapeutic Club started to use the name Lambda. Under this name it was accepted in the summer of 1989 as a member of the International Gay and Lesbian Association (ILGA). The main political activities of Lambda were oriented toward withdrawal of the prohibition on homosexual acquaintance advertisements and, together with some sexologists and lawyers, preparation of changes to the Penal Code to eliminate paragraph 244. After the political change, Lambda was officially registered by authorities in February 1990. A similar gay and lesbian movement developed, with the help of sexologists, in Slovakia. In 1990, the more radical Movement for the Equality of Homosexual Citizens was founded. It lasted 1 year, but increasing numbers of gay and lesbian groups have since appeared outside of Prague.

Today, sexologists support the efforts of gay and lesbian movements to obtain official recognitions of registered partnerships, not just in the interests of preventive medicine, but also as an important expression of the human rights of minorities (Weiss, Zvěřina, & Procházka, 1994).

Conclusion

We can characterize the legal position of homosexual men and women in the Czech and Slovak Republics as better than it is in the other countries of Central and Eastern Europe, with the exception of the former German Democratic Republic and Poland. The main social oppression of gays and lesbians in the communist period was not based so much on the legal statutes as on public ignorance of the needs and rights of homosexuals and other minorities and on the prohibition of the free circulation of information and the consequential invisibility of gays and lesbians.

Even after the political changes of 1989, the scientific approach to homosexuality has been largely limited to medical and sexological studies, with little interest in gay and lesbian issues on the part of the social sciences. The short time that democracy has been in place has not yet sufficed to change neither negative social attitudes toward gays and lesbians nor homosexuals' poor self-esteem, lack of social experience, and inadequate integration of sexual orientation issues into daily life.

References

Bártová, D. (1979). Skupinová psychoterapie pacientů s poruchami psychosexuální identifikace. *Moravskoslezský referátový sborník*, 11, 92–94.

Bianchi, L. (1973). *Dejiny štátu a práva 2*. Bratislava, Czechoslovakia: SAV (Slovak Academy of Sciences).

Bondy, H. (1926). K trestnosti homosexuality. Druhý sjezd čsl.právníků 1925 [II.-IV.sekce], otázka 3b, práce 1. Brno, Czechoslovakia.

Boswell, J. (1980). *Christianity, social tolerance and homosexuality*. Chicago: The University of Chicago Press.

Bruns, M., & Beck, V. (1991). Die Ehe für Lesben und Schwule aus rechtpolitischer Sicht. *Zeitschrift. für Sexualforschung*, 4 (3), 192–204.

Brzek, A., & Hubálek, S. (1988). Homosexuals in Eastern Europe: Mental health and psychotherapy issues. *Journal of Homosexuality*, 15 (1/2), 153–162.

Brzek, A., & Šípová. I. (1983). Transsexuelle in Prag. *Sexualmedizin*, 9 (13), 110–112.

Čeřovský, F. (1926). K otázce trestnosti homosexuality. Druhý sjezd čsl. právníků 1925 (II.-IV. sekce), otázka 3b, práce 2. Brno, Czechoslovakia.

Dobai, P. (1990). *Aféra plukovníka Redla*. Praha, Czechoslovakia: Máj NV.

Dvořák, J., (1992). *Ve stínu AIDS*. Praha, Czechoslovakia: Academia.

Freund, K. (1962). Homosexualita u muže. Praha, Czechoslovakia: SZdN.

Frolík, J. (1990). *Špión vypovídá*. Praha, Czechoslovakia: Index Orbis.

Hanušová, J. (1989). AIDS. *Mladý svět*, 31 (8), 6–21.

Hubálek, S. (1988). Skupinová psychoterapie homosexuálních pacientů. *Prakt. lékař*, 68, 187–188.

Hudec, V. (1926). Trestnost homosexuality. Druhý sjezd čsl.právníků 1925 (II.-IV. sekce), otázka 3b, práce 3. Brno Czechoslovakia.

Jelínek, F. (1924). *Homosexualita ve světle vědy*. Praha, Czechoslovakia: Obelisk.

Malý, K. (1979). *Trestní právo v Čechách v 15.-16. století*. Praha, Czechoslovakia: Univerzita Karlova.

Mezinárodní klasifikace nemocí (10. revize) [The International Classification of Disease (tenth revision)]. (1992). WHO Geneva, Praha, Czechoslovakia: Ústav zdravotnických informací a statistiky.

Molčan, J., Bardoš, A., Hynie, J., Izakovič, V., Kočiš, Ľ., Lábady, F., Oravec, D., Sklovský, A., Stančák, A., Valent, M., & Žigo, Ľ. (1989). *Vybrané kapitoly zo sexuológie a hraničných odborov*. Bratislava, Czechoslovakia: Osveta.

Oosterhuis, H. (n.d.). The guilty conscience of the left. *The European Gay Review*, 72–80.

Procházka, I. (1989). Über den Soziotherapeutischen Klub der Homosexuellen in Prag. In *Psychosoziale Aspekte der Homosexualität* (pp. 125–126). Jena, German Democratic Republic: Friedrich Schiller Universität Jena.

Procházka, I., Bobřík, S., & Kodl, P. (1991). LAMBDA Prag im Jahre 1989. In *Psychosoziale Aspekte der Homosexualität* (pp. 26–27). Jena, Democratic German Republic: Friedrich Schiller Universität Jena.

Šejda, J. (1993). *Prevence, léčba a další aspekty nákazy HIV/AIDS.* Praha, Czechoslovakia: Galén.

Stehlíková, D., Procházka, I., & Hromada J. (1995). *AIDS, homosexualita a společnost.* Praha, Czechoslovakia: ORBIS.

Tuček, P., & Holub, J. (1994). *Epidemiologicko-sociologické šetření názorů občanů České republiky na onemocnění AIDS.* Praha, Czechoslovakia: Nadace Společně proti AIDS.

Weiss, P., Zvěřina, J., & Procházka I. (1994). K výskytu homosexuality v obecné populaci. *Prakt. lékař, 12,* 573–576.

Zemek, P. (1973). Žijí mezi námi. *Mladý svět, 15* (4), 20.

Zvěřina, J. (1994). *Lékařská sexuologie.* Praha, Czechoslovakia: H + H.

16

Germany

RAINER HOFFMANN, JÖRG HUTTER, and RÜDIGER LAUTMANN

Lesbians

This chapter primarily concerns same-sex relations between men. Initially, we planned to include contributions from lesbian sociologists and lawyers but then failed to enlist their help, possibly because the social concerns of male and female homosexuals are different, the latter not being so rooted in matters of penal law.

The official nonpunitive stance on lesbianism bears a Janus-like face. Historically, the differences in control of the two homosexualities are striking: cruel and wide-ranging in the case of men, negligent and intolerant in the case of women. On the one hand, lesbian relationships could go on without much official interference, which was beneficial for participants. On the other hand, the sexual character of such relationships remained unrecognized, even sometimes by those involved. To a certain degree, this put the love between women on an unstructured level. Romantic feelings came to the fore; but sexual meanings often stayed latent. Consequently, sexual science preferred to study male homosexuality. Sexual policy and public opinion have been very concerned with male homosexuality, tending to consider female homosexuality a minor problem. A more balanced account can be found in Lautmann (1993), which gives a comprehensive review of the lesbian and gay history of ideas 1900 to the present.

In theoretical discourse lesbians have caught up with gay men, and, at the present time, lesbian authors have taken the lead in discussing gender and sexuality. Lesbians do not solely look back at their former invisibility and tend to concern themselves with more than drawing up a list of current disadvantages (which are changing fast in a more egalitarian direction). Lesbian issues are also inseparably interwoven with the feminist struggle for equality of rights. It is in such unplanned and unforeseen ways that social change for gay men as well as lesbians takes place, as the former take advantage of the advances made in the human rights field by the latter without having themselves contributed to the effort.

The Background of Social Control

Institutional responses to homosexual activity have had a changeable history. Christianized German tribes repressed it with capital punishment, but from the Middle Ages onward there were meeting places for homosexuals in some metropolitan areas such as Cologne. However, unlike Paris or London, German cities were too small to develop a real

RAINER HOFFMANN, JÖRG HUTTER, and RÜDIGER LAUTMANN • Department of Gay and Lesbian Studies Fachbereich 8, University of Bremen, D-28334 Bremen, Germany.

Sociolegal Control of Homosexuality, edited by West and Green, Plenum Press, New York, 1997.   255

urban subculture. From the early nineteenth century Swiss and German writers gave expression to the idea of love between men and the term *homosexual* was created. Interpretations of same-sex relations were published, and demands for civil liberties for homosexuals arose. The foundations for the modern concepts of "lesbian" and "gay" were laid down. In 1933 the Nazi government suddenly interrupted this development. The persecution of gays, enforced with jail and concentration camps, was based on racial–biological and demographic beliefs and was the fiercest ever seen in modern times. It was not until the 1970s that the gay and lesbian movement could recover.

Today homosexuality is established in society as never before. Not even the menace of AIDS has reversed the trend. Despite the numbers affected by HIV, the quality of life for homosexual and bisexual people continues to increase. In the German-speaking world, same-sex relations between consenting adult men were completely decriminalized some 20 years ago. Sexual contact among women had not ever been criminalized, except in Austria in earlier decades. Currently, any distinction between homosexual and heterosexual behavior has been removed from the German Penal Code, as it had been in Switzerland in 1992 and in the former East Germany in 1988. Contemporary political demands have extended to include an antidiscrimination amendment to the constitution and the legalization of marriages for same-sex couples.

The state has long since abstained from open discrimination (e.g., against teachers or civil servants, in the judiciary, public administration, and social security). Many politicians, mainly conservatives, hasten to confirm that they won't "discriminate." This does not mean that politicians are willing to grant equal rights to homosexuals. They concede just enough equality as is necessary to be regarded as tolerant, but not as much as is needed for full homosexual integration.

Homosexuality enjoys a high degree of social visibility, which was increased, though not initiated, by the public reaction to AIDS. There are more occasions than ever before to learn about homosexuality, to discuss it, and to make contact with it. Questions of homosexuality are addressed in many sectors of everyday life: at school, in the family and peer group, at work, and during leisure activities. People can thus develop any latent feelings and find possible partners.

Residual discrimination remains in niches like the military and the churches, although even here homosexual lifestyles are possible as long as they are kept discreet. Legal pressure is also difficult to bring against intolerant private sector landlords, employers, and the like. This leaves homosexual liberation essentially incomplete, superimposed as it is upon a quite solid foundation of antihomosexual prejudice. As several surveys between 1970 and 1990 using identical questions have shown, at least one-third of the German population hold very unfavorable attitudes toward homosexuals, and only one-third is genuinely tolerant (Bochow, 1993; Wienold & Lautmann, 1977). Nevertheless, there are considerable opportunities for gay men and lesbians. Many newspapers, mainstream as well as subcultural, have a section for same-sex contact ads. Special guides list the commercial and the covert meeting places for homosexuals, and today each city with over 50,000 inhabitants has at least a gay bar and an anonymous meeting point in a public park or lavatory ("tea room"). Bigger cities have baths, numerous bars for special sexual interests, book shops, voluntary groups, and a "gay switchboard." The lesbian and gay community is thus well developed.

Historical Development of the Penal Code

Antihomosexual criminal law in Germany went through periods of strong politicization and has developed from offenses threatening the death penalty to complete deletion from the Penal Code.

Early Developments

Until almost the middle of the sixteenth century there was no standard criminal law. Town, country, market, and other local laws often differed strongly from one to another and had rules partly based on orally communicated legal customs. With a gradual loss of centralist power by the German kings and the consequential deterioration in any unified German legal system, local rulers made their own laws, which increasingly led to uncontrolled criminal persecutions (Langbein, 1974). Brutal and summary criminal proceedings, as well as a great increase in offenses attracting the death penalty, stimulated endeavors to reform and strengthen criminal law and procedure. Under Charles V the Reichstag convened in the assemblies of Regensburg (1530) and Augsburg (1532) and established a new law of the Reich, the Constitutio Criminalis Carolina (CCC).

The CCC defined sodomy as follows: "If a human being with an animal, man with man, woman with woman have unchaste intercourse, they have forfeited life and one should, as is generally the custom, execute them by fire from life to death" (art. 116). In formulating new law the legislator of this time used the Italian law as his model, but he followed the Franconian legal tradition in selecting the punishment of death by fire.

In the second half of the eighteenth century Frederick the Great of Prussia ordered extensive criminal law reforms and more precise regulations so that judges, when interpreting the law, had no discretionary powers. The result was the Allgemeines Landrecht (ALR) enacted on June 1, 1794 (Steakley, 1989). Current legal practice was put on the statute book by substituting imprisonment or banishment for the death penalty.

At the beginning of the nineteenth century the ideas of the liberal criminal law theoretician and philosopher Immanuel Kant became influential throughout the German states. He differentiated sharply between offenses against morals and acts that violate the rights of a third party. The idea of keeping rights and morals strictly separated was also the theoretical foundation for one of Kant's pupils, Paul Johann Anselm von Feuerbach, when he drafted the Bavarian Criminal Code. This came into force in 1813 and decriminalized same-sex contacts between adults for the first time. In those days the reality of German law was marked by great regional variation: The Kingdom of Bavaria and the Duchy of Hannover, for instance, provided no punishment for homosexual acts, whereas judges in the city-state of Bremen and the Duchy of Mecklenburg, even as late as 1869, could pass the death sentence according to the CCC of 1532.

Prussia and the Kaiser Reich

Brisk revisionist activity began in Prussia only a few years after the ALR had come into force in 1794 and culminated with the enactment of the Prussian Penal Code in 1851. The lines of conflict, however, ran not between liberal southern Germans and Prussians, but between Prussian and liberal French legal tradition. In areas west of the Rhine, annexed by Prussia in the 1815 Vienna Congress after the breakdown of Napoléonic France, the Code Pénal of 1810 was in force, in which punishment for consensual homosexual acts among adults (simple homosexuality) was unknown. Consequently, the representatives of the Rhineland Provinces fought against the impending adoption of the relevant articles from the Prussian Penal Code. The prosecution of homosexual acts was thought to have a negative effect. If "these cases are made the subject of criminal investigations," the "harmful effect of the news of these abominations" (Lautmann, 1992, p. 156) would be to spread them further among the public. This is why in the first Prussian drafts at the beginning of the nineteenth century simple homosexuality went unpunished.

An order of King Frederick William IV of Prussia brought a clear end to this wrangling over the impunity of "unnatural fornication." He instructed the Criminal Law Commission to follow the ALR and not to limit the maximum penalty. The discussion was not about criminalization, but about the form of punishment. The term *fornication* in the ALR had been interpreted as the "widespread vice of pederasty," which appears to have motivated the draft of 1833. The reference in Article 143 in the Prussian Penal Code to "unnatural fornication between persons of the male sex or of humans with animals" automatically limits its application to male homosexuality, in line with the common interpretation of the nature of these cases. *Emmissio seminis* [ejaculation] and *immissio penis* [penile penetration] were components of the offense, which women, for reasons of their anatomy, could not commit (Hutter, 1992a).

During the civil uprising of 1848 and 1849 two further drafts came into being with remarkable provisions concerning sexual offenses. There were no homosexual offenses, and the terms *same-sex* and *unnatural* had disappeared. With the collapse of the uprising this liberal interpretation of moral law was reversed. A revision of the law in 1850 reverted to the draft of 1847 (Lautmann, 1992). When the King approved the new Prussian Penal Code on April 14, 1851, the homosexuality article read: "Unnatural fornication which is practised between persons of the male sex or by humans with animals is to be punished with imprisonment from six months to four years and by temporary forfeiture of civil rights" (art. 143).

With the founding of the North German Union in 1866, Prussia, under Chancellor Otto von Bismarck, was able to assert political supremacy over its Austrian rivals. Since the regional variation of German criminal law was an obstacle to a unified nation-state, the creation of a common criminal law was regarded as vital. Representations from the medical profession and numerous petitions by those affected, led by the jurist and author Karl Heinrich Ulrichs, had little influence (Féray & Herzer, 1990). Thus, von Mühler, the Prussian Minister for religious, educational, and medical affairs, was able to assert that in the interests of "public morals," sodomy and pederasty could not go unpunished. As a consequence, Article 143 of the Prussian Penal Code was transferred almost unchanged to become Article 173 of the Penal Code of the North German Union (Taeger & Lautmann, 1992).

Following the Franco-German war and German unification, Article 173 became Article 175 of the German Penal Code of the new Reich in 1871. The penalty was now imprisonment and possible loss of civil rights (Höinghaus, 1870). This remained law until 1935, notwithstanding various attempts for reform that ranged from a wish to include lesbian sex to proposals to abolish the offense of simple homosexuality altogether. Although successive criminal law commissions worked out drafts of a new Penal Code, reform attempts were frustrated first by the onset of World War I and then by Nazi seizure of power. The code of 1871 remains in force today. In a draft in 1909, penologists, citing results of psychiatric research, wanted to see "unnatural fornication" between women punished, but the draft of 1922 took a more liberal approach.

The Inter-War Period

By 1898 the first homosexual rights movement, the Scientific Humanitarian Committee led by Dr.med. Magnus Hirschfeld, had already petitioned many times for the abolition of Article 175 (Fähnders, 1995). With the collapse of the Kaiser's Reich after World War I and the advent of democracy in the Weimar Republic, hopes for a reform of the moral criminal law and for decriminalization rose but were not fulfilled. In Article 325 of the draft of 1919 an offense of "sexual intercourse and similar acts" between men was maintained. Thus, the Commission suggested a formulation that would put on the statute book what the Reich Supreme Court had already read into Article 175 by expansive interpretation.

With the appointment of the Social Democrat Gustav Radbruch as justice minister, the pendulum swung once more toward a more liberal approach. He had in the past petitioned against Article 175 of the Penal Code of the Reich, and now he suggested impunity for simple homosexuality in his draft for a new code in 1922. The later draft of 1925, under a new conservative justice minister, once again, in Article 267, penalized homosexuality. In October 1929, in a vote on the Reichstag's draft of 1927, the Reichstag Committee for Justice decided to delete the homosexuality offense by a narrow majority (Herzer, 1995; Mende, 1990).

The Nazi Era

The homosexual civil rights movement celebrated prematurely this decriminalization. The general political situation had changed in the face of ever-worsening social and economic conditions, and when the National Socialists took over the trend was reversed. With the help of the emergency decree of February 28, 1933, Adolf Hitler suspended basic rights guaranteed by the constitution. The National Socialists demanded an interpretation of the laws orientated less toward their literal wording and more toward a "highest possible value of life for the German National Community" or "sane National Sentiment," as they called their own ideology (Schoppmann, 1991, p. 85).

Try as they might to fulfil Hitler's demands for mass convictions, the judicial authorities, who made an effort to give an impression of legality, found themselves competing with the police and the Schutzstaffel, a party-owned special police force. These forces could circumvent the courts by holding suspects in preventative or protective custody, which meant dispatch to a concentration camp.

Immediately after the seizure of power by the National Socialists, jurists started redrafting the criminal law according to the new ideology, with "national community" as its central theme (Frank, 1934). The political character of National Socialist law was clearly revealed in the words of the Party jurist Rudolf Klare: "The criminal law is first and foremost a law of battle. Its enemy is anyone who threatens the existence, power and peace of the People" (Klare, 1937, p. 122). While harsher penalties for male homosexual acts were discussed by the law commission, the National Socialist jurists examined whether same-sex intercourse among women should be punished. In the end the majority of the commission refrained from making lesbian sex a crime. In their image of women they could see no major threat to their politics; women were excluded from the corridors of power, so there was no fear of lesbianism "distorting public life." What is more, whereas homosexual men might withdraw from the reproductive process and thus be a threat to Nazi ideas of Germanic world population, women could be submitted to intercourse whatever their sexual preferences.

In 1934 Ernst Röhm, the Chief of Staff of the Sturmabteilung, the party's Storm Troopers, and Hitler's rival, was murdered by Hitler loyalists when he was allegedly found in the middle of an all-male orgy. This served as a pretext for the immediate tightening of the articles of the Penal Code governing homosexual acts, thus preempting the review of the whole code, which was planned, but never passed. Racist arguments served as a justification for a drastic increase in sentencing and the expansion of what constitutes a crime to cover all homosexual acts, including mutual masturbation. It was argued that, in striving for a strong and morally healthy nation, it was necessary to fight all "unnatural acts" with vigor (Criminal Law Amendment Act, 1935, p. 9). New Article 175a imposed stronger penalties for special aggravating circumstances.

The courts made full use of the expanded definition of homosexual offenses and of a new catch-all provision that made everything an offense that according to "sane National Sentiment" deserved punishment (Criminal Law Amendment Act, 1935, p. 8). In later court rulings even homosexual behavior not involving physical contact was held to be included (Supreme Court of the Reich, 1938, 1939). The tightening of the laws resulted in some 50,000 convictions for homosexual offenses in the period between 1933 and 1944. The number of those sent directly to concentration camps without judicial authority can only be estimated today: It could have been 5000–15,000, of which few can have survived (Grau, 1995b; Lautmann, 1981).

The Federal Republic of Germany

After the collapse of Hitler's regime, German law remained valid under Allied occupation. Although Law 1 of the military government in the western occupied zones expressly abolished a whole range of National Socialist laws, it left Articles 175 and 175a untouched, and the West German courts continued to use them against homosexuals after May 1945. The West German Federal Supreme Court (Bundesgerichtshof) confirmed the unlimited validity of the Nazi homosexuality offenses in a whole series of rulings at the beginning of the 1950s (Schultz, 1994). The Federal Constitutional Court (Bundesverfassungsgericht) held in 1957 that the two articles were not unconstitutional. Although enacted by an undemocratic government, the law was still formally correct. Points showing typical National Socialist injustice were not discernible. Finally, the regulations did not infringe upon the right to free development of personality, which is guaranteed by the constitution, nor did they violate the principles of equal treatment for men and women by criminalizing only male homosexual sex (Federal Constitutional Court, 1957). The tone of the courts' judgments showed that the West German constitutional judges did not intend to break with a legal tradition that in principle put a fictitious "national sentiment" above individual rights.

The official draft for a new Penal Code, which was based on the findings of a criminal law commission appointed in 1954, once again limited the offenses of simple homosexuality to intercourse and similar acts that required the physical union of the genitals. It also moderated the range of sentences, but apart from this stuck to the three-part distinction of *simple fornication* between males, *serious fornication* between males, and *fornication with animals*, as used by the National Socialists. In effect, the whole moral criminal law was to be expanded to 31 offenses. The draft came under a fire of criticism from penologists and, in 1966, 17 renowned experts of jurisprudence published an alternative draft suggesting that, as far as sexual offenses are concerned, certain offenses should be deleted since the prohibited behavior did not violate any rights protected by law. The alternative draft intended to decriminalize simple homosexuality when those concerned are over 18 years of age and to abolish all offenses of "aggravated cases" of homosexual sex (Schultz, 1994).

In the Criminal Law Reform Act 1969 West German legislators for the first time decriminalized simple homosexuality if the partner was over 21 (lowered to 18 soon thereafter). However, they retained the offenses that had been introduced by the Nazi Article 175a, that is, the abuse of dependence, seduction and homosexual prostitution, and the broad definitions of fornication. It was not until the Criminal Law Reform Act of 1973 that sexual offenses were based on the principle of legally protected rights as called for by the alternative draft. The relevant chapter of the Penal Code, which had hitherto been called "Immoral Offenses" was now renamed "Offenses Against Sexual Self-determination," and the term *fornication* was replaced by the more value-neutral expression *sexual act*. Aggravating offenses involving an abuse of dependency and prostitution were abolished.

As there is a separate offense for sexual acts with children under 14, the remaining Article 175, sexual acts by a male with a male under 18 years of age, was purely discriminatory. Despite repeated demands for its abolition during the 1980s from sectors of the Social Democrats, Liberal Democrats, and especially the Green Party, all the attempts were opposed by the governing Christian Democrats, who argued that the article was required for the protection of children and young people. Only after German reunification was there a sign of further movement.

The German Democratic Republic

In the (East) German Democratic Republic (GDR) the politics of criminal law took a different path. After the collapse of Hitler's Reich, the Nazi version of the homosexuality articles remained formally in force in East Germany, as in West Germany. As early as 1948, however, the Provincial High Court of Halle ruled that the expanded definition of the offenses under Article 175 and the heavier sentences enacted by the Nazis had to be regarded as National Socialist injustice. In 1950 the Supreme Court of the GDR found that Article 175 of the Penal Code was to be applied in its old form, in which only sexual acts involving penile penetration of a bodily orifice were punishable. On the other hand,

Article 175a was still in force in the new version, which, in contrast to Article 175, punished acts falling short of penetration (Schultz, 1994).

A total of three drafts for a new Penal Code were produced in the GDR between 1952 and 1968, all containing modifications to homosexuality offenses. The draft of 1967 planned their deletion and in 1968 became law (Grau, 1995a). The crime of simple homosexuality thus finally disappeared. The new Article 151, which now included men and women, penalized sexual acts carried out by an adult with a juvenile under 18 of the same sex (Röhner, 1988; Thinius, 1990).

On August 11, 1987, the Supreme Court of the GDR, in quashing a conviction under Article 151 on appeal by someone who had been sentenced to a term of probation by a lower court, held that "homosexuality, just as heterosexuality, depicts a variation of sexual behavior. Homosexual people therefore are not outcasts of the socialist society, but are entitled to civil rights in the same way as all other citizens" (Grau, 1988, p. 162). After this the Volkskammer, the East German parliament, deleted Article 151 from the Penal Code and from June 30, 1989, onward, East German courts have treated homosexuality and heterosexuality equally under criminal law. The equalized protective age was now 14, but in Article 149 the Penal Code retained an offense of seduction of a person over 14 and under 16 of either sex by an adult, punishable with imprisonment up to 2 years (Thinius, 1990; Bach & Thinius, 1989).

Unification

During negotiations about the unification of Germany the last government of the GDR fought vigorously against the threatened adoption of the West German Article 175. They succeeded in having a special article written into the unification treaty that rendered Article 175 invalid in the East German states until a common provision had been adopted by Parliament (Schultz, 1994).

After unification on October 3, 1990, and the first all-German elections, a coalition of Liberal Democrats and Christian Democrats was formed. The Liberal Democrats insisted that Articles 175 and 182 (seduction of a girl under 16 to intercourse) of the Penal Code and East German Article 149 be abolished and replaced by a uniform offense to protect male and female juveniles under 16. The consultant draft article, which ensued on October 21, 1991, abolished the term "same sex." However, for the first time it also criminalized sex by an adult woman with boys or girls between 14 and 16 years of age (Hutter, 1993). Despite initiatives by the opposition for the total abolition of all three articles, the government's "compromise" proposal prevailed after a hearing of experts by a committee of the Bundestag (the lower house of the federal parliament) and was finally passed into law. The new Article 182, covering sexual abuse of juveniles, creates two offenses: (1) sex with a person over 14 and under 16 by a person over 18 exploiting a vulnerably placed minor or for payment (up to 5 years imprisonment) and (2) sex with a minor in the same age group by a person of over 21 if he or she takes advantage of the victim's incapability of sexual self-determination (up to 2 years imprisonment). When the new law came into force on June 11, 1994, Article 175 finally disappeared from the Penal Code.

The homosexual movement had been fighting for this for almost 100 years. Liberal jurists, sexologists, and other intellectuals had committed themselves to it. Alone, they would not have been able to prevail against the inertia of an adverse public opinion, but the historical coincidence of German unification created a favorable moment for liberalization.

The Effects of Decriminalization

In light of the long tradition of penalizing homosexuals, the effect of decriminalization is not to be underestimated. In West Germany the law reforms of 1969 and 1973 had produced a social climate in which those affected could form interest groups, openly show their sexuality, and create a new homosexual movement. Decriminalization went further in its influence on public opinion. As empirical studies confirm, although Article 175 of the Penal Code was not consistently enforced, it worked to maintain negative views in the consciousness of the population (Wienold & Lautmann, 1977; see also the survey by Lautmann, 1984).

In the former GDR no special groups for lesbians, gays, feminists, environmentalists, and the like were permitted. The state professed to know what was expedient for the individual and for society. Homosexuals therefore had no place in public life (Dietrich, 1995). Groups from the East German homosexual movement, which had formed clandestinely since the beginning of the 1980s, were subject to spying and suppression. Security enforcers applied the same methods against lesbians and gays that were normally used against political dissidents. In the large cities spies under contract with the Ministry of State Security (Stasi) or the Criminal Investigation Department of the police infiltrated the gay scene, kept meeting places and apartments under surveillance, and kept records of partnerships. The organizers of the movements were dealt with in "operative personal checks" (Grau, 1995a, p. 137).

SAME-SEX COUPLES

Recent Efforts for Same-Sex Partnerships

In West German society, decriminalization greatly reduced legal discrimination in civil areas. Wide discussion on homosexual marriage shows that the greater part of the population has become aware of the areas of discrimination still in existence. A trend toward liberalization in other legal areas is also beneficial (Bruns, 1996). In the social sciences decriminalization has thrown up, among other things, the question of whether same-sex couples can count as a family. German academic discourse has concentrated mainly on whether gay men and lesbians are capable of sufficient commitment to form lasting partnerships and on the internal structures and dynamics of such relationships (Akkermann, Betzelt, & Daniel, 1990; Dannecker, 1990; Hoffmann, Lautmann, & Pagenstecher, 1993; Pingel & Trauvetter, 1987). The public debate concerning marriage between homosexuals first came into prominence in 1989 when neighboring Denmark passed a law regarding registered partnerships for gays and lesbians (Bech, 1991). Interest focused on the question of the right of the state to limit marriage to opposite-sex couples.

Around 55 percent of gays and lesbians in the Federal Republic of Germany live in a committed same-sex relationship (Akkermann et al., 1990; Bochow, 1988; Starke, 1994). Many lesbians and gay men view their partnerships not just as a form of cohabitation but as long-term relationships based on inner bonds and the mutual assumption of responsibility.

Heterosexual couples in long-term relationships are always free to marry. This is denied to gay and lesbian partners, who in law remain strangers. For example, same-sex partners have no right to refuse to give evidence as witnesses against their partners, no right to information or to visit in cases of accident or illness and no right to arrange a funeral. In contrast, opposite-sex partners have all these rights if they are only engaged to be married. What is more, marriage secures tax advantages and is beneficial for both partners when claiming pension, maintenance, retirement, and inheritance rights as well as for immigration purposes for partners of a different nationality (Bruns & Beck, 1991).

In order to remove these disadvantages the party of Union 90/The Greens brought a motion for the "abolition of legal discrimination against homosexuals" into the Bundestag (Negotiations of the German Parliament, 1990). After this, in a campaign called Registry Office Action promoted by the Gay Association of Germany and the Gay Lawyers, same-sex couples went to registry offices all around the country and attempted to take out banns. Following rejection they filed complaints about an infringement of the Constitution with the Federal Constitutional Court on the grounds of breaches of the right to marry, which is guaranteed by the Constitution, and the implied right to select a partner of one's own choice (Federal Constitutional Court, 1972, 1974). However, the court rejected the complaint (Federal Constitutional Court, 1993). In its judgment, the court held that there was insufficient ground for a fundamental change to the concept of marriage as a union between one man and one woman in a life-long relationship. Change could not be justified by the argument that the union of marriage is not dependent on the reproductive capability of the partners, that the number of childless marriages is increasing, or that more and more children are born illegitimate. Marriage was protected by the Constitution because it facilitated legal protection of the partners when founding a family and having children together. Nevertheless, the court acknowledged that same-sex couples are legally disadvantaged in many ways and that the constitutional right to equality before the law could commit the legislators to introduce legal protection for this form of living. However, this could be done in other ways than by granting same-sex couples marriage rights.

The Federal Constitutional Court's interpretation of the term *marriage* as being a community of life exclusive to people of different sexes met with much criticism (Wegner, 1995). It was pointed out that in law marriage was not confined to any special form, that it was protected in itself and not because of children. The relevant article of the Constitution says nothing about the actual requirements of civil marriage. Thus, it is undisputed today that marriages that are childless for whatever reason should enjoy equal constitutional protection.

Changes in social structure have increased the proportion of childless marriages. In 1957 47.2 percent of families in the Federal Republic of Germany were married couples with children; in 1991 the proportions were 29.8 percent in West and 33.5 percent in East Germany (Fifth Governmental Family Report, 1994). Today, the period of child-rearing can be seen as just a transitory stage. The phase when married couples live alone, because of longer life expectancy, is on the increase. It would be contrary to modern understanding to refuse legal protection to childless married couples or those with adult offspring. Marriages have the function of stabilizing the partners, channelling their sexuality, and mobilizing their solidarity in the vicissitudes of life and in old age. Marriage today is not just a "germ cell," but a "building block" in society (Bruns, 1996, p. 19).

Arguments have developed about whether the ruling of the Federal Constitutional

Court had precluded in principle the extension of marriage to same-sex couples or whether it had merely identified the existing limits. Various legal drafts have reflected this confusion. While the parliamentary Green Party has proposed a bill in the Bundestag for the "introduction of the right of persons of the same sex to marry," the state government of Lower Saxony has proposed one in the Bundesrat (the federal upper house) creating "registered same sex communities of life" (Regional Government of Lower Saxony, 1995). The Green Party suggested changing the relevant article in the Civil Code as follows: "Marriage may be entered into by two persons of differing or same sex for a lifetime" (Negotiations of the German Parliament, 1995). In contrast, the Lower Saxon draft suggests the alternative of "registered partnership" based on the Scandinavian model. The cabinet of Lower Saxony has said that it will cooperate with other federal states with the aim to create a legal status of registered same-sex communities of life through federal law (Regional Government of Lower Saxony, 1995). It is suggested that registered same-sex partnerships shall be treated similarly to childless married couples, except regarding rights to mutual maintenance, a common surname, and adoption of children.

Unlike the draft by the Green Party, the Lower Saxon draft assumes that gay and lesbian marriages cannot be possible under the Constitution (an interpretation that has been sharply criticized by the Gay Association of Germany) and instead seeks to create a special alternative status in which gay and lesbian couples would to some extent have the same rights as heterosexual couples. The draft is less radical than the system enacted in neighboring Denmark, Norway, and Sweden, where a registered partnership secures the same rights as marital status save for adoption.

Is Gay Marriage Desirable?

A debate has erupted among gay men and more so among lesbians about whether demands for same-sex marriage are appropriate. A large section of the lesbian movement supports the elimination of patriarchal, heterosexual family structures. Some representatives of the gay movement oppose the importation of heterosexual concepts into gay sexuality and fear a heterosexualization of gay relationships. Supporters of gay marriage on the other hand insist that nobody should be entitled to special rights because of their sexual orientation. In reality, it seems that the argument is not so much one between gays and lesbians as between two political strategies, namely, those of "integration" and those of "revolt" (Lautmann, 1992). Pragmatists of the moderate solution (favoring gay marriage) and fundamentalists favoring the radical solution have formed opposing camps. The latter characterize the pragmatists' position as intrinsically assimilatory (Oesterle-Schwerin, 1991). In addition, they fear that in joining the mainstream of society minority status would be lost (Elfering, 1991). Added to all this, suspicions arise that discussing this subject may provoke a flaring up of antihomosexual prejudices (Bleibtreu-Ehrenberg, 1991). The integrationist position insists on the basic right and freedom of choice to marry, which can be reduced to the formula: "They are free to chose to have it. They are free to chose not to have it." (Roggenkamp, 1991, p. 197) The question of assimilation can be looked at differently: "Is assimilating yourself conforming at all? Are not gay men and lesbians conforming to the expectations and demands of heterosexual society exactly when they relinquish the right to marriage?" (Roggenkamp, 1991, p. 200). The famous feminist Alice Schwarzer recognizes a far-reaching principle at the social level. Desire to marry can be seen as conformist at the individual level, yet at the same time it is outright revolutionary at the social level. In a heterosexually dominated world it is an outrage to take homosexual love as seriously as heterosexual love, but that is exactly what is being expressed in the desire to marry (Schwarzer, 1991).

REFERENCES

Akkermann, A., Betzelt, S., & Daniel, G. (1990). Nackte Tatsachen, part II. *Zeitschrift für Sexualforschung, 3*, 140–165.

Bach, K., & Thinius, H. (1989). Die strafrechtliche Gleichstellung hetero- und homosexuellen Verhaltens in der DDR. *Zeitschrift für Sexualforschung, 2*, 237–242.

Bech, H. (1991). Recht fertigen. Über die Einführung "homosexueller Ehen" in Dänemark. *Zeitschrift für Sexualforschung, 4*, 213–224.

Becker, W. (1937). Die richterliche Rechtschöpfung in der strafrechtlichen Praxis. *Deutsche Justiz, 99*, 457–461.

Bleibtreu-Ehrenberg, G. (1978). *Tabu Homosexualität. Die Geschichte eines Vorurteils.* Frankfurt/Main: S. Fischer Verlag.

Bleibtreu-Ehrenberg, G. (1991). Eheschließung gleichgeschlechtlicher Partner und Vorurteil. In K. Laabs (Ed.), *Die Debatte um die Homoehe: Lesben, Schwule, Standesamt* (pp.135–139). Berlin: Links Verlag.

Bochow, M. (1988). *AIDS: Wie leben schwule Männer heute?* Berlin: Deutsche AIDS-Hilfe e.V.

Bochow, M. (1993). Einstellungen und Werthaltungen zu homosexuellen Männern in Ost-und Westdeutschland. In C. Lange (Ed.), *Aids — eine Forschungsbilanz* (pp. 115–128). Berlin: Edition Sigma.

Bruns, M. (1996). *Überlegungen zu einem Antidiskriminierungsgesetz für Lesben und Schwule.* Unpublished manuscript.

Bruns, M., & Beck, V. (1991). Die Ehe für Schwule und Lesben aus rechtspolitischer Sicht. *Zeitschrift für Sexualforschung, 4*, 192–204.

Criminal Law Amendment Act (1935) (Die Strafrechtsnovellen vom 28 Juni 1935) und die amtlichen Begründungen zu diesen Gesetzen). (1935). *Gesetz zur Änderung des Strafgesetzbuches* (pp. 27–30, 38–40). Berlin: Decker's Verlag.

Dannecker, M. (1990). Homosexuelle Männer und AIDS. Eine sexualwissenschaftliche Studie zu Sexualverhalten und Lebensstil. In *Schriftenreihe des Bundesministers für Jugend, Familie, Frauen und Gesundheit* (vol. 152). Stuttgart: Kohlhammer-Verlag.

Dietrich, C. (1995). *Lesbische Identität im Kontext heterosexueller gesellschaftlicher Bedingungen.* Unpublished manuscript.

Elfering, R. (1991). Bald alles wie nur sonstwo auch. In K. Laabs (Ed.), *Die Debatte um die Homoehe: Lesben, Schwule, Standesamt* (pp. 217–222). Berlin: Links Verlag.

Fähnders, W. (1995). Anarchism and homosexuality in Wilhelmine Germany: Senna Hoy, Erich Mühsam, John Henry Mackay. *Journal of Homosexuality, 29*(2/3), 117–153.

Federal Constitutional Court (Entscheidungen des Bundesverfassungsgerichts). (1957). The Constitutionality of Penal Regulation against Male Homosexuality, (vol. 6). Tübingen: J.C.B. Mohr Verlag.

Federal Constitutional Court (Entscheidungen des Bundesverfassungsgerichts). (1971). (vol. 29). Tübingen: J.C.B. Mohr Verlag.

Federal Constitutional Court (Entscheidungen des Bundesverfassungsgerichts). (1972). (vol. 31). Tübingen: J.C.B. Mohr Verlag.

Federal Constitutional Court (Entscheidungen des Bundesverfassungsgerichts). (1974). (vol. 36). Tübingen: J.C.B. Mohr Verlag.

Federal Constitutional Court (Entscheidungen des Bundesverfassungsgerichts). (1993). *Neue Juristische Wochenschrift, 47*, 3058–3059.

Féray, J.-C., & Herzer, M. (1990). Homosexual studies and politics in the 19th century: Karl Maria Kertbeny. *Journal of Homosexuality, 19*(1), 23–47.

Fifth Governmental Family Report (Fünfter Familienbericht der Bundesregierung). Verhandlungen des Deutschen Bundestags. (1994). (12. election period, number 7560, vol. 499). Bonn: German Parliament.

Frank, H. (1934). Zur Strafrechtsreform. *Deutsches Recht, Zentralorgan des Bundes Nat.-Sozialistischer Deutscher*

Juristen (vol. 4). (Journal of the German National Socialist Jurists Association) Berlin: Deutsche Rechts- und Wirtschaft Verlags-Gesellschaft.

Grau, G. (1988). Entscheidung des Obersten Gerichts der DDR zur Homosexualität. *Zeitschrift für Sexualforschung, 1,* 162–165.

Grau, G. (1995a). Sozialistische Moral und Homosexualität. In D. Grumbach (Ed.), *Die Linke und das Laster. Schwule Emanzipation und linke Vorurteile* (pp. 85–141). Hamburg: MännerschwarmSkript-Verlag.

Grau, G. (1995b). Hidden Holocaust? Gay and lesbian persecution in Germany, 1933–1949. In The Cassell (Ed.), *Lesbian and gay Studies List.* London: Cassell.

Herzer, M. (1995). Communists, social Democrats, and the homosexual movement in the Weimar Republic. *Journal of Homosexuality, 29*(2/3), 197–226.

Hoffmann, R., Lautmann, R., & Pagenstecher, L. (1993). Unter Frauen-unter Männern: homosexuelle Liebesbeziehungen. In A. E. Auhagen, & M. von Salisch (Eds.), *Zwischenmenschliche Beziehungen* (pp. 195–211). Göttingen: Hogrefe.

Höinghaus, R. (1870). *Das neue Strafgesetzbuch für den Norddeutschen Bund mit den vollständigen amtlichen Motiven.* Berlin: Gustav Hempel.

Hutter, J. (1992a). *Die gesellschaftliche Kontrolle des homosexuellen Begehrens. Medizinische Definitionen und juristische Sanktionen im 19. Jahrhundert.* Frankfurt/Main: Campus Forschung.

Hutter, J. (1992b). Die Entstehung des § 175 im Strafgesetzbuch und die Geburt der deutschen Sexualwissenschaft. In R. Lautmann & A. Taeger (Eds.), *Männerliebe im alten Deutschland. Sozialgeschichtliche Abhandlungen* (pp. 187–238). Berlin: Verlag rosa Winkel.

Hutter, J. (1993). Abschaffung des § 175 StGB. Diskussion um die Schutzaltersgrenze. In Senatsverwaltung für Jugend und Familie (Ed.), *Pädagogischer Kongreß: Lebensformen und Sexualität. Was heißt hier normal?,* (pp. 179–189). Berlin: editor.

Klare, R. (1937). *Homosexualität und Strafrecht.* Hamburg: Hanseatische Verlagsanstalt Hamburg.

Laabs, K. (Ed.). (1991). *Die Debatte um die Homoehe: Lesben, Schwule, Standesamt.* Berlin: Links Verlag.

Langbein, J. H. (1974). *Prosecuting crime in the Rennaissance.* England: Cambridge.

Lautmann, R. (1981). The pink triangle: The persecution of homosexual males in concentration camps in Nazi Germany. *Journal of Homosexuality, 6*(1/2), 141–160.

Lautmann, R. (1984). *Der Zwang zur Tugend. Die gesellschaftliche Kontrolle der Sexualitäten.* Frankfurt/Main: Suhrkamp-Verlag.

Lautmann, R. (1992). Das Verbrechen der widernatürlichen Unzucht. Seine Grundlegung in der preußischen Gesetzesrevision des 19. Jahrhunderts. In R. Lautmann & A. Taeger (Eds.), *Männerliebe im alten Deutschland. Sozialgeschichtliche Abhandlungen* (pp. 141–186). Berlin: Verlag rosa Winkel.

Lautmann, R. (1993). *Homosexualität. Handbuch der Theorie- und Forschungsgeschichte.* Frankfurt/Main: Campus-Verlag.

Lautmann, R., Grikschat, W., & Schmidt, E. (1977). Der rosa Winkel in den nationalsozialistischen Konzentrationslagern. In R. Lautmann (Ed.), *Seminar: Gesellschaft und Homosexualität.* (pp. 383–139). Frankfurt/Main: Suhrkamp-Verlag.

Mende, B. (1990). Die antihomosexuelle Gesetzgebung in der Weimarer Republik. In Freunde eines Schwulen Museums in Berlin e.V. (Eds.), *Die Geschichte des § 175. Strafrecht gegen Homosexuelle.* (pp. 105–121). Berlin: Verlag rosa Winkel.

Negotiations of the German Parliament (Verhandlungen des deutschen Bundestages). (1990). (11. election period, no. 7197, vol. 406). Bonn: German Parliament.

Negotiations of the German Parliament (Verhandlungen des deutschen Bundestages). (1995). (13. election period, no. 2728, vol. 538). Bonn: German Parliament.

Oesterle-Schwerin, J. (1991). Assimilation oder Emanzipation. In K. Laabs (Ed.), *Die Debatte um die Homoehe: Lesben, Schwule, Standesamt* (pp. 28–38). Berlin: Links Verlag.

Pingel, R., & Trautvetter, W. (1987). *Homosexuelle Partnerschaften.* Berlin: Verlag rosa Winkel.

Regional Government of Lower Saxony (Niedersächsische Landesregierung). (1995). *Abbau rechtlicher Diskriminierungen lesbischer Frauen und homosexueller Männer; Gesetzliche Regelungen für gleichgeschlechtliche Lebensweisen.*

Roggenkamp, V. (1991). Spaltpilz Ehe. In K. Laabs (Ed.), *Die Debatte um die Homoehe: Lesben, Schwule, Standesamt* (pp. 195–200). Berlin: Links Verlag.

Röhner, K.-H. (1988). Die Bewertung des homosexuellen Verhaltens durch das Strafrecht der DDR. In H.

Schmigalla (Ed.), *Psychosoziale Aspekte der Homosexualität* (pp. 188–195). Jena: Verlagsabteilung der Friedrich-Schiller-Universität Jena.

Schoppmann, C. (1991). *Nationalsozialistische Sexualpolitik und weibliche Homosexualität*. Pfaffenweiler, Germany: Centaurus-Verlagsgesellschaft.

Schultz, C. (1994). *Paragraph 175. (abgewickelt)*. Hamburg: MännerschwarmSkript Verlag.

Schwarzer, A. (1991). Auch das noch? In K. Laabs (Ed.), *Die Debatte um die Homoehe: Lesben, Schwule, Standesamt* (pp. 19–22). Berlin: Links Verlag.

Starke, K. (1994). *Schwuler Osten. Homosexuelle Männer in der DDR*. Berlin: Links Verlag.

Steakley, J. D. (1989). Sodomy in Enlightenment Prussia: From execution to suicide. *Journal of Homosexuality*, 16(1/2), 163–175.

Strafgesetzbuch für die Preußischen Staaten (1851). *para 143 (Paragraph 143)*. Berlin: Albert Nauk and Comp.

Supreme Court of the Reich (Reichsgericht). (1935). Widernatürliche Unzucht. Bindung an frühere Urteile. In Members of the Court (Eds.). *Entscheidungen des Reichsgerichtes in Strafsachen* (vol. 69, pp. 273–276). Berlin & Leipzig: Walter de Gruyter & Co.

Supreme Court of the Reich (Reichsgericht). (1938). Der § 175 a Nr. 3 StGB ist entsprechend anzuwenden, wenn ein Mann über einundzwanzig Jahren eine männliche Person unter einundzwanzig Jahren durch Verleitung zum Alkoholgenuß in einen willenlosen und bewußtlosen Zustand versetzt und dann zur Unzucht mißbraucht. In Members of the Court (Eds.), *Entscheidungen des Reichsgerichtes in Strafsachen* (vol. 72, pp. 50–53). Berlin: Walter de Gruyter & Co.

Supreme Court of the Reich (Reichsgericht). (1939). Das Merkmal des Unzuchttreibens mit einem anderen im Sinne der §§ 175, 175 a RStGB kann auch durch Handlungen erfüllt sein, bei denen keine körperliche Berührung stattgefunden hat. In Members of the Court (Eds.), *Entscheidungen des Reichsgerichtes in Strafsachen* (vol. 73, pp. 78–81). Berlin: Walter de Gruyter & Co.

Sweet, D. M. (1995). The church, the Stasi, and Socialist integration: Three stages of lesbian and gay emancipation in the former German Democratic Republic. *Journal of Homosexuality*, 29(4), 351–367.

Taeger, A., & Lautmann, R. (1992). Sittlichkeit und Politik. § 175 im Deutschen Kaiserreich. In R. Lautmann & A. Taeger (Eds.), *Männerliebe im alten Deutschland. Sozialgeschichtliche Abhandlungen* (pp. 239–268). Berlin: Verlag rosa Winkel.

Thinius, H. (1990). Verwandlung und Fall des Paragraphen 175 in der Deutschen Demokratischen Republik. In Freunde eines Schwulen Museums in Berlin e.V. (Eds.), *Die Geschichte des § 175. Strafrecht gegen Homosexuelle* (pp. 145–164). Berlin: Verlag rosa Winkel.

Wegner, J. (1995). Die Ehe für gleichgeschlechtliche Lebensweisen. *Zeitschrift für Rechtssoziologie*, 16(2), 170–191.

Wienold, H., & Lautmann, R. (1977). Antihomosexualität und demokratische Kultur in der BRD. In R. Lautmann (Ed.), *Seminar: Gesellschaft und Homosexualität* (pp. 383–439). Frankfurt/Main: Suhrkamp-Verlag.

17

Austria

HELMUT GRAUPNER

"Against the Order of Nature" — a History of Persecution

Among the countries that do not generally criminalize homosexual conduct as such, Austria has the most restrictive legislation on homosexuality[1]. Each year more than 60 criminal proceedings are instituted and more than 20 people are convicted. Most are given prison sentences solely on the basis of their sexual orientation. Discrimination in other areas of the law is manifold. The Austrian constitution does not provide effective protection against discrimination on the basis of sexual orientation. The discriminatory legal system seems to be out of touch with public attitudes, which are rather tolerant, especially among young people.

The Time before 1768

Initially, homosexual relations — like all the other deviations from Christian moral teaching — came exclusively under the jurisdiction of the ecclesiastical courts. These courts radically mitigated the Teutonic practice, which applied the death sentence for certain (passive) forms of homosexual contact. In the main they imposed lenient punishment, mitigated even further by the possibility of substituting penitence (Graupner, 1995a).

It was not until the ninth or tenth centuries that criminal justice reverted to its former severity. As "sodomy" or "lewdness against the order of nature" became a matter for the secular courts, death by fire became the penalty for this "abominable sin." Initially, the courts interpreted sodomy as meaning homosexuality or bestiality, but later they included intercourse with corpses or with statues made of wood or stone and even masturbation to fall under this same capital offense. The Hexenhammer of the year 1487, and the subsequent evolution of judicial practice, declared sodomy to be the central characteristic of witchcraft, thereby causing massive intensification of criminal persecution (Graupner, 1995a).

In those days, children and adolescents were treated not as victims but as accomplices. Youth did not eradicate criminal liability but merely (and only sometimes) led to more lenient sentences than those imposed on adults (Graupner, 1995a).

Later on, certain German criminal codes, like the Constitutio Criminalis Bambergensis (1507) and the Constitutio Criminalis Carolina (1532), retained the death penalty

---

[1]Only Liechtenstein kept a similarily strong antihomosexual legislation after basic decriminalization (cf. Graupner, 1995a).

HELMUT GRAUPNER • Rechtskomitee LAMBDA, Austrian Sexological Society, Linke Wienzeile, 102, A-1060 Vienna, Austria.

Sociolegal Control of Homosexuality, edited by West and Green, Plenum Press, New York, 1997.

for homosexuality and bestiality, but decriminalized other kinds of sodomy (Graupner, 1995a).

Generally it can be said that up to as late as the eighteenth and nineteenth centuries the law focused essentially upon penetration, primarily upon anal intercourse. In the main, medieval people understood "voluptuous acts" to be just the "gross forms" of what we understand as "sexuality" today, namely, varieties of sexual penetration ("carnal knowledge"). We do not know why nearly all of the reported court cases deal with anal intercourse only; it may be that the reason for the rarity of oral sex in court practice reflects the rarity of this kind of sex in the community, due to the state of hygiene then prevailing. The medieval understanding of sexuality cannot be analyzed here further, but it may be connected both to the generally franker attitude toward the body and nudity and to the "rough" circumstances of living those days, leading to a similar roughness in understanding of sexual acts (Graupner, 1995a).

Constitutio Criminalis Theresiana (1768)

The Criminal Code promulgated by empress Maria Theresia — the first to be enforced over the whole of the Austrian territory — following medieval tradition understood *sodomia, feu luxuri contra naturam* [unchastity against nature] to be: (1) sexual contact with animals, or (2) with corpses; (3) "lewdness against the order of nature between persons of the same sex, be it man with man or woman with woman, but also woman with man" and (4) "unchastities against the order of nature committed alone" (s. 74).

Bestiality was liable to death by fire, lewdness between human beings to decapitation and subsequent burning of the corpse, and all other forms of sodomy to a penalty at the discretion of the judge. If *immissio seminis* did not occur, death by fire could be reduced to decapitation or decapitation to reasonable corporal punishment. Torture was explicitly admissible (s. 74).

Offenses not punishable as sodomy but nevertheless punishable by severe corporal punishment were (1) incest [vaginal intercourse between certain relatives: "disgrace of the blood"(s. 75)], (2) intercourse between the unmarried, (3) concubinage, and (4) debauchery by an unmarried woman (all as "common fornication," (s. 81). In the case of incest in the direct line, the punishment was decapitation. All of these offenses were liable to intensified punishment if committed between Christians and "Jews, Turks or other unbelievers" on the other side ["a particular abomination" (s. 82)].

Constitutio Criminalis Josephina (1787)

With the advent of the French Revolution, Joseph II instituted radical sex law reform. He decriminalized masturbation, intercourse between the unmarried, "lewdness against the order of nature" between man and woman, incest,[2] and intercourse between Christians and "unbelievers."

---

[2]Resistance against the decriminalization of incest seemingly has been underestimated. Only 9 months after the promulgation of the Constitutio Criminalis Josephina the offense was introduced again by imperial decree (Justizgesetzammlung 744, cf. Graupner, 1995). Penile vaginal intercourse between certain close relatives remains criminal [Criminal Code (s. 211)].

In contrast to French legislators 5 years later, and to all lawmakers influenced by the French revolutionary legislation, Joseph II retained the offense of "carnal knowledge of a beast or of someone of his own sex" (2nd part, s. 71), but drastically mitigated the sentences for this offense (2nd part, ss. 10, 72), reducing the offense from a felony to a misdemeanor punishable by the political authority. When dealt with as public nuisance the penalty was public whipping and public labor from 1 day to 1 month followed by banishment from the site of the act; in all other cases the penalty was "severe jail" (i.e., iron on the feet, lying on boards, no visits without supervision, no drinks except water, and "reasonable" work) from 1 day to 1 month, accompanied by whipping (2nd part, ss. 10ff, 72).

Criminal Code (1803)

The Criminal Code of 1803 (CC), the first after the advent of the French Revolution, decriminalized solicitation for "lewdness" on a public street [Constitutio Criminalis Josephina (CCJ), 2nd part, ss. 67F, 69], permitting "lewdness" on one's own premises (CCJ, 2nd part, s. 73) and prostitution (CCJ, 2nd part, s. 75: "lewdness for gain"),[3] but reintroduced the offense of "lewdness against the order of nature" (CC, ss. 113ff), without, however, providing a specific definition. This enabled some commentators to interpret it according to medieval tradition as covering all kinds of lewdness that do not serve procreation, including, for example, masturbation. However, an imperial decree of 1824 finally made clear that this provision was in place of the earlier CCJ Section 71 and therefore covered homosexuality and bestiality only (Graupner, 1995a). In contrast to the 1787 CCJ the offense was classified as a felony, with the penalty drastically raised to confinement from 6 months to 1 year [with no drink other than water and supervised visits only (s. 12 CC)].

Criminal Code (1852)

The Criminal Code of 1852 — which was in force until 1975 — largely adopted the sex offenses from the 1803 CC and renumbered them, but the penalty for homosexual conduct (and conduct with animals, which always has been regulated in the same provision) was again dramatically raised to severe imprisonment from 1–5 years (ss. 129, 130 CC).

Unlike the German Empire, the Austrian Empire never restricted the offense to males and always interpreted "lewdness against the order of nature" to cover all kinds of same-sex conduct, not limiting it to acts analogous to sexual intercourse. The Supreme Court repeatedly held that any sexual act constituted the offense, although mere touching of the genitals did not (OGH 22.10.1937, 4 Os 690/37; OGH 27.11.1928, 4 Os 774/28).

The Austrian Criminal Code remained in effect during the time of unification with Germany (1938–1945). The German Criminal Code was never introduced into Austria (Hoyer, Geller, & Metzler, 1944).

[3]Prostitution remained an offense punishable with up to 3 months if it caused public nuisance, if young people were seduced, and if the prostitute knew that she suffered from venereal disease [1803 CC (s. 254); 1852 CC (ss. 519ff)]. In 1885 this offense was taken out of the Criminal Code and the penalty was raised to 6 months imprisonment [Act on Forced Labour and Correctional Institutions (s. 5)]. In 1975 all of these forms of prostitution were decriminalized (The Act on Forced Labour and Correctional Institutions was abolished by the Criminal Law Adaption Act of 1974).

Criminal Law Amendment Act (1971)

In 1971 Austria basically decriminalized homosexual conduct. It abolished the general ban on homosexual relations, but introduced four new discriminatory criminal laws.

The age of consent (minimum age) for male homosexual relations was set at 18 (ss. 129, 130), and gay male prostitution (s. 500a), "public approval of same-sex lewdness" (s. 517), and forming "associations promoting same-sex lewdness" (s. 518) were made new offenses.

By introducing these laws Austria enacted significantly stricter legislation on homosexuality than the Austrian Criminal Law Reform Commission had recommended in 1956. The draft elaborated by that commission of experts had set the age of consent for all homosexual contact at 14 (equal to the traditional age limit for heterosexual conduct) and established only three discriminatory offenses: (1) seduction of a male minor under 18 by another male, (2) gay male prostitution, and (3) public approval of homosexuality (Graupner, 1995a). Parliament did not follow these earlier recommendations.

But even homosexual relations that had been basically decriminalized in 1971 (contacts between women over 14, between 14- and 18-year-old male adolescents, or between men over 18) could still be prosecuted under Section 516. This provision made it an offense to "violate morals and modesty in a gross way causing public nuisance."[4] The courts did not require that nuisance had in fact been caused (it sufficed that the concrete act was able to cause public nuisance) or that the nuisance had to have been caused by the act itself (nuisance caused by subsequent knowledge sufficed). In effect, therefore, nearly all of the previously decriminalized homosexual behaviors could be punished on the basis of this offense. It was scarcely an effective restriction that the courts required the offender to be aware that the act could come to public knowledge (Graupner, 1995a).

Criminal Code (1975)

It was not until the introduction of the Criminal Code of 1975, which is still in force, that the general ban on homosexual behavior was effectively lifted. The code looked over the four discriminatory provisions (ss. 129f, 500a, 517, and 518 of the Criminal Code of 1852) as ss. 209, 210, 220, and 221 of the Criminal Code of 1975 but no longer included any provision equivalent to Section 516 of the 1852 Criminal Code (Graupner, 1995a).

Criminal Law Amendment Act (1988)

Since 1988, when the age of liability for violations of the age of consent of 18 for male homosexual relations (s. 209) was raised to 19, sexual contact with 14- to 18-year-olds by 18-year-olds has not been punishable (Graupner, 1995a).

---

[4]This offense has been introduced by the Criminal Code of 1852 and strongly resembles the former Spanish offense *grave escándalo ó transcendencia* (abolished in 1988), which traditionally has been used to punish sexual contacts not expressly covered by the criminal law (Graupner, 1995). Neither the Criminal Code of 1803, the Constitutio Criminalis Josephina, nor the Constitutio Criminalis Theresiana contained such a provision (Graupner, 1995).

Criminal Law Amendment Act (1989)

Whereas previously the Criminal Code had contained much more lenient penalties for homosexual violence than for heterosexual violence, this 1989 act equalized the penalties by raising those for homosexual violence (BGBl. 1989/242).

Moreover, the ban on gay male prostitution was also repealed in this year (heterosexual prostitution had been decriminalized in 1803, lesbian in 1975) following strong representations by the public health authorities that the ban massively hindered effective AIDS prevention (JA 928 Blg.NR XVII. GP; BGBl. 1989/243).

The other three discriminatory criminal provisions remain in effect.

THE CRIMINAL LAW

The Minimum Age

The relevant statute (s. 209; "Same Sex Lewdness with Persons under 18 Years") reads: "A man over 19 years of age who engages in same sex lewdness with a person who has attained the age of fourteen but not yet the age of eighteen years shall be punished with imprisonment from six months to five years."

In contrast, the minimum age for heterosexual and lesbian relations is fixed at 14 (ss. 206, 207). It does not eradicate criminal liability if both partners are consenting or if the adolescent is a hustler (Graupner, 1995).

Although there are today only one-fourth the number of criminal proceedings and convictions that there were in the early 1970s, nevertheless each year there are still about 60 criminal proceedings (59 in 1994) instituted on the basis of the 1975 code; more than 20 men (24 in 1994) are normally convicted. Altogether, by 1994, 2153 criminal proceedings had been instituted and 886 people sentenced since the introduction of this offense in 1971 (Graupner, 1995). Typically, it is men between the ages of 18 and 39 (men over 40 are underrepresented), but sometimes even women and adolescents themselves (as accomplices; e.g., in the case of group sex), who are reported to the police for this offense (Graupner, 1995a). In 1994 more than one third of suspects in reported cases were under 25, one tenth under 20 (Graupner, 1996b).

The percentages given prison sentences generally, or prison sentences without suspension, have fallen continually since 1971 but still amount to 65 to 75 percent and 15 to 25 percent of all convictions, respectively. Prison sentences of up to 3 years are common. The last time imprisonment of more than 3 years was inflicted was in 1985, but compared to other sexual offenses court practice for this offense seems harsh. Until the late 1980s the percentages of prison sentences and of unsuspended prison sentences were as high as those for cases of sexual contact with children under 14 (ss. 206) and until the mid-1980s a shorter imprisonment of under 3 months was being imposed less often than for this offense. As for (heterosexual) misuse of a relationship of authority over a minor,[5] in 25 to 50 percent of the cases only fines are imposed, and since 1988 imprisonment without suspension has been imposed only once (Graupner, 1995a). Moreover, the courts count (same-sex) consensual

---

[5]The age of majority is 19 [General Civil Code (s. 21)].

sex with an adolescent between 14 and 18 as being indicative of the same harmful inclinations as sexual violence, even (heterosexual) rape. Consequently, especially harsh sentences are inflicted where there is a prior criminal record of (even heterosexual) rape or sexual violence (OGH 28.11.1995, 14 Os 114/95).

It seems particularly remarkable that after the introduction of the new Criminal Code in 1975 the proportion of prison sentences of more than 1 year increased considerably from about 2 percent before 1975 to about 7 to 15 percent after. This trend seems to reflect an affirmation of the criminality of homosexuality inherent in the decision to retain this provision in the new code. Although sentencing became less harsh after the mid-1980s, even today the prison sentences inflicted are considerably longer than they were before 1975. This seems inconsistent with the drastic decline in reports and convictions and suggests a lack of response on the part of the courts to the development of public attitudes on these matters (Graupner, 1995a).

As recently as 1990 the Upper Regional Court of Graz held that the punishment (of 6 months to 5 years) laid down in Section 209 had to be imposed in proportion to the degree of wrongdoing involved and to the public sense of justice. Therefore (on appeal) it significantly increased the sentences imposed on two defendants by a Corinthian court. One was given a suspended imprisonment of 7 months for manual and oral (in one case also anal) sex with three boys, the other a suspended sentence of 1 year for manual and oral (in one case also anal) sex with seven boys. The boys were all between 15 and 17 years old at the time and consenting willingly to the sexual relations, some even initiatating them. The Upper Regional Court increased these sentences to 14 months and 18 months, respectively, on the ground of an alleged general increase of such offenses and the high number of unreported incidents. For the same reasons the court also quashed the total suspension of the sentences and directed parts of the imprisonment to be unsuspended (4 and 6 months, respectively), noting that the first defendant, in particular, as a teacher should have been aware of the "danger of a homosexual development against which adolescents have to be protected" (Upper Regional Court of Graz 19.06.1990, 11 Bs 181/90; 29.10.1990, 10 Bs 385/90).

Typically, proceedings nowadays are instituted when police are able to capture a couple caressing or engaging in sex at a public site or in a car; when persons, cars, or homes are being searched (very often illegally); or when police exert pressure on adolescents, especially hustlers, to confess to a sexual relation with one or more men [cf. Lambda Nachrichten 4/89 (47f); 1/90; 2/90; Jus Amandi 1/93 (23f); 2/93 (24); 3/93 (24f); 4/93 (26); 1/94 (20); 2/95 (3)].

In 1990 a Corinthian court went so far as to sentence an adolescent to (suspended) imprisonment of 10 months for false testimony in court and attempted aiding and abetting his adult partner. This was on the basis that in court he had retracted his confession to the police that he had had sexual contacts with the man. The boy claimed that police had subjected him to considerable pressure and that he had been coerced to testify against his partner by threats to make his future life unbearable in Corinthia. The court dismissed these claims solely on the basis of the assurance by the detective concerned that the interrogation was carried out correctly and no pressure had been exerted on the boy [Regional Court of Klagenfurt 20.06.1990, 14 EVr 216/90; cf. Regional Court of Klagenfurt 20.06.1990, 14 EVr 651/90 (8); Upper Regional Court of Graz 29.10.1990, 10 Bs 385/90 (5f)]. In 1989 a Viennese court sentenced a man to 3 months (suspended) imprisonment for an attempt at this offense. He had propositioned a 15-year-old to have sex with him in a public lavatory nearby (Regional Criminal Court of Vienna, 3aE Vr 6530/89, Hv 3825/89).

In the process of enforcing Section 209 of the Criminal Code, fundamental principles of justice are often breached. For example, on February 8, 1996, the Regional Criminal Court of Vienna sentenced a 28-year-old gay man to 1 year (suspended) incarceration for allegedly engaging in consensual sex with young men ages 15–17. The penalty was imposed despite the absence of any prior criminal record for a sex offense. The extraordinary terms of the charge were "same-sex lewdness with a multitude of unknown, no longer identifiable adolescents, at unknown, no longer identifiable, places in Austria, Slovakia, the Czech Republic, the Netherlands and Italy." The court rejected counsel's application for an investigation into the age and identity of the young men, whose first names and ages, as only guessed by the defendant, were all that was known about them. The case had been brought on the evidence of a notebook found in a house search in which the defendant had recorded dates and his partners' first names and apparent ages, which were mostly over 18. Since it was only Austria in which his conduct was prosecutable, counsel sought an inquiry into where the contacts took place and the relevant laws in those places. That, too, was rejected (Graupner, 1996a). The Supreme Courts quashed the judgment with regard to the contacts abroad only and upheld it as far as the alleged contacts in Austria are concerned (OGH 05.11.1996, 11 Os 128/96). Therefore, the Regional Criminal Court of Vienna on January 29th, 1997, again sentenced the man to 11 months (suspended) incarceration for the contacts in Austria (Graupner, 1997).

This was not the first time that decisions incompatible with a fair trial have been made in the enforcement of Section 209. In 1995, after having been mistreated by police, a man signed a statement confessing that over the past 14 years he had also had sex with males aged 15–17. (The time limit for prosecution is 5 years.) He gave a name and address for two boys. In the course of intensive investigations the police interrogated 13 youths, but found no evidence of criminal relations. One of the identified boys was found not to exist, and the existence of the second was not verified. Nevertheless, the Regional Criminal Court of Vienna sentenced the man to 6 months (suspended) imprisonment for allegedly having sex with the adolescent he had named in his "confession," whose identity the police and the court failed to verify (Graupner, 1996b). The Upper Regional Court of Vienna upheld the conviction (Graupner, 1996d).

Approval of Homosexuality

The relevant statute (s. 220: "Advertisement for Lewdness with Persons of the Same Sex or with Animals") reads: "Whosoever, in printed matter, in a film or otherwise, promulgates same-sex lewdness or lewdness with animals or who approves of it in a manner which is able to suggest such acts, shall, if he is not himself, as a participant to the lewdness, liable to a more severe sentence (§ 12), be punished with imprisonment of up to six months or with a fine of up to a rating of 360 days."

According to the explanatory notes of the Criminal Law Amendment Act (1971) this provision should cover printed matter or films that "surround the homosexual inclination and behavior with the nimbus of the noble or the culturally valuable, which praise the homosexual way of living as being superior to the heterosexual" (39 BlgNR XII.GP). Also "oral propaganda, for instance for membership in a homosexual group" (39 BlgNR XII.GP) should come under this law, but not "scientific treatment of the issue for the purpose of research or doctrine" (39 BlgNR XII.GP). According to some commentators, however, this restriction does not apply to "pseudoscientific" publications "propagating same-sex lewdness under the cloak of scientific discourse" (Leukauf & Steininger, 1992, p. 1258, Section 220 annotation 3), and the law also forbids support through the "enumeration of the merits of same-sexual behavior without expressely recommending it" (Pallin, 1980, s. 220 annotation 4).

So far there have only been three convictions under this law, and it is not determinable from the criminal statistics if these cases concerned "advertisement" for homosexuality or for bestiality. Because of the small number of convictions there is no case law on this provision. However, in 1981 the Supreme Court held that the law does not require that the propaganda be aimed at arguing a large crowd of people out of their hitherto heterosexual inclination (SSt 51/51).

Even if currently the courts do not convict under this law, authorities regularly use it to seize AIDS prevention (safe-sex) material, especially when imported from abroad. In 1992 the Regional Criminal Court of Vienna ordered the permanent confiscation of the safe-sex brochure "Schwuler Sex.Sicher" of the German Aids-Hilfe Wien for its positive representation of homosexuality by the enumeration of the merits of certain homosexual behaviors and the reference to its "harmlessness" (Regional Court of Vienna 07.07.1992, 9aE Vr 10701/90, Hv 2858/92). In 1994 the Regional Court of Wels ordered the confiscation of a safe-sex video shown by Aids-Help of Upper Austria at an AIDS prevention event (*Der Standard*, 1994).

In 1990/91 an issue of *Tabu*, the magazine of the youth group of the gay/lesbian association Homosexuelle Initiative Wien (HOSI-Wien), was confiscated because of its positive representation of homosexuality (Upper Regional Court of Vienna 29.04.1991, 21 Bs 20/91). The court of first instance confiscated letters from the youth group to student representatives at Viennese secondary schools in which the group pointed to the problems of gay and lesbian teenagers, presented itself, and offered to provide informative material and organize discussions and other events. The court even held that the true presentation of the homosexuality of historical persons should constitute punishable "advertisement" for homosexuality (Regional Criminal Court of Vienna 18.09.1990, 9b E Vr 3083/88, Hv 5746/89), but these parts of the verdict were quashed on appeal. Section 220 of the Criminal Code also causes side effects in other areas of the law. Gay and lesbian pornography remain illegal as a result of this offense (see later in this chapter).

In 1988 a communal advertising agency, appealing to Section 220, refused to attach to Viennese trams labels with the words "Lesbians Are Always and Everywhere." The gay and lesbian movement went to court and won. The Commercial Court of Vienna held that the sentence stated a mere fact: Lesbians ARE always and everywhere. Today such a statement would not constitute "advertisement" in the sense of Section 220. The advertising agency concerned was obliged to attach the labels and for some weeks Viennese trams carried this slogan (Commercial Court of Vienna 19.12.1989, 1 R 302/89; County Court for Commercial Affairs 15.06.1989, 11 C 2979/88y).

In 1994 the Austrian postal service also appealed to Section 220 to justify its refusal to grant pages to the organization Homotext, who wanted to establish a gay and lesbian service in the Austrian post-administrated BTX network. Only after an order by the Minister of Public Industries and Transport was the postal service granted the pages and Homotext allowed to establish its electronic communication service (*BTX-Bildschirmtext*, 1995).

Groups Promoting Homosexuality

The relevant statute (s. 221, "Associations Promoting Same Sex Lewdness"), reads: "Whosoever founds an association of a greater number of people, whose aim, even if not the predominant one, is to promote same sex lewdness and which is able to cause public nuisance; furthermore whosoever is a member of such an association or solicits members for it shall be punished by imprisonment of up to six months or a fine of up to 360 day rates."

There have been no convictions under this law and there is no case law on it. According to commentators, a "great number of people" shall mean at least 10 (Foregger & Serini, 1988; Leukauf & Steininger, 1992; Pallin, 1980); according to others at least 30 (Bertel & Schwaighofer, 1992).

In 1980 the Federal Police Authority of Salzburg, appealing to Section 221, prohibited the formation of the organization Homosexuelle Initiative (HOSI) Salzburg; on appeal the decision was quashed by the Ministry of Interior, as such a prohibition is possible only within 6 months from the day authorities are notified of the formation of a group, and the decision had been made 1 day after the expiration of this period (Dr. R. Brandstätter personal communication).

As long ago as 1928 the Austrian authorities prohibited the formation of the gay and lesbian organization Bund für Menschenrechte [Association for Human Rights], the Austrian division of the then biggest gay rights organization in Germany (Hauer, 1989).

Pornography

The Austrian Pornography Act (1950) in its Section 1 bans all commerce in "indecent" publications, films, and other media for pecuniary profit.

Until 1977 all sexually explicit material was held to be indecent and therefore banned under the Pornography Act. In 1977 the Supreme Court reversed its jurisdiction and stated that only material depicting criminal sexual behavior can be understood as indecent (cf. Mayerhofer & Rieder, 1992, Section 1 PornoG Z. 5). Since that decision, only pornography involving persons under 14 (the general age of consent) or depicting sexual violence has been banned (so-called "hard pornography").

However, where homosexual pornography is involved, the court also decided that while homosexual behavior is not criminal as such, the propagation of it is [Criminal Code of 1975 (hereafter CC), s. 220]. And since pornography always contains an element of propagation, gay and lesbian pornography (and pornography involving animals; cf. CC, s. 220) as such is classified as hard pornography (cf. Mayerhofer & Rieder, 1992, s. 1 PornoG Z. 5ff).

In 1987 final decisions on pornography cases were removed from the Supreme Court to the four Upper Regional Courts (BGBl. 1988 No. 599). From these four, the Upper Regional Court of Innsbruck, having jurisdiction over the western states of Tyrol and Vorarlberg, reversed the former decisions and legalized commerce in gay and lesbian pornography (Upper Regional Court of Innsbruck 13.09.1989, 7 Bs 332/89; Regional Court of Innsbruck 30.06.1989, 37 Vr 882/89, Hv 96/89). The other three Upper Regional Courts did not [but the Regional Criminal Court of Vienna did so on February 3, 1994 (13a Bl 61/94)].

Currently, in Vienna, courts try to avoid convictions, while still complying with the jurisdiction of the Upper Regional Court, by staying the criminal proceedings and just seizing the pornographic material. But since this still infringes the freedom of information and the right to possession, Rechtskomitee LAMBDA, the Austrian gay and lesbian legal advice organization, is currently supporting a test case to go before the European Commission of Human Rights. They contend that a ban on homosexual pornography violates the right of freedom of information (Scherer, 1993) and are appealing against a verdict confiscating lesbian pornography (personal communication).

Sadomasochism

According to the Criminal Code assault is not illegal if the injured party consents and the injury as such does not conflict with good morals (s. 90).

In 1977 the Supreme Court in a gay sadomasochism case held that, in principle, sadistic and masochistic assault and battery does conflict with good morals. Consent therefore cannot eradicate criminal liability (OGH 10.03.1977; 12 Os 180/76). In contrast, the Supreme Court has never declared assault and battery in boxing or other combat sports to be, in principle, "conflicting with good morals."

THE CIVIL LAW

A short overview of the treatment of homosexuality by Austrian civil law is given in this Section. Because of the nearly endless number of (potentially) discriminatory provisions, this account does not in any way claim completeness.

Partnership

History.   Sexual intercourse between the unmarried ("debauchery", "simple fornication", "fornicationes simplices", "concubinage") was punishable until 1787. In the Middle Ages, however, this offense could not easily be distinguished from the institution of "marriage by consensus", that is, marriage simply by sexual intercourse with the intent to marry (Graupner, 1995a).

Only after the reform of matrimonial law by the Trientinian Council in the year 1563 did the offenses of simple fornication and concubinage gain increased practical importance. This reform repealed the institution of marriage by consensus and prescribed that henceforth a valid marriage could only be contracted in a formal ceremony before a priest. From then on intercourse between the unmarried and concubinage could be readily identified and therefore sanctioned without involving major practical (evidentiary) problems (Graupner, 1995a).

In the sixteenth century the offense came under the jurisdiction of the secular courts (cf. Police Regulations of the Reich 1548, Constitutio Criminalis Theresiana 1768, s. 81). In 1787 Joseph II repealed the offense (Graupner, 1995a).

Though concubinage was thereafter not expressly mentioned in the Criminal Code, nevertheless it was still considered illegal. Consequently, the partners could be liable under a decree of 1857. This made it an offense to commit acts that were "declared illegal by law or decree without establishing a certain penalty for contraventions" (RGBl. 198). For such acts the decree established a fine or detention from 6 hours up to 14 days. Domestic servants, journeymen, apprentices, and day laborers, in lieu of detention or as aggravation, could be beaten. Beating consisted of 20 strokes with a stick, but boys under 18 and women were caned (Graupner, 1995a).

Since the authorities regarded concubinage as illegal and constituting an offense under this decree, without it being expressly made an offense in any law, it seems highly probable that not only concubinage but also intercourse between the unmarried (simple fornication) could be punished under this decree (Graupner, 1995a).

Case law on this offense has not been uniform. Sometimes the authorities restricted it to "acts conflicting with public morals which entail negative effects by causing public nuisance" (The Supreme Political Authority, 1828, cited in Graupner, 1995a).

The decree of 1857 was repealed in 1925 (Art. II. pr. 2 lit. 10 EGVG, BGBl. 1925/273). Since then concubinage has definitely not been punishable (Graupner, 1995a). On the contrary, legislation in the 1920s and 1930s placed (heterosexual) companions of life (in law termed "house-keepers") on the same footing with spouses regarding some areas of social security rights, thus mitigating the social problems of couples who could not marry because one partner had already been married (divorce was not available at that time). With the introduction of divorce in 1938 this social need for recognizing (heterosexual) companions of life decreased, and corresponding legal development slowed (Schneider, 1965).

Same-sex partnerships never have been legally put on a par with marriage, nor even with heterosexual companions of life. The courts even exclude same-sex partners from normal partnership rights where the text of the law just mentions "partnership" or "community of life" without specifying partners' gender. A striking example is in Section 14 of the Tenancy Rights Act. This provision grants the right of succession to the partner if he has been living with the deceased tenant "in a community of life economically arranged like marriage." The courts — in sharp contradiction to the word of the law — held that only partners of different sex could economically arrange their partnership like marriage (OGH 05.12.96, 60b2325/96, cf. Würth, 1992).

Definition of "Relations."   The law and the courts understand an opposite-sex partner but not a same-sex partner to belong to the category of one's *relations*. This causes manifold discrimination.

Testimony in Criminal Courts.   Same-sex partners do *not* have the right to refuse to give testimony against their partner in a criminal court. Partners of different sex do have this right (Act on Criminal Procedure, s. 152; CC, s. 72; see also CC, s. 290).

Aiding and Abetting.   Partners of the same sex are punishable if they aid and abet their partner who has committed an offense. Heterosexual partners are not punishable (s. 299 par. 3, s. 72 CC). The same is true for nonprevention of the commission of a criminal offense, if the crime has not been prevented to protect the partner from damage (CC, s. 286).

Offenses against the Property of the Partner.   Offenses against the property of the partner in a homosexual partnership are punishable in the same way as such offenses between strangers. However, such offenses committed without violence in a heterosexual partnership cannot be prosecuted by the public prosecutor, but only by the victim (with a strict 6 week time limit), and the offender is liable to imprisonment of not more than 6 months regardless of the value of the possessions taken (CC, s. 166). For example, theft with damage of more than Austrian Schilling 500.000, is normally punishable by imprisonment from 1 to 10 years. A heterosexual companion of life, however, can steal millions from his partner and is not liable to more than 6 months imprisonment; if his partner does not prosecute within 6 weeks from his knowledge of the deed, he cannot be punished at all. Moreover, purloining [i.e., theft with minor damage committed out of destitution, thoughtlessness, or to satisfy a desire (CC, s. 141)], fraud with minor damage out of destitution (CC, s. 150), and unauthorized use of motor vehicles (CC, s. 136) are not punishable at all if committed between heterosexual partners [the same is true for negligently causing minor bodily harm (CC, s. 88)]. In 1996 a man had been sentenced to 6 months imprisonment (without suspension) by the Regional Court of Leoben for unauthorized driving the car of his partner. On appeal, the Upper Regional Court of Graz reduced the sentence to 2 months (unsuspended) incarceration. The case prompted an outcry by the Austrian lesbian and gay movement. Due to massive lobbying by Rechtskomitee LAMBDA and other organizations, the Austrian president pardoned the convict and changed the sentence to a fine. This was the first time an Austrian president pardoned a (discriminated) homosexual (Graupner, 1996e).

Succession Rights in Tenancy Legislation. Same-sex partners are not allowed to succeed into the tenancy of their deceased companion of life. Heterosexual partners succeed by law if they do not expressly waive this right [the waiver is possible only after the death of their partner (Tenancy Rights Act, s. 14)].

Leave to Nurse. Homosexual employees do not have a claim to leave to nurse a same-sex partner who is ill. Heterosexual employees can claim paid leave of up to 40 hours per year for nursing their sick companion of life.

Coinsurance in Social Insurance. Same-sex partners cannot claim benefits out of the public health insurance of their partner. Heterosexual partners can do so if the social insurance company incorporates such a regulation into its statute. All public insurance companies did so. Social insurance companies, however, are restrained by law from granting benefits to (noninsured) same-sex partners of their clients [General Act on Social Insurance (s. 123); Act on Social Insurance for the Tradespeople (ss. 10, 83); Act on Social Insurance for Independent Professions (s. 3); Act on Health and Accident Insurance of Civil Servants (s. 56)].

Benefits in Unemployment Insurance. Unemployed persons who live in a community of life with a partner of the opposite sex who is dependent on them can claim increased unemployment benefit, but an unemployed homosexual living with a dependent partner of the same sex cannot [Act on Unemployment Insurance (s. 20)]. On the other hand, the income of a same-sex partner reduces the "emergency aid" (i.e., the relief after expiration of the unemployment benefit) of an unemployed person [Act on Unemployment Insurance (s. 36)]. Occasionally, benefits from unemployment insurance can even be claimed directly by the heterosexual partner of an unemployed person in lieu of the insured person himself [Act on Exceptional Relief (s. 2)]. Same-sex partners never are allowed to do so.

Tax Privileges.   According to the Act on Income Tax, communities of life partnerships with children can claim tax reductions (s. 106). The Austrian Ministry of Finance insists that only partners of different gender who raise a child can claim this privilege (Rechtskomitee LAMBDA, personal communication).

Testimony in Civil Courts and in Administrative Procedures.   The right to refuse testimony against one's partner in civil courts or before administrative authorities is restricted to spouses [Code of Civil Procedure (s. 320); Act on Administrative Procedure (s. 49)]. This is even true in administrative penal procedures [Act on Administrative Penal Procedure (s. 24; see also CC, s. 290)].

Inheritance.   Inheritance in the absence of a will is limited to spouses [General Civil Code (s. 758)]. If a will has been made, unmarried partners have to pay the same amount of inheritance tax as strangers (cf. Donation and Inheritance Tax Act).

Freehold Flats.   Common property with regard to freehold flats is restricted to spouses [Act on Freehold Flats (ss. 8ff)].

Assignment of Tenancy.   The right to assign a tenancy to one's partner without the consent of the lessor is restricted to married partners [Tenancy Rights Act (s. 12)].

Unification of Families.   Facilitated entry and immigration of a partner of an Austrian citizen or of a foreigner legally residing in Austria is restricted to married partners [Residence Act (s. 3); Foreigners Act (ss. 8, 28, 29)].

Assignment of Citizenship.   Facilitated assignment of citizenship by a partner of an Austrian citizen is limited to spouses [Citizenship Act (s. 11a)].

Dependents' Relief.   Dependents' relief in the social insurance system is limited to spouses (e.g., widows' and widowers' pensions; cf. General Act on Social Insurance; Act on Social Insurance of Tradespeople; Act on Social Insurance of Independent Professions; Act on Social Insurance of Farmers; Act on Insurance of Notaries; Act on Health and Accident Insurance of Civil Servants). In the law of torts [General Civil Code (s. 1327), it is also limited to spouses.

Hospitals.   Same-sex partners can encounter problems visiting their partners in the hospital. When the patient cannot decide himself (e.g., if he is in a coma), visitation rights are often limited to heterosexual partners, sometimes even to spouses (Rechtskomitee LAMBDA, personal communication).

Funerals.   Problems can arise if the deceased did not specify who should make funeral arrangements. In such a case the family of the deceased often excludes the same-sex (sometimes even the opposite-sex) partner from the arrangements (*XTRA!* 23/95, 29).

Annulment and Divorce.   Marriage can be dissolved if one partner has been mistaken in circumstances concerning the other partner where the information and a correct assessment of the true meaning of wedlock should have prevented the marriage [Marriage Act (s. 37)]. According to case law, a homosexual inclination is such a circumstance and entitles a claim for dissolution of marriage [EvBl 1963/466, Pichler, 1992; Marriage Act (s. 38)].

Moreover, divorce can be claimed if the other partner committed acts seriously inconsistent with the true sense of matrimony [Marriage Act (s. 49)]. The courts held that a homosexual relationship is such an act and is thus grounds for divorce if it has irreparably disrupted the foundations of marriage [RZ 1978/25; Pichler, 1992; Marriage Act (s. 49)]. Nevertheless, the homosexual behavior of one spouse in the absence of the other is not considered so unbearable for the partner as to justify eviction from domestic premises during a divorce suit [Code of Execution (s. 382); Upper Regional Court of Vienna 19.12.1986, 11 R 266/86 = EF 52.413].

Custody

Residence of the Child.   When custody of a child is assigned after the divorce of his parents, the best interests of the child are of paramount importance in this decision. Even if the parents agree on the future care of the child this agreement has to be approved by the court [General Civil Code (s. 177)].

In the courts a partner known to be homosexual is in a weak position to claim custody of the child. The knowledge that a mother is homosexual can override the generally stronger position of mothers compared to fathers in care proceedings. Gay men are especially unlikely to be assigned the care of their children (Rechtskomitee LAMBDA, personal communication).

Adoption.   Adoption is possible only for single persons or married couples. Joint adoption by unmarried couples is impossible [Civil Code (s. 179)]. Adoption of a minor must further the best interests of the child, and his parents must consent to the adoption. In the case of unjustified refusal the court can give consent [Civil Code (s. 181)]. Adoption of adults has to further a justified interest of the adoptive parent or the adoptee [Civil Code (s. 180a)]. Courts have recognized the securing of a residence permit or Austrian citizenship as such a justified interest. (Rechtskomitee LAMBDA, personal communication).

Adoption of adults is common, but there is no case known where anyone living openly as a lesbian or a gay man has been granted adoption of a minor (Rechtskomitee LAMBDA, personal communication).

An adoption can be declared null and void if it primarily served as a cover for unlawful sexual relations [Civil Code (s. 184)]. There is no case known where a court tried to annul an adoption by a homosexual on this basis (Rechtskomitee LAMBDA, personal communication); such an attempt might not be successful since homosexual relations (between men over 18 or women over 14) are no longer unlawful.

Fostering.   In some exceptional cases homosexual couples have been allowed to foster minors (Rechtskomitee LAMBDA, personal communication).

Artificial Insemination

Artificial insemination is available for heterosexual companions of life only. Women living in a lesbian community of life are not entitled to it. If they engage in it they (or the physician carrying out the insemination) can be punished with an administrative fine of up to ATS 500.000 or, in default of payment, with detention of up to 14 days [Act on Reproductive Medicine (s. 22f).

Inheritance Law

Children (and parents) can be disinherited if they "pertinaciously lead a way of life conflicting with public morals" [General Civil Code (s. 768)]. Bequests to such people can be reduced to the level of bare necessity [General Civil Code (s. 795)]. These provisions seem especially harsh in comparison with prison sentences for felonies, which can constitute a ground for disinheritance (or reduced benefit) only if the sentence amounts to 20 years or life [General Civil Code (s. 768)]. However, there is no case known where a homosexual has been disinherited or his benefits reduced on the basis of these provisions (Rechtskomitee LAMBDA, personal communication).

Persons convicted of adultery or incest cannot appoint each other to be their heirs [General Civil Code (s. 543)], but homosexual partners can, since homosexual relations do not constitute adultery or incest (which require penile penetration of the vagina).

Industrial Law

Notice to Quit.   Termination of employment on the basis of sexual orientation is not absolutely illegal, but it can be contested successfully in court if the employee has been employed at least 6 months and if he can prove that he could not easily find another equivalent job. In such cases, the employer must prove that the homosexuality of the employee adversely affected the interests of the company. However, if a works council consents to dismissal on the basis of homosexuality it cannot be contested in court [Labour Code (s. 105)].

Equal Opportunity.   The Equal Treatment Act covers discrimination on the basis of sex, but so far the authorities do not accept the notion that discrimination on the basis of sexual orientation always amounts to sex discrimination.

Neither the law nor collective agreements nor staff agreements contain equal opportunity policies on the basis of sexual orientation. That is alien to Austrian labor law.

Insult

The Supreme Court has held repeatedly that a homosexual insult is always defamatory, since homosexual acts still cause massive discrimination in society. Therefore, if any property damage has been sustained, the person defamed is entitled to apply for an injunction and claim compensation and the perpetrator is criminally liable for defamation. This holds true even if the allegation made by the perpetrator is true, unless there is shown to be a compelling public interest in making known the sexual orientation or behavior of the person concerned (OGH (Supreme Court) 04.05.1995, 6 Ob 11/95; OGH 26.01.1984, 13 Os 214/83). In summer 1995 an Austrian gay activist "outed" four Austrian bishops as being gay. The four brought actions and in December 1995 a court of first instance ordered the outer to revoke his statement and to refrain from it in the future, since he could not prove the truth of his allegations. The Supreme Court upheld the verdict (Krickler, 1997).

THE ADMINISTRATIVE LAW

Security Forces

Police. In 1993 the Minister of Interior issued a decree ordering *(inter alia)* that the police must abstain from behavior that could be perceived as discrimination on the basis of sexual orientation (Decree of Guidelines). This is the first antidiscrimination ruling to protect homosexuals in Austrian law. Nevertheless, police still occasionally and illegally film visitors to public parks and carry out raids on gay pubs (cf. Graupner 1993c; 1994b; 1995b; personal communication).

Army. In 1990 and 1993 the Minister of Defense stated that the army keeps records on the (real or supposed) homosexuality of its members. This is necessary, he claimed, to avoid blackmail and to protect young recruits. Since no affected person has brought a petition, neither the Commission for the Protection of Data nor the courts could decide on the legality of this practice (Jus Amandi 1/94 [12]).

Asylum

In enacting the Asylum Act (1991) the legislature stated that persons who are persecuted on the ground of their sexual orientation are entitled to asylum because — in the sense of the Geneva Convention — they are persecuted as members of a "distinct social group" (RV 270 Blg.NR XVIII. GP, § 1 Z. 1). Thus far no one has been granted asylum on the basis of persecution solely because of sexual orientation.

Compensation for Victims of National Socialism

Persons persecuted by the national socialist authorities on the grounds of their homosexuality — in contrast to other victims of persecution — have never been granted compensation. As late as 1980 this law was stiffened. From 1971, the year of decriminalization, until 1980, the possibility of claiming times of incarceration for homosexual acts as accountable times for the right to claim a pension. In 1980 this possibility was repealed. Since then, Nazi detention for committing the crime of "lewdness against the order of nature" (§12954G) has not counted toward pension rights (Ivansits, 1990).

In 1995 Parliament (by a tiny majority) again refused to grant to homosexual victims — along with other victims — a right to compensation under the Act on Public Relief for Victims. Instead they can only receive compensation from the National Fund for Victims of National Socialism established by Parliament in 1995. However, there are no automatic rights to benefits from this fund (BGBl. 1995/432).

Tax Law

In 1989 finance authorities refused to grant status of a nonprofit organization to the lesbian and gay rights organization Homosexuelle Intiative (HOSI) Wien since a substantial portion of society showed significant reservation about the aims of the group (Regional Financial Authority for Vienna, 1989, 6/2-2209/83-05).

The Constitution

In 1989 the Constitutional Court held that the Austrian constitution protected the basic rights of homosexuals regarding a private life free from discrimination on the basis of sexual orientation. Simultaneously, however, it decided that the higher age of consent for male homosexual conduct did not give rise to discrimination since it was justified by the need to protect the youth against sexual maldevelopment (Constitutional Court 03.10.1989, G 227/88, 2/89; cf. Graupner, 1995).

Public Opinion

About one-fourth (27 percent) of the Austrian population still favors the reintroduction of the general ban on homosexuality. Among teenagers the proportion is very low (6 percent), among pensioners it seems significantly high (45 percent) (Fritsch & Langbein, 1991).

The considerable amount of tolerance among young people was also shown in another study, which found that only 29 percent of 16- to 24-year-olds, as opposed to 44 percent of the adults, placed homosexual acts among things one is not allowed to do under any circumstances. Only killing in self-defense and divorce were treated with less taboo (Österreichisches Institut für Jugendkunde, 1991). Among Viennese teenagers, 78 percent agreed that for some people homosexuality is as important and normal as love between man and woman is for others (Dür & Haas 1991).

Outlook

In 1979 a gay and lesbian movement fighting for equal rights emerged in Austria. In 1989 a large number of youth organizations petitioned Parliament to repeal the anti-homosexual criminal laws (Graupner, 1995). In 1991 the Platform Against § 209 was founded to develop an effective lobby for the repeal of the discriminatory age of consent and the other two antihomosexual criminal laws. This platform today consists of 38 associations, including nearly all organizations of the Austrian gay and lesbian movement as well as all AIDS organizations, the Austrian AIDS Committee, the Austrian Sexological Society, the Austrian Probationary Service, the Austrian Federal Youth Council, the National Students Union, and the National Conference of the Austrian Children and Youth Attorneys (Graupner, 1995).

The Social Democratic Party and the Liberal Party have incorporated the principle of equality and nondiscrimination of homosexuals into their statute. In 1995 proposals were introduced in Parliament to repeal the three antihomosexual laws, to introduce registered partnership, and to amend the constitution with an effective prohibition of discrimination on the grounds of sexual orientation. In October 1995 the justice committee of Parliament heard representatives of the lesbian and gay movement and experts on the discriminatory age of consent; 11 of the 13 experts who were heard called for the immediate equalization of the age of consent at age 14 (Jus Amandi 2/95, 3/95, XTRA! 21/95 [10] Grauper, 1995c).

Meanwhile, the lesbian and gay movement became involved in election campaigns.

In 1994 and 1995 Vote Pink — the platform for Lesbian and Gay Human Rights — launched a campaign to vote only for parties that respect the human rights of lesbians and gay men (*Jus Amandi* 3/95). In the parliamentary elections of 1995, for the first time in Austrian history, an openly lesbian woman, supported by the Green Party, ran for election. She only narrowly missed winning a seat.

These developments suggest that in the future persecution and discrimination against homosexual and bisexual women and men will come to an end in Austria.

On November 27, 1996, the Austrian Federal Parliament voted on the antihomosexual provisions of the Criminal Code. The Social-Democratic Party (SPÖ), the Liberal Forum (LIF), and the Green Party had submitted proposals to repeal Articles 209, 220, and 221 of the Criminal Code completely. The right-wing Freedom Party (FPÖ) proposed to lower the age limit in Article 209 to 16, to repeal Article 221, and to revise Article 220. The conservative People's Party (ÖVP) proposed to keep the age limit of 18 in Article 209, amending it, so that relations with an age difference of not more than 2 years would not be punishable, and to revise Articles 220 and 221. The proposals to equalize the minimum age at 14 were rejected by a tied vote of 91-91. All Member of Parliaments (MP) of the SPÖ, LIF, and the Green Party and one MP of the OVP (the well-known actor Franz Morak) and one of FPÖ (former Minster of Justice Dr. Harald Ofner) voted for the repeal; the rest of the ÖVP and FPÖ MPs voted against it. The proposal to lower the age limit to 16 was rejected by a vote of 138-41; the proposal of ÖVP regarding Article 209 was rejected by a vote of 131-48. Thus Article 209 remains as it was. Article 220 has been repealed by a vote of 90-89; the aforementioned MP from FPÖ again voted with SPÖ, LIF, and the Green Party (two FPÖ MPs and one ÖVP MP left the plenary). Finally, Article 221 was repealed by a vast majority vote of 127-52. The ban on advertisement for bestiality (formerly included in the now repealed Article 220) has been reintroduced in a new Article (220a).

REFERENCES

Bertel, Ch., & Schwaighofer, K. (1992). *Österreichisches Strafrecht: Besonderer Teil II (§§ 169 bis 321 StGB)*. Vienna: Springer-Press.

Dür, W., & Haas, S. (1991). *Aids-Aufklärung und sexuelle Kommunikation bei Jugendlichen*. Vienna: Ludwig-Boltzmann-Institut für Medizin- und Gesundheitssoziologie.

Foregger, E., & Serini, Eu. (1988). *Strafgesetzbuch samt den wichtigsten Nebengesetzen: Kurzkommentar*. Vienna: Manz.

Fritsch, S., & Langbein, K. (1991). *Land der Sinne — Die große Analyse: Liebe, Sex und Partnerschaft in Österreich*. Vienna: Orac.

Graupner, H. (1989, No. 4). Schwulenhatz in Kärnten, *Lambda Nachrichten*, pp. 47–49.

Graupner, H. (1993a, No. 1). Die Mühlen der Justiz…, *Ius Amandi*, p. 23–25.

Graupner, H. (1993b, No. 2). Rechtskomitee LAMBDA - Rechtsfälle, *Ius Amandi*, pp. 24–25.

Graupner, H. (1993c, No. 3). Rechtskomitee LAMBDA - Rechtsfälle, *Ius Amandi*, pp. 24–26.

Graupner, H. (1993d, No. 4). Rechtskomitee LAMBDA - Rechtsfälle, *Ius Amandi*, p. 26.

Graupner, H. (1994a, No. 1). Rechtskomitee LAMBDA - Rechtsfälle, *Ius Amandi*, p. 20.

Graupner, H. (1994b, No. 2), Queer Klagenfurt-datenermittlung durch die Polizei, *Ius Amandi*, p. 18.

Graupner, H. (1995a). *Sexualität, Jugendschutz und Menschenrechte: Uber das Recht von Kindern und Jugend-lichen auf sexuelle Selbstbestimmung* (doctoral dissertation, vols. 1 & 2). Vienna: University of Vienna. [to be published in 1997 (Peter Lang)]

Graupner, H. (1995b, No. 2). Polizeiübergriffe & Haftstrafen - § 209 wird bis zuletzt mit aller Härte exekutiert!, *Ius Amandi*, p. 3.

Graupner, H. (1995c). Expertenanhörung zu § 209, *Ius Amandi*, 2/95, p. 2–3.

Graupner, H. (1996a, February 15). "Kalender-Urteil: Homophobe Justiz auf frischer Tat ertappt." *Der Standard*, p. 25.

Graupner, H. (1996b, No. 1) RKL-Fälle. *Ius Amandi*, p. 3.

Graupner, H. (1996c, No. 2). RKL-Fälle. *Ius Amandi*, p. 3.

Graupner, H. (1996d, No. 4). RKL-Fälle. *Ius Amandi*, p. 2–3.

Graupner, H. (1996e, No. 5). Als erster Präsident: Klestil begnadigt Homosexuellen. *Ius Amandi*, p. 1.

Graupner, H. (1996f, No. 5). Sonderstrafgesetze: Vor der Entscheidung. *Ius Amandi*, p. 2–3.

Graupner, H. (1996g, No. 6). Polizei schlägt schwulen Jugendlichen. *Ius Amandi*, p. 1–2.

Graupner, H. (1996h, No. 7). Der Pyrrhus-Sieg der ÖVP!, *Ius Amandi*, p. 1.

Graupner, H. (1997, No. 1). Ungebrochene Repression –Die Verfolgung nimmt wieder zu, *Ius Amandi*, p. 2–3.

Hauer, G. (1989). Lesben- und Schwulengeschichte— Diskriminierung und Widerstand. In M. Handl, G. Hauer, K. Krickler, F. Nussbaumer, & D. Schmutzer (Eds.), *Homosexualität in Österreich* (pp. 50–67). Vienna: Junius.

Hoyer, H., Geller, H., & Metzler, Ph. (1944). *Das Strafgesetz vom 27. Mai 1852*. Vienna: Manz.

Ivansits, H. (1990). Das Wiedergutmachungsrecht für Opfer politischer, religöser oder rassischer Verfolgung. *Das Recht der Arbeit (DRdA)*, 1990, 185–195.

Krickler, K. (1997). Outing: Verfahren in Straßburg, *Lambda Nachrichten*, 1/97, 30–31.

Leukauf, O., & Steininger, H. (1992). *Kommentar zum Strafgesetzbuch*. Vienna: Prugg.

Mayerhofer, Ch., & Rieder, S. (1989). *Das österreichische Strafrecht: Erster Teil, Strafgesetzbuch*. Vienna: Österreichische Staatsdruckerei.

Mayerhofer, Ch., & Rieder, S. (1992). *Das österreichische Strafrecht: Dritter Teil, Nebenstrafrecht*. Vienna: Österreichische Staatsdruckerei.

Osterreichisches Institut für Jugendkunde. (1991). *Österreichische Jugendwertestudie*. Vienna: Author.

Pallin, F. (1980). §§ 201-221 StGB. In E. Foregger & F. Nowakowski (Eds.), *Wiener Kommentar zum Strafgesetzbuch*. 4.Lieferung Vienna: Manz.

Pichler, H. (1992). Das Ehegesetz. In P. Rummel (Ed.), *Kommentar zum Allgemeinen Bürgerlichen Gesetzbuch* (vol. 2, pp. 1519–1634). Vienna: Manz.

Schneider, F. (1965). Die rechtliche Stellung der Lebensgefährten. *Österreichische Juristenzeitung*, 7, 174–179.

Würth, H. (1992). Das Mietrechtsgesetz. In P. Rummel (Ed.), *Kommentar zum Allgemeinen Bürgerlichen Gesetzbuch* (vol. 2, pp. 1635–1869). Vienna: Manz.

BTX-Journal: *Die Zeitschrift für Bildschirmtext*. Vienna: ProBTX.

Der Standard: *Austrian Daily*. Vienna.

Euroletter: *Newsletter of the Euro-Working-Party of the International Lesbian and Gay Association (ILGA)*. Copenhagen: The National Danish Organisation for Gays and Lesbians (LBL).

Jus Amandi: *Zeitschrift für gleichgeschlechtliche Liebe und Recht*. Vienna: Rechtskomitee LAMBDA.

Lambda-Nachrichten: *Zeitschrift der Homosexuellen Initiative Wien*. Vienna: Homosexuelle Initiative (HOSI) Wien.

XTRA!: *Österreichs größtes Schwulen- und Lesbenmagazin*. Vienna: Safe Way.

Belgium

ALAN REEKIE

Introduction

Criminal and civil laws in Belgium are largely derived from the French Civil and Penal Codes of 1804 and 1810, respectively, which were intended to embody the revolutionary ideals of liberty, equality, and fraternity. Initially they were applicable throughout what has since become Belgium. Although their provisions have been amended substantially since Belgium became an independent constitutional monarchy in 1830, continuing strong cultural and economic links with France have constrained the natural tendency toward divergence. Furthermore, the Belgian electoral system, which combines compulsory voting with party-list proportional representation ballots, generally results in coalition governments that reflect a broad consensus of public opinion. Thus, legislation on sexual behavior is not a purely pragmatic and rational framework intended to facilitate the coexistence of people with diverse opinions. On the other hand, it is not simply an application of traditional moral principles with the aim of maintaining harmony in a homogeneous, hierarchical society. In effect, it is a compromise containing elements from both approaches. A corresponding compromise existed in France during much of the same period, and the situation in Belgium then was similar to that in France as described shortly before the discriminatory law introduced there during the Nazi Occupation was repealed by the Law of 21 July 1982 (Gury, 1981).

Belgian society comprises the relatively right-wing Catholic, but associative, Flemish and the relatively left-wing, free-thinking , but often individualistic, Walloons. Possibly because most political effort in Belgium has long been concentrated on trying to find a satisfactory balance between the priorities of these two groups, there has been little pressure for fundamental reform of the criminal law, particularly where the texts provide adequate scope for the exercise of judicial discretion. For example, for more than a century after the last execution in Belgium except for crimes committed during wartime had taken place on 2 July 1863, Belgium Courts were still sentencing serious offenders to death under Art. 7–11 of the Penal Code. Despite repeated proposals to repeal these archaic provisions long after they had in practice been replaced by imprisonment for life, they remained in the Code until 1995. Indeed, the first part of an initial draft of a fundamentally revised Penal Code was prepared in the 1980s at the instigation of one Minister of Justice, but, like so many others, this dossier is now collecting dust in the archives.

ALAN REEKIE • International Gay and Lesbian Association, Brussels B-1000, Belgium.

Sociolegal Control of Homosexuality, edited by West and Green, Plenum Press, New York, 1997.

The Criminal Law and Its Application

The opinions of individual Belgians regarding homosexuality have been as diverse as they are elsewhere in Europe, even though the law originally embodied no explicit discrimination of homosexuality. Legal nondiscrimination persisted through important changes in subsequent legislation. In particular, the age of sexual majority, embodied in the definitions of certain sexual offenses, remained in step with the age of criminal responsibility, which was raised in 1912 from 14 to its present level of 16 in the context of child welfare legislation. Incidentally, the minimum age at which women can marry, set since 1803 at 15 (Art. 144 of the Civil Code) was raised to 18, the same as it is for young men, by the Law of 19 January 1990. There was an exception to the equality principle, however, in the Child Protection Act of April 8, 1965, Article 87 (which subsequently became Art. 372 bis of the Penal Code). This made it an offense for a man or woman over 18 to perform homosexual acts with a consenting person under 18 years of age. This law was presumably based on similar provisions with cut off ages of 21 that had been enacted much earlier in France by the Law of 16 August 1942 (Gury, 1981). Other than the two decades up to the repeal of Article 372 bis in 1985, the legal situation of homosexuals in Belgium has been determined by a somewhat selective enforcement of apparently nondiscriminatory, gender-neutral legislation. The following review discusses the situation in this context.

The first impact of the so-called sexual revolution, triggered by the development of the contraceptive pill, was felt in 1973 with the decriminalization of the publication of information about contraception. Adultery remained a criminal offense under Article 387 until June 22, 1987, although in the years preceding prosecutions for it had become very rare. Rape, defined in Article 375, has included since 1912 the legal fiction of statutory rape, or mutual genital contact with a person younger than 14. In 1988 the scope of rape was expanded, following debates lasting several years, to include anal rape and rape within marriage. Medically supervised and authorized abortion was decriminalized in 1990, after a long campaign that had received new impetus on each arbitrary occasion the law was enforced. Organizations providing information about clinics abroad were favorite targets. Provisions against nudity in public have not been relaxed; Belgians wishing to swim or sunbathe in the nude, who do not have access to suitable private facilities, have to travel to one of the neighboring countries, as there is nowhere at home they can do so publicly without risk of prosecution.

Liberalization in the neighboring countries, and the relaxation of border controls in the context of closer European integration, ultimately led to Belgian Court decisions holding that the display or sale to adults of explicit depictions of sexual acts not involving violence, minors, or bestiality was no longer deemed to amount to the offense of "outraging public morality" under Articles 383–386 of the Penal Code (Brussels Appeal Court, 1991). On the other hand, enforcement of the provisions of Article 379 et seq, which define various offenses associated with prostitution and the dangerously imprecise term *debauchery*, has continued sporadically. Some clarification was provided by the judgment in the *Macho* case, in which the owner and manager of a private club for homosexuals, after a series of trials, were ultimately acquitted of "providing opportunities for debauchery." It was held that the provision of facilities for consenting adults to perform homosexual acts in private could not in itself amount to an offense without necessarily implying that all homosexual acts are prohibited, which was clearly not the intention of the legislation (*Belgian Crown v. Haenen and Vincineau*, 1986; Vincineau, 1985). A campaign intended to persuade Parliament to remove all reference to debauchery from the Penal Code has so far been unsuccessful (*Tels Quels*, 1994).

As already mentioned, the discriminatory Article 372 bis of 1965 was deleted from the Penal Code in 1985. This followed a campaign based on the arguments that it was irrational, making existing consensual teenage homosexual relationships illegal as soon as the elder partner reached the arbitrary age of 18, and unnecessary, because adequate protection against exploitation was already available through other provisions. Since 1985 the main source of gay and lesbian discontent with the criminal law has focused on the interpretation of the legislation on debauchery, Article 379 *et seq*, which assimilates it to prostitution. Notwithstanding various contradictory precedents, the present situation is that the term must be interpreted according to its everyday meaning, but on this opinions vary widely. In the absence of a precise legal definition, those definitions given in dictionaries, such as *habitual immorality* or *punishable sexual behavior* are excessively imprecise guides where sentences of many years of imprisonment can be at stake. The situation reflects the lack of consensus in society on where to draw the line between personal freedom and the protection of vulnerable individuals. On the one hand, the Catholic Church, in agreement with other religious bodies, has repeatedly urged that the law should embody its belief that all sexual acts except those open to procreation within marriage are sinful, while accepting a minimum age limit for marriage close to puberty. On the other hand, supporters of free-thinking philosophy, including Belgian gay/lesbian/bisexual groups, have argued that, at least in the case of adults, the law should forbid only those acts that are objectively harmful or not desired by somebody directly involved. In practice, law enforcement has inevitably become arbitrary and inconsistent, in part because the authorities have become heavily overloaded in dealing with other, less controversial, offenses. When most, if not all, allegations concerning some minor offense are left on file (*classé sans suite*) the public receives an impression of official tolerance.

ISSUES CONCERNING YOUNG PEOPLE

In practice, the legislators have mainly focused their attention on the protection of young people, who are not just recognized as especially vulnerable, but are also apparently widely believed to be liable to moral corruption by exposure to explicit information about human sexuality. Under Article 386 the punishment for making obscene material available is increased if minors are involved and any film for exhibition to persons under 16 must pass a certification committee. When sexually stimulating messages first become available via the so-called "telephone rose," anyone such as adolescents could easily access them. One irate parent faced with a large bill took the telephone company to court on the grounds that there had been a breach of Article 386. Since then, legislation has been enacted (new Article 380 quinquies, by Law of 27 March 1995) to prohibit such commercial sexual services from being addressed specifically to minors.

Although the provisions against sexual contact with the young may make no formal distinction, it is likely that in practice protection from homosexual experiences may be regarded as of particular importance. Notably in the enforcement of Article 372, which requires a punishment of at least 5 years imprisonment for having sexual relations with a freely consenting partner of either sex even a few days before their 16th birthday. That age limit, set in 1912, is now well above the average age of puberty. Indeed, it is higher than the minimum age for consensual sexual relationships (in the absence of a relationship of authority or dependency) in Belgium's main neighbors. Belgian law contains no explicit recognition that many young people become sexually active well before 16.

The lack of any evidence to show that young persons had allegedly been involved was of crucial importance when the editor of the gay/lesbian/bisexual monthly magazine *Tels Quels* was prosecuted in 1989 for the publication of personal gay contact advertisements that allegedly contravened the provisions of Article 380 quater against publicly announcing opportunities for debauchery, even if only obliquely. This politically inspired prosecution was all the more surprising because similar heterosexual personal contact advertisements had long been appearing in numerous commercial "soft porn" magazines that are much more widely available than *Tels Quels*, with no apparent concern being shown by law enforcement agencies or the general public. The court ruled that, in the absence of prostitution or the involvement of minors, homosexuality in itself does not fall within debauchery. The decision did not, however, settle the issue of how far this widely disregarded law is now effectively defunct in other contexts (*Tels Quels*, 1988).

As a further example of the great concern to protect the young, an official with special responsibility for protecting children's rights was appointed recently. This followed extensive media coverage of the topic of "sex tourism" in Southeast Asia and allegations of official corruption in the enforcement of laws against the white slave trade. On the basis of Article 34 of the United Nations Convention on the Rights of the Child, a campaign was organized to collect signatures for a petition calling for stricter legislation against the sexual exploitation of children. Although most of the proposed new legislation amounts to reinforcement and expansion of existing provisions on offenses associated with prostitution and debauchery and some of it would be very difficult to enforce, it was eventually enacted in the Law of 13 April 1995. The new offenses consist of being knowingly in possession of "pornographic images of minors under sixteen" and allows prosecutions in Belgium for sexual offenses committed against young persons anywhere else in the world. In such cases the limited statutory period for bringing a prosecution is now deemed to restart when the young person involved reaches 18.

BELGIAN GAY/LESBIAN/BISEXUAL GROUPS

Although, like most Belgian organizations, gay and lesbian groups are organized on a linguistic basis, they collaborate in many ways, notably in the international context. The headquarters of the Dutch-speaking Federation of Working Groups on Homosexuality (FWH) is in Ghent, and the main French-speaking group, Tels Quels, is located at the Gay and Lesbian Meeting Point in central Brussels, where, since September 1990, the offices of the International Gay and Lesbian Association (ILGA) have also been housed; ILGA provides facilities for the worldwide exchange of information among lesbian and gay groups and represents their interests in various international contexts.

PUBLIC AND PRIVATE DISCRIMINATION

Article 6 of the 1831 Constitution states that all Belgians are equal before the law, but, in contrast to French and Dutch law, for example, the Belgian Penal Code contains no provisions specifically directed at prohibiting arbitrary discrimination. Consequently, any-one claiming to be a victim of discriminatory treatment has the burden of proving that the other party acted unreasonably. Most people are unwilling to incur the substantial risk, expense, and delays of civil litigation. The best-known cases are those where teachers have been dismissed after doing something considered by the authorities to be incompatible with their professional duties. In the case of Elaine Morrissens, for example, her dismissal after coming out as a lesbian in a television broadcast was upheld by the courts.

The frequency of such arbitrary discrimination is of course impossible to quantify, but the Minister of Justice, Stephan de Clerck, in an interview on the relations between the press and the legal profession, gave a revealing reply to the question, "Are you aware that a barrister in Brussels has just been punished [by the bar council] simply because he was involved in a homosexual relationship?": I find that surprising. I know a lot of barristers who are homosexual, without being punished as such. (Clerck, 1995). Given an unemployment rate of over 10 percent in Belgium, it is not surprising that so few gays and lesbians are willing to be open about their sexual orientation, and thus run the risk of finding themselves without a job for months or even years.

The Belgian Gay/Lesbian Bisexual (GLB) movement is working towards the enact-ment of a broad antidiscrimination law. However, experience of parliamentary debate in neighboring countries has shown that such legislation attracts claims for "exemptions" coming from religious groups and other organizations concerned about young people. Until there is a sufficient parliamentary majority committed to the prevention of such loopholes, it would be unproductive to press too hard for what might amount to less than equal rights and no more than statutory recognition of what is now only (nonbinding) jurisprudence. This issue is discussed further in the next section.

PUBLIC OPINION

For reasons already explained, homosexuality as such is not high on the political agenda in Belgium. While this has generally rendered unsuccessful the occasional at-tempts by individual members of right-wing parties to introduce their discriminatory opinions into legislation, it has also ensured that little attention has been paid to the par-ticular concerns of the gay and lesbian community. During the general election campaign of 1995, Belgian GLB groups took the opportunity, by means of a questionnaire, to ask the democratic political parties to state their position on the resolution on equal rights for homosexuals in the European Union that was adopted by the European Parliament on February 8, 1995, and also on the related issues of civil partnerships and anti-discrimination legislation (*Tels Quels*, 1995).

Responses from democratic parties all expressed at least some degree of willingness to support the enactment of a law prohibiting discrimination on grounds of sexual orientation and introducing the legal status of civil partnership. The responses from the Socialist and

Green parties had the fewest reservations, whereas those from the other main parties emphasized that their members were free to make up their own minds on such ethical matters, which made it impossible to give an opinion on behalf of the whole party. On the issues of allowing homosexual couples to adopt children or giving out information on homosexuality in secondary schools, the spokesman from the right wing Parti Reformateur Liberal (PRL) party was unable to accept full equality. An absence of any response from the center-right Christian Social Party (which is the dominant partner in the coalition govern-ment formed after the 1995 elections) probably reflects the diversity of opinion within it. No information was obtained from the far right Vlaams Blok, but its position is clear from the slogan it has adopted: "Eigen volk eerst" ("Our Own People First").

Nevertheless, some political response has taken place. On May 15, 1996, the Flemish Christian Social and Socialist parties within Belgium's governing coalition tabled a bill intended to outlaw discrimination on grounds of sexual orientation, with penalties similar to those under the 1981 law against racial discrimination. The bill does not address issues of gay marriages or civil partnerships.

CIVIL PARTNERSHIPS (*CONTRAT DE LA VIE COMMUNE*)

In 1993, at the instigation of the Belgian GLB groups, the text of a proposed legislation to create the status of civil partnership, analogous to heterosexual marriage, was drafted by the lawyers Jacques Hamaide and Michel Pasteel (*Le Soir*, 22 Oct.). As in similar legislation already in force in Denmark, Norway, Sweden, Iceland, and Hungary it would enable partners to acquire this status by making a formal declaration at the registry office, accompanied by a certified inventory of each partner's property. Registered partners would be expected to live together and to share their resources, including any social security benefits, and to accept liability for each other's household expenses and payments. This new status would presumably not appear on the identity card that everybody in Belgium must show on request and would only be revealed to third parties, such as employers, when necessary. The present proposals would not confer any new immigration rights, and legal recognition of the status outside of Belgium would not be automatic.

The financial impact of such legislation on government revenue and expenditure is likely to be trivial and a bill has already been tabled, but it seems unlikely that the new government will be in any hurry to enact it. One influential factor may be that there are no openly homosexual members of the national or regional parliaments and that openly gay or lesbian candidates for public office have so far been unsuccessful (*Tels Quels*, May 1995). However, following the example of their counterparts in the Netherlands, several Flemish city councils have recently announced that they are willing to register civil partnerships by couples who are unable to marry under current legislation. The author Tom Lanaye and the politician Rene Los from the "A different life" (AGALEV) party were the first homo-sexual pair to express their commitment to each other in this way in Antwerp on January 20, 1996. As yet, such contracts are essentially symbolic, without legal impact.

As far as can be gathered from press reports, gay-bashing assaults (hate crimes) moti-vated by homophobia are relatively rare in Belgium. That impression could be unreliable, due in part to the lack of official statistics and in part to the care taken by most gays and lesbians to remain discreet. A typical scenario involves an assault at night by a group of young males on a man found in an open-air "cruising place" and thought to be looking for anonymous same-sex activity. The assailants do not expect the victim to report the assault to the police because, if he does, he may risk being prosecuted himself for public indecency (Homosexuels agressés a Namur, 1995). As long as reports of such incidents are virtually the only references to homosexuality in the mainstream media, it is scarcely surprising that schoolchildren use slang terms for homosexuals as convenient insults. The increase in popular support for far-right parties like the National Front and Vlaams Blok, both of which have blamed AIDS and other social problems on immigrants and homosexuals, show that gays have little reason for complacency.

As recently as 1995 the Belgian Pharmaceutical Association refused to allow pharmacies to display a poster produced by the official AIDS Prevention Agency Info-SIDA on the grounds that it would involve committing the offense of "incitement to debauchery." It carried the message "at only 20 francs for 3 condoms [less than 25 US cents each] you can afford to use them whether you are in love or not." Likewise, the newspaper *La Libre Belgique* refused to publish an Agency advertisement on the same theme, an action criticized by the director in another newspaper (Petijean, 1995). On the other hand, coin-operated condom dispensers are already widely available and the announcement of a program to install them in state secondary schools provoked relatively little controversy (Letters to the editor, June, July 1995).

THE STAMFORD CASE AND THE DUTROUX AFFAIR

How several of the foregoing issues work themselves out in actual court cases is well illustrated by the affair of John Stamford, former editor and publisher of the *Spartacus Guide for Gay Men*. He was prosecuted recently under Articles 380.4 and 383 of the Belgian Penal Code, which prohibit the publication of information about opportunities for prostitution or debauchery as well as the commercial production, importation, public distribution and the like of publications that are *contraire aux bonnes moeurs* [indecent]. According to the newspaper *Le Soir* (Vandemeulebroucke 1994) the charges concerned only Mr. Stamford's activities since he came to Belgium in 1987, after ceasing to be responsible for *Spartacus*. His alleged offenses consisted of correspondence with individuals outside Belgium about the topics covered by the *Spartacus Guide* and involvement in the preparation of material for publication outside Belgium that dealt with various sexual topics, including pedophilia. The prosecution was apparently undertaken in response to complaints made by three international Non-Governmental Organizations (NGOs) concerned with child welfare, which claimed that Mr. Stamford was part of an international pedophile conspiracy. They sought to have him charged under Article 379 (corruption of minors and prostitution), for which the maximum sentence is 20 years' imprisonment where the child is less than 10 years old.

The situation was complicated by provisions in the Belgian Constitution regarding freedom of the press, requiring that political and press offenses be tried before a jury, which had made such prosecutions extremely rare. Furthermore, in accordance with public opinion, which has become more liberal since the legislation was enacted, it has long been the practice in Belgium to enforce the articles on indecent publications and public announcements of opportunities for prostitution or debauchery (even if disguised) only in the most flagrant cases (Ost & Kerchove, 1981). This tolerance has enabled the mainstream media to publish sensational reports, including detailed information on where to find young prostitutes in Belgium and abroad, without risk of prosecution.

The Stamford case, which has been commented on by P. David (1995) of Children's Defence International, was brought to trial before the Turnout Correctional Tribunal in November 1994. Press reports of the hearing referred repeatedly to Mr. Stamford's former role in publishing *Spartacus*. Although that guide is not concerned with pedophilia, *Le Soir* (24 Nov. 1994) carried a headline "Spartacus? C'était pour décourager la pédophilie." The court eventually decided, in April 1995, that it was not competent to deal with the case, since the issue of whether it was a "press offense" which required a jury trial, needed to be determined. The NGOs concerned with child welfare, who were civil parties in the proceedings, expressed surprise and accused the state prosecution of being extraordinarily lax in view of the criminal nature of the *Spartacus* network (*La Libre Belgique*, 22 & 23 April, 1995).

It seems probable that this case influenced the new legislation, enacted at the beginning of 1995, allowing prosecution of anyone in Belgium found knowingly in possession of pornographic images of children under 16 or accused of sex offenses against minors committed abroad. The allegations against Mr. Stamford were not against *Spartacus* itself, but rather that he used his contacts to circulate information about child prostitution; the way the case was treated in the media, however, was calculated to reinforce the public perception of homosexuality as inevitably associated with child sex abuse. Mr. Stamford's guilt or innocence was never established. He died suddenly on December 27, 1995. An official of Terre des Hommes, one of the organizations pressing charges, was reported as stating, "We regret it because we wanted to make an example of him" (*Guardian*, 30 Dec. 1995).

In August 1996, after this chapter was thought to be complete, Marc Detroux, a second-hand car dealer living near Charleroi with his wife and children, was charged with murders and abductions of a number of young girls, two of whom were the subject of a dramatic rescue from their place of incarceration. The affair received massive publicity, with much criticism of the law enforcement authorities for at first failing to realize the crimes were in progress and then failing to arrest the offender, a man who had been released early from a long prison sentence for previous sex offenses. When the investigating magistrate, suspected of partiality toward the prosecution, was taken off the case a great outcry ensued and a quarter of a million people marched in protest through the center of Brussels. A telephone line was set up for anyone to call with worries about "pedophiles" (which is being used widely as the generic term for anyone having a sexual relationship with a minor, regardless of age or consent). Thousands did so, but only a handful produced concrete information.

In the climate of suspicion and anonymous denunciations that developed, concerns soon spilled over from the actual events, which involved only heterosexual attacks on girls, to alleged male homosexual activity. The Deputy Prime Minister of Belgium, Elio di Rupo, who was widely known to be homosexual, was reported in the press to have been guilty of pedophile crime. Such was the extent of moral panic that Marie-France Botte, a prominent campaigner against sex tourism and child sex abuse, was moved to appeal for calm and for homosexuals not to be confused with pedophiles (*Le Soir*, 20 Nov., 1996, p. 2). On the instructions of Parliament, the allegations against di Rupo were investigated by the Cour de Cassation [Supreme Court] and declared unfounded. Apparently, they had originated in enforced police interrogation of a thief in his 20s who said he had had sexual contact with di Rupo. Allegations against another minister and allegations against other homosexual men are still being pursued. One could hardly have a clearer example of how easily and illogically the homosexual minority can come under public suspicion once emotions have been aroused by sensational press coverage of sexual atrocities.

The Outlook for Individuals

Belgian law and custom give adequate protection against breaches of privacy, so it is virtually unknown for anyone to be publicly identified as homosexual unless they have themselves already taken the initiative. Belgium is a small country, sharing its languages and freedom of movement with neighboring European Union states. It is relatively easy for anyone finding the local environment in Belgium too constricting to move to large cities abroad, such as Paris or Amsterdam. The larger Belgian towns, however, do have gay bars and a few have similar establishments for lesbians. The two main GLB groups each publish monthly magazines. For several years one of the noncommercial (community) radio stations in Brussels broadcast a weekly program of GLB material intended to inform and entertain both the homosexual community and the general public. Since 1996, the Flemish public broadcasting company BRTN has allocated two teletext pages (762 and 763) for news of particular interest to the GLB community, supplied by the FWH. There is no central telephone information service of the kind known elsewhere as gay and lesbian "switchboard," but the telephone counseling service Telegal has been provided in recent years. Several unsuccessful attempts have been made to launch commercial magazines intended to appeal mainly to gays and lesbians in Belgium, but it seems that those imported from France and the Netherlands suffice to meet local demand.

Conclusions

The situation of gays and lesbians in Belgium is relatively satisfactory, at least when compared with that in many other countries. Certainly, some discrimination does occur, but mainly as a result of individual aberrations of enforcement practice rather than as systematic implementation of a deliberate policy. The opportunity for this to happen is caused by the failure of successive governments to bring the Penal Code up-to-date in accordance with the evolution of public opinion about sexual matters and, in particular, the failure to eliminate the term *debauchery*, or at least to define it in a clearly limited sense. The legal provisions for consensual sexual behavior by adolescents appear unnecessarily stringent in comparison with those in neighboring countries. Because of its central location within the European Union, the impact of increasingly close European integration may be expected to reinforce Belgium's long tradition of gender-neutral, nondiscriminatory legislation and perhaps to stimulate reform of the Penal Code. In the short term, however, the political will seems to be lacking.

Cited Case

Belgian Crown v Haenen and Vincineau, Liège Appeal Court (1986, March 23).

References

Brussels Appeal Court, 11th Chamber. (1991, April 24). Pornographie — evolution des moeurs. *Journal des procès*, *185*, 30.
Clerck, S. de. (1995, November 2) *Télémoustique*, p. 29.
David, P. (1995). *Enfants sans enfance*. Paris: Hachette Pluriel. pp. 57–60.
Gury, C. (1981) *L'homosexuel et la loi*. Lausanne: Editions de l'Aire.
Homosexuels agressés a Namur. (1995, September 4). *Le Soir*.
Letters to the editor. (1995, June 28). *Le Soir*, p. 2.
Letters to the editor. (1995, July 12). *Le Soir*, p. 2.
Ost. F., & Kerchove, M. van de. (1981) *Bonnes moeurs, discours pénal et rationalité juridique*. Brussels: Faculté Universitaires St-Louis.
Petijean, P. (1995, July 12) Carte blanche. *Le Soir*, p. 2.
Tels Quels (1994) *126*, 7–9.
Tels Quels (1988) *70*, Dec. et seq. "Nos Libertés … bientôt les vôtres!"
Tels Quels (1995) *135*, 4–9. "En mai, vote comme il te plaît …"
Vandemeulebroucke, M. Spartacus? (était pour décourager la pédophile. (1994, 24 November). *Le Soir*, p. 15.
Vincineau, M. (1985) *La débauche en droit et le droit à la débauche*. Brussels: Editions de l'Université de Bruxelles.

19

THE NETHERLANDS

MARTIN MOERINGS

INTRODUCTION

In the eyes of many foreigners, the Netherlands is a very tolerant country — sometimes *too* tolerant. The number of prisoners is proportionately among the lowest in the world and the policy of tolerance with regard to soft drugs annoys several European countries, particularly France. The social climate is friendly toward homosexuals, and Amsterdam has been portrayed as the gay capital of the world. Indeed, it probably has the largest number of gay bars of any city worldwide. All kinds of groups, including political parties, have gay/lesbian segments among their members. At the same time, however, the fact that there are so many gay segments in organizations for male homosexuals and lesbians means that homosexual emancipation cannot yet be taken for granted and that equal treatment has not yet been realized.

In this chapter, a brief sketch of Dutch society centers on the position of homosexuals. A picture of the tolerance as well as the rejection and reservations existing in the Netherlands is provided.

Against this background a description is given of relevant legislation and law enforcement, with the focus primarily on the developments designed to combat discrimination. On this issue the Netherlands undoubtedly plays a leading role. The question is, however, whether such legislation is indeed effective, or merely cosmetic.

That much inequality has been built into existing legislation is shown, with marriage as the most obvious example because of the legal consequences automatically attached to the institution of marriage. Currently, there is a public debate on marriage for homosexual and lesbian couples. It was received enthusiastically by a majority motion in parliament, but has not yet come to a bill of law. Also, within social institutions such as healthcare, much inequality is still to be found through practices that are only partly or not at all hindered by laws or law enforcement

HOMOSEXUALS IN DUTCH SOCIETY

Social survey statistics, reproduced in Table 1, show that tolerance has increased enormously in the last 15–20 years. In 1968, 64 percent of the population agreed that homosexuals should be able to live the way they themselves wanted. By 1991 that figure had risen to 95 percent. However, being left free to live in any way is not the same as having

---

MARTIN MOERINGS • Institute for Criminal Sciences, University of Utrecht, Utrecht 3512 BM, The Netherlands.

Sociolegal Control of Homosexuality, edited by West and Green, Plenum Press, New York, 1997.

TABLE 1. Attitudes toward Homosexuals[a]

Percent agreeing that	Year					
	1968	1975	1980	1985	1987	1991
Homosexuals should be left as free as possible to lead their own lives	64%	83%	93%	93%	94%	95%
Homosexuals should have the same rights as ordinary married couples to adopt children	—	—	35%	43%	44%	47%
Homosexual couples should have the same rights as ordinary married couples to inherit from each other	—	—	89%	92%	94%	93%

[a]From Sociaal en Cultureel Planbureau Rijswijk (1992).

equal rights. In 1991 only 47 percent thought that homosexuals should be allowed to adopt children. The reservations with respect to adoption are undoubtedly based on the idea that children should be able to grow up in a family with both a father and a mother. Acceptance of the right of same-sex couples to inherit from each other is much greater (93 percent).

The biggest leap in tolerance took place in the 1970s. A high point seems to have been reached in the mid-1980s. Since then attitudes have remained more or less stable. This is in conformity with the general tendency toward liberalization in Dutch society, which is evident from the growing opinion that divorce should be permitted. Dutch tolerance toward drug use, but also toward such issues as euthanasia, has received much attention. In this regard, the Netherlands has built up a certain reputation internationally. Again, for many years the low percentage of incarcerations in Dutch prisons, while crime figures rose no higher than in the surrounding countries, was regarded as exemplary, although of late this headstart is fast being eradicated.

This image of the Netherlands as a country where many things are tolerated is not a recent one. Writers often refer to the sixteenth-century when the Dutch opened their borders to the Hugenots fleeing France during the persecutions of Protestant thinkers. It should be observed, however, that today the Dutch are by no means remarkable in their willingness to receive refugees and on this do not compare particularly favorably with neighboring countries.

Tolerance toward homosexuals did not become manifest until the end of the 1960s. Those were the years when leaders of the gay movement and a number of important social scientists began to emphasize that homosexuals are *gewoon hetzelfde* [just like anyone else] (Sengers, 1971) — differing only in their sexual preference, but otherwise ordinary people. This idea was also predominant within the COC, the Dutch organization for the integration of homosexuals that was, for many years, their mouthpiece. Integration in society, as the name suggests, was its aim, not to be different because one was gay, but to be part of society. During that period there was a preference for the term *homophiliac*, rather than homosexual, in order to demonstrate that what is at stake is not merely sexuality, but love and affection for a person of the same sex.

During the 1970s, reaction set in, starting within certain student circles. A number of radical gay groups appeared, with names like Red Gays, for whom homosexuality also had political significance that meant more than one's choice of sexual partner being different from that of heterosexuals (Warmerdam, 1991). These groups were inspired by Marxist and feminist ideas. During demonstrations they wore women's clothes and makeup to challenge gender stereotypes. They were not presenting themselves as women or transvestites, but emphatically as men in women's clothes. The aim was to spread confusion, in which they were singularly successful. They met with a great deal of resistance and their influence on the emancipation of homosexuals has remained limited, although it cannot be ignored entirely.

In any event, and despite the fact that it has not changed its name, the COC has exchanged integration for emancipation. It has changed to an emphasis on the uniqueness of a person's development and identity as a homosexual and the special position of the homosexual in society — where, for example, marriage need not, and may not, be copied as a way of giving shape to a same-sex relationship.

During the past 10–15 years, the gay movement — insofar as it has ever been possible to speak of a united front — has fragmented. The approach, moreover, is more pragmatical. In most sectors of society, gay groups have arisen that take a pragmatic stand in their fight for their own specific concerns within their own field (Schedler, 1992). Most political parties have their own gay groups; there are groups within the trade unions, including the union of government employees; the army has its foundation for homosexuality and armed forces; and there is a national group of lesbian doctors. These are just a few examples. Only industry and commerce have lagged behind and appear to have no gay groups. To this extent, the emancipation, acceptance, and furthering of the interests of homosexuals in the Netherlands is only relative, although in comparison with most, if not all, other countries it may seem remarkable.

The relatively favorable position of homosexuals is not entirely due to their own effort. It is fairer to say that they were active on a modest scale, originally through providing the public with information, lobbying by leaders, and later through large demonstrations by groups of homosexual men and lesbians. Such action needs a fertile soil in which to flourish (Stolk, 1991). During the 1960s a number of leading figures in the field of public morals were instrumental in influencing thinking about sexual issues in general, such as contraception and abortion, as well as homosexuality. They were able to lift homosexuality from the sphere of sinfulness and perversity, at first by explaining it as the result of sickness and deviance and later by regarding it as a variation of sexuality. These men and women brought their influence to bear on the moral climate and created an openness that allowed homosexuals to speak and be heard.

It is characteristic of Dutch society that it remains open to moderate action groups in general, listens to them, takes them in, and, in doing so, manages to neutralize them to a certain extent.

Antihomosexual Violence and the Police as Friends

For years criminal law was an instrument to maintain discrimination against homosexuals. An example of such legislation was the notorious Section 248 bis of the Criminal Code, which prohibited homosexual contact with anyone under the age of 21 while allowing heterosexual contact at a much earlier age. This section was repealed in 1971. Although this unequal law was abolished, inequality in law enforcement continued. Heterosexual couples making love in cars and in parks were left alone, while young men having sex in public places still ran the risk of being arrested for an offense against public decency.

For a long time homosexuals were looked upon first and foremost as potential offenders. For years, the standard reaction of the police to a complaint of antihomosexual violence — if the victim could bring himself to report it — was that the victim simply should not have gone to that park or that parking place. Cruising areas for men seeking homosexual contacts, such as parks and, increasingly in recent years, parking areas along the motorways, especially when there is access to woods behind them, meet this need. The police used to patrol cruising areas to see if they could catch anyone committing an indecent act, or they drove with bright headlights along the wooded areas to hunt down and terrorize persons who had made a contact there. Now police use-on-the spot patrols to prevent violence against homosexuals. In Rotterdam, two police officials, one homosexual and one heterosexual, have been appointed for this purpose. They patrol the city park.

Only recently have the judicial authorities become aware that homosexuals can also be victims, for example, of antihomosexual violence. Men who seek sexual contact with other men in cruising areas are often beaten up by "queer-bashers," youths operating in groups who beat up homosexuals, steal their money, or blackmail them if they can. Married men seeking anonymous homosexual contacts are the easiest to blackmail.

For the police the tide is turning, certainly in the larger cities. A few police forces recruit some of their staff via job advertisements in gay magazines. There is a working group within the police service, Police and Homosexuality, of which homosexual police staff are members. Practically all of them are men. Women are more reserved about this, but undoubtedly there are quite a few lesbians in the police force.

In 1984 the first antihomosexual violence project was started by police in Groningen. This has since been copied throughout the country. Several years later the first victim survey was conducted among lesbians and homosexual men (Tuijl & Arts, 1987). Victims' reports are now often being taken seriously and result in the prosecution of queer-bashers for such crimes as extortion, blackmail, acts of violence in public places, threatening behavior, assault, or, in the most serious instances, murder or manslaughter.

Lesbians are sometimes assaulted or raped by men who want to "make a real woman out of them" or "let them experience what it is like to have sex with a man." In these instances nothing is mentioned in the indictment about the antihomosexual nature of the violence. However, the public prosecutor and the courts may take this into account in demanding and passing sentences. There are several instances where the court has handed down a more severe sentence than usual because of the antihomosexual nature of the offense. Of course, this does not exceed the statutory maximum punishment for the offense charged.

It is not always clear whether the (assumed) homosexuality of the victim has played a part. This is sometimes apparent from an offender's remarks [e.g., "I went to the park in the hope of being approached by a homosexual. Then, if I was approached I had an excuse to beat up that homo" (Haveman & Moerings, 1992, p. 41)].

In other cases it is the circumstances that lead one to suspect that antihomosexual offenses have taken place. Some cruising grounds are located such that it is not easy to get there unintentionally. And if the approach ritual has been performed, there is little room for doubt. ["That business of driving around each other, I don't think a hetero would do that. He wouldn't be so interested in my car that he thinks, hey! I want to see it three more times." (Haveman & Moerings, 1992, p. 41)].

Antihomosexual crime happens everywhere, not just in cruising areas. Crimes against lesbians seem to occur more often in private than crimes against homosexual men.

The fact that antihomosexual crime occurs is indisputable. What is not clear is *how often* it happens. During recent years studies have been carried out on its nature and scope, but these studies have been too small-scale to draw reliable conclusions. Statistics from the police do not give the impression that gigantic numbers are involved. Some writers suspect that the "dark figure" of crimes that are not brought to the attention of the police and therefore remain unrecorded in police statistics is more than 90 percent. From a survey conducted by the Eindhoven police among (potential) victims, researchers conclude that this estimate is "unfortunately more than confirmed" (Van Tuijl & Arts, 1987, p. 145). Many victims are very reluctant to report the crimes, undoubtedly because so many of them are married men who frequent the cruising areas, where sexual contacts can take place in anonymity. They are the last ones to go to the police as victims of an antihomosexual crime. As is evident from the survey of victims, other reasons may also deter them from going to the police. Sometimes the victims do not find it worth the effort to report the crime or they find it a waste of time because the police do nothing about it anyway. More specific reasons may be fear of reprisals by the perpetrator or the strained relations that still exist between police and homosexuals, which leads to unfriendly treatment. The impression that the Netherlands is a paradise for homosexuals is not really true.

Antihomosexual violence has become more visible. During the period of 1974–1983 an average of 63 cases a year were recorded, versus 138 in 1989. The greater visibility is especially evident in the forms of violence involving public order and/or related to (un)paid sexual contacts at meeting places. Forms of violence that take place in the victim's immediate living environment (i.e., where perpetrator and victim know each other) are much less visible. Antilesbian violence goes practically unnoticed. During the period 1974–1989 only 45 instances of anti-lesbian violence were recorded, versus 655 of anti-male homosexual violence (Dobbeling & Koenders, 1985; Veen & Dercksen, 1990). Little is known about the perpetrators (Boogaart & Stolk, 1992).

PROVISIONS AGAINST DISCRIMINATION IN THE CRIMINAL LAW

Antihomosexual violence can be inspired by an aversion to homosexuals. Such an aversion will express itself first in verbal remarks and discrimination against homosexuals in everyday life. Since 1992, already existing provisions of the Criminal Code that ban racial discrimination have been expanded to include gender, religion, personal convictions, and homosexual or heterosexual preference.

The government also wants to demonstrate via criminal law that homosexual behavior is not reprehensible, or at any rate that it is the business of individuals between themselves in which others, including the state, should not interfere. In this regard the government is distancing itself more and more from pornography, as long as adults are not confronted with it unexpectedly.

The state is also taking more of a back seat when it comes to other sexual behavior. Sex between an adult and a young person between the ages of 12 and 16 is permitted by law, as long as the young person consents. It may only be prosecuted by complaint from the young person or the young person's parents. The question remains whether the public prosecutions department would proceed to prosecute if the young person himself had consented and his parents filed the complaint. Sadomasochistic sexual relations are not punishable. Where children are involved in sexual relations in which they had no choice, then the government acts forcibly. The penalties for child pornography are being toughened, and merely having child pornography in stock now carries a penalty.

If the government steps aside where people enjoy sexual pleasures with mutual consent, the next logical step seems fairly obvious — namely, that the citizens who want to keep their fellow citizens from doing so should be restrained by law. This may be embodied in criminal law (in which the Netherlands, Sweden, and some other countries have taken the lead), but it may also be included in civil law, as in de Algemene Wet Gelijke Behandeling [the General Equal Treatment Act].

Although the criminal law aims to deter homosexual discrimination, many situations experienced by the victims as discrimination remain outside the scope of the law because the legal provisions have the nature of a compromise and require very specific conditions. When acts do fall under the criminal law, there are still factors that make enforcement very difficult, even though criminal law officials are taking discrimination more and more seriously.

It is now prohibited under criminal law to incite publicly (e.g., via the distribution of pamphlets) hatred, discrimination, or violent acts against persons because of their homosexual preference (s. 137d). An example might be a pamphlet saying: "It's about time that homosexuals in cruising areas whose filthy acts drive mothers with children out of parks were taught a good lesson." It does not matter whether or not the inciter has actually had success through the distribution of his pamphlet.

Participation in or support of activities aimed at discriminating against people because of their homosexual preference is also prohibited (s. 137e). Participation in a demonstration in which hatred of homosexuals is incited is also prohibited. Anyone who provides financial support for such activities while staying out of sight is also liable to punishment.

The most important provisions are those that penalize insults and prohibit discrimination in the workplace. It is thus an offense to utter insults intentionally, either verbally or in writing, in public against a group of people because of their homosexual preference (s. 137c). You may not call someone a "filthy queer" in public. Remarks made in newspapers and books and radio and television messages are always "public." An insult in a personal letter stating, for example, "They should have gassed all of you during the war," does not fall under this provision. The general insult provision (s. 266), which has been in force for some time, does not require a public insult. This is actually a complaint-based offense for which prosecution can only take place after a complaint has been filed by the person insulted. In the new Section 137c the circle of people who may complain to the police has been expanded considerably. Although the actual "victim" may not have felt himself insulted, a hurtful remark may be a reason for the COC to report it to the police.

This new section requires the *intention* to insult. In the past it has often been brought forward in cases of racial discrimination that there was no intention to insult because no one knew that such a remark would be hurtful to a certain group of people. This is also not necessary, according to the courts. If one knowingly takes the risk that a remark might be hurtful, intention is present (doctrine of recklessness). What is relevant is whether a remark like "filthy queer" can be considered insulting to homosexuals in general.

The penalty the courts may impose for violation is imprisonment for up to 1 year or a fine not exceeding 10,000 guilders (about $US6000). Moreover, the court seldom imposes the maximum penalty. It usually remains far below.

The other important provision is Section 429 quater, which prohibits discrimination in the exercise of one's office, profession, or business. Neither public officials nor private employers and institutions may discriminate. An employer may not reject an applicant because of his or her sexual orientation, and a building society is not allowed to refuse homosexual tenants. A bank may not refuse a permanent position to an employee for making known the fact that he is homosexual, for example, by wearing a pink triangle, the symbol of the homosexual movement. This section is aimed at the exercise of a profession. A private individual who wants to rent a room may refuse to rent it to a lesbian girl or homosexual young man. It is obvious that here the government again remains in the background where private matters are concerned. Other than in the criminal provisions described here, infractions are *misdemeanors*. Intention or guilt need not be proved. For the perpetrator to be liable to punishment it is not required that his purpose was to discriminate. Indirect discrimination also falls within the scope of this section, as the Supreme Court has so ruled in cases of racial discrimination.

Direct discrimination is unequal treatment on one of the grounds of discrimination listed earlier in this chapter. If someone is not allowed to rent a certain house or apartment because he is gay, then he is a victim of direct discrimination. Indirect discrimination occurs when a certain requirement that cannot be justified (i.e., is not *justifiable*) is made that seems neutral, but leads indirectly to discrimination. A job advertisement for bulb peelers that specifies fluency in Dutch as a requirement is an example. It may seem like a neutral requirement, but it leads indirectly to discrimination of ethnic minorities, which cannot be justified: Fluency in Dutch is not necessary for an adequate fulfillment of the job.

Does indirect homosexual discrimination occur? An example would be an insurance company that refuses to insure people who are HIV-positive. This policy affects homosexual men in particular, but is probably justifiable objectively because of the increased insurance risk. Or, suppose that a building society in a certain neighborhood will only rent houses to families with children because this provides a friendly atmosphere. The result is that homosexuals are indirect victims of this policy, without there being a clear objective justification for this. Discrimination on the grounds of this section carries a lighter penalty than breach of the aforementioned criminal provisions. The sentence is at most 2 months detention or a fine of up to 10,000 guilders.

As far as is ascertainable, since its introduction no one has yet been criminally convicted of discrimination on the ground of homosexuality. Several reports that were indeed filed by the public prosecutor have been dismissed for various reasons. The following are two examples.

> In the dunes at Zandvoort two young men are sunbathing in an area that is known as a meeting place for homosexuals. One is naked, the other wearing bathing trunks. They are startled by a policeman on horseback who gallops towards them and fires a battery of curses at them, including "get out of here, you dirty sods." Then, with his horse, the policeman forces them into the thorny bushes. The two young men file a report, which does not lead to prosecution. The police officer is reprimanded by his superior and receives a mark on his conduct record, which will for the time being probably cost him a promotion. This has more effect on him than a fine of $US120.

> In Zwolle a police report was made against an alderman who had uttered discriminating remarks against homosexuals outside the council meeting. The public prosecutor finds that proof of discrimination can be furnished. He decides to settle the matter with an oral warning, because the municipal council has condemned the remark in public.

SCOPE OF THE EQUAL TREATMENT ACT

As mentioned earlier, the criminal court has not yet had to give any interpretation of the concept of *homosexual discrimination*. If cases are put before it, it will no doubt be guided by the General Equal Treatment Act. According to the reasoning of the former Minister of Justice, what is allowed under this act may not then be punished via criminal law.

The act came into force on September 1, 1994. The Equal Treatment Commission, an independent, professional organization, reviews the complaints it receives to see if the regulations on equal treatment have been violated. It deals with unequal treatment involving religion, personal convictions and views, political orientation, race, gender, nationality, marital status, and sexual preference (i.e. homosexual or heterosexual preference, pedosexuality is excluded). The act stated that it is forbidden to treat people differently on these eight grounds of discrimination in the following situations:

1. In working relationships between employers and employees, unequal treatment is forbidden in any area that is related to work, from job advertisements to actual employment. These regulations also apply to people in the liberal professions, such as lawyers, civil law notaries, and doctors
2. When goods and services are offered, everyone should be treated equally when taking out insurance policies, renting houses, and opening bank accounts

Not all forms of discrimination fall within the scope of this act. It is a typical example of the Dutch policy of accommodating political compromises, the result of accommodation of the Christian Democrats on one side and the Social Democrats and liberals on the other. Dutch liberals, unlike liberals elsewhere, are the more conservative party. No single party in the Dutch Parliament has a majority. The three mentioned have almost equally strong representation in the Dutch Parliament. That means that legislating is always a process of negotiation. The result is a compromise, as in this act, where discrimination is prohibited, but not under all circumstances. A debate went on for almost 10 years before the Christian Democrats were willing to let the act pass, but with some important exceptions. For example, the Church is exempt on the grounds of religious freedom. Priests and ministers may preach family life from the pulpit, may label homosexuals as sinners, and may portray homosexuality as a sickness. Such statements may only be made during church services and not outside them.

Not all church congregations are going to make eager use of this freedom. There are tolerant Christian movements, within both the Catholic and Protestant churches, for whom a homosexual pastor is not a problem and who are willing to sanctify a homosexual relationship in a church service.

The Church as an institution does not fall under the law and under certain circumstances exceptions are made for Christian schools. Debates on this issue in particular have been going on for years both in and out of Parliament. Christian Democrats are holding fast to their demand that schools should be able to bar homosexual teachers and students from their school on religious grounds.

The compromise reached is that such schools may bar gay teachers if this is necessary for the fulfillment of their functions. This means that a distinction may be made between gay teachers who teach physics and those who teach religion or social studies. Such teachers may be barred if they express their feelings at school, such as by kissing their partner in public or wearing a pink triangle, thereby identifying themselves with a group that does not recognize marriage as the cornerstone of society. However, a teacher may never be rejected solely for *being* gay if he or she has not expressed this in any way. The commission will have to decide how far special schools may go in making a distinction. So far, there has been only one complaint from a homosexual teacher.

The commission deals with complaints about direct as well as indirect discrimination. Anyone who feels that he is being treated unequally may request a decision from the commission. An individual may submit a request only if some personal disadvantage has been suffered. If he prefers not to file a complaint personally, he may ask someone else to do it as his representative, which could be a family member or a friend, but also a pressure group such as the COC, the major organization for homosexuals in the Netherlands. Pressure groups may also file complaints to the commission independently, but only if they are organizations or societies officially founded to promote the interests of the people to whom the regulations on equal treatment apply.

The commission will question the complaining party and the person or organization that is allegedly discriminating. The commission can also call third parties as witnesses to give information about the case. It could be said that the commission acts like a judicial organization, but with one important difference: It can itself search for the information that it feels it needs.

The commission's decision is not legally binding. It cannot force the party who is found guilty of discrimination to cooperate with its ruling. However, after the decision has been made the commission often contacts representatives of the organization in which the case occurred, hoping that good communication will help to prevent unequal treatment in the future.

Up to the time of this writing (April 1996), the commission has received only a few complaints about homosexual discrimination, all of them concerned with the exclusion of a homosexual partner from spousal pension rights. These complainants could not be helped because pension schemes are excluded from the equal treatment law.

There are still some complaints waiting to be handled. One came from a homosexual teacher who felt that his chances for promotion were hindered and that he had received signs of discrimination from colleagues and students. Another came from someone who had applied for a teaching position at a Christian school and had to sign a statement saying that he condemned extramarital forms of cohabitation. This could become a "classic" case, as during the years of preparation and passing of the act, this issue was the subject of debate. Two other complaints (analogous to the Grant case from the United Kingdom, which has been referred to the European Court of Human Rights) came from homosexual partners of staff members who work at transport companies. They state that they are not able to travel at the same reduced rates as heterosexual partners are.

The scarcity of complaints about homosexual discrimination, 1½ years after introduction of the act, raises questions. Do too few people know about the commission? Do people hesitate to complain because the commission cannot make binding decisions? Or is homosexual discrimination not such a problem after all? Several years after the relevant section was introduced, the criminal courts have not had to deal with a single case of homosexual discrimination. Internationally, the Netherlands is still considered one of the most tolerant countries with regard to homosexuality, as it is on most social issues.

MARRIAGE ONLY FOR HETEROSEXUALS

The restriction of marriage to heterosexual relationships is the most important remaining antihomosexual legislation in the Netherlands. The exclusion of couples of the same sex from marriage cannot be found in so many words in the law, but this exclusion is read into it by the courts, who conclude from the legal system that the law only governs marriages between man and wife. The consequence of this is that lesbian women and homosexual men are denied both the social status and an important set of legal consequences that are attached to marriage (Waaldijk, 1992).

Marriage imposes a duty upon the partners to support each other; unless otherwise arranged, their possessions become community property and they become each other's heir. By way of a cohabitation contract or the making of a will a number of these legal consequences can also be regulated outside marriage, but that does not apply to *statutory dependents' pension or parenthood*. It is precisely in these areas where homosexual couples are discriminated against concretely in comparison with heterosexual couples.

According to the statutory pension scheme for public servants,[1] the wife of the deceased is entitled to a pension when her husband dies. The survivors of a cohabitation relationship have no right to this pension.[2]

[1]Private business pensions have similar schemes, although not on a statutory basis. They may — and sometimes do — institute pension schemes for the surviving partners of unmarried employees. Insofar as they refuse to do so, they are not acting in contravention of the General Equal Treatment Act, which excludes pension schemes. If a statutory pension scheme is concerned, such as for public servants, the Equal Treatment Act and the provisions of the Criminal Code do not conflict. The courts cannot test one law against the other.
[2]Amendment is forthcoming.

If a married woman has a baby, her husband is automatically the father and shares parental authority over the child. He also has the duty to maintain the child. If an un-married woman has a baby, her female partner does not acquire the rights and duties of fatherhood. Two lesbian mothers cannot have joint parental authority. The same applies to two homosexual fathers. In other words, by law, partners of the same sex cannot both be parents. Legal parenthood has many consequences for the relationships between the child and his legal parents regarding inheritance, duty of maintenance, parental authority, and visiting rights after divorce. Same-sex partners who are not legal parents do not have these rights and duties with respect to the children they help to raise.

A married couple may adopt a child and through this be charged with the rights and duties of parenthood. An unmarried couple may not adopt. On these and other points there is no difference between unmarried but cohabiting heterosexual couples and cohabiting homosexual couples. The issue does not seem to be the distinction of sexual preference as much as the form of living together/civil status. But this is not altogether true, because heterosexual couples may make a conscious choice to live together without getting married. Homosexual couples have no choice; they can only cohabit.

Some types of inequality between marriage and other forms of relationship have already been abolished through cohabitation contracts and wills. A cohabitation contract open to same-sex couples offers a solution for, among other things, the following: commu-nity of goods, the costs of running a household, the housing rights of the partners if the relationship is ended, the duty of the one with the highest income to contribute toward maintenance of the other at the end of the relationship, and, perhaps most importantly, the survivorship clause. This last provision is more or less an agreement that one or more items from the *community of goods* will become the sole property of one of the two partners as soon as a specific circumstance occurs, such as death. This is important, for the surviving partner, who, for instance, would become the owner of a house registered in both names that might otherwise fall within the inheritance entitlement of other surviving relatives.

If a married person dies, his or her spouse, in addition to the children, is the heir. Until the beginning of 1996 the parents of an unmarried person became automatically the heirs if he or she died. It might happen in the case of a homosexual man, who, for example, died as a result of AIDS and for this reason had been rejected by his parents years before, that his estate would still go to those parents. Even if a beneficiary in his will, his partner would only have a right to a small part. At the beginning of 1996, this form of inequality was abolished: Parents no longer have the automatic right to inherit a portion of the estate. A homosexual man or lesbian may leave the entire estate to his or her partner, unless there are children from a marriage.

SPECIAL HOMOSEXUAL MARRIAGE OR TRADITIONAL MARRIAGE PERMITTED?

The inequality between married and unmarried people (of the same sex) who live together can be abolished by making marriage available to partners of the same sex. The legal consequences of marriage would then automatically apply also to gay and lesbian couples. It has not yet come to that. The (junior) minister of justice with the approval of the Council of Ministers did put forward the *Nota Samenlevingsregistratie* [Policy Docu-ment on Partner Registration]. This will be debated in widely representative social quarters and should result in a bill. Under this proposal, after official registration, unmarried people who live together — thus also gays and lesbians — would acquire the same rights and duties in a number of areas as married people: They may inherit from each other and have the right to dependents' pension, but also have a mutual duty of maintenance. This may also have consequences for the children in their relationship. The parent and his or her partner may acquire joint parental authority over the children. It is possible for the children to take on the family name of the partner of their parent, and possibly his or her Dutch nationality, and they may inherit directly from him or her.

The only thing still excluded from partner registration is adoption. This is defended by the argument that adopted children in the Netherlands often come from countries where homosexual couples are regarded with suspicion and where adoption by homosexual or lesbian couples is considered sinful. There is the fear that this would severely limit the possibilities of Dutch citizens to adopt children. Is this a just argument or merely one enabling the (junior) minister easily to avoid a decision? If the present plans go through, single-parent adoption will indeed become possible. A homosexual will then be able to adopt a child and will then be able, together with his or her partner, to acquire joint parental authority over the child.

These plans have led to extensive debate in the media and in Parliament. A parliamentary majority (by a vote of 81–60) considered that the (junior) minister's plans do not go far enough and wants to allow actual marriage for homosexual and lesbian couples. The (junior) minister is not willing to agree and has appointed a committee to examine the pros and cons of allowing persons of the same sex to marry and to propose a bill of law. At least two prominent members of the gay movement sit on this committee, which has led the Church to comment critically that the committee is biased and the outcome determined from the start.

Those who oppose the idea of homosexual marriage in this public debate regard it as an insult to the institution of marriage, as subverting our culture. A leading solicitor and notary public who is also a university professor declared publicly that he would divorce if marriage between homosexuals were made possible.

Another regularly heard argument has it that homosexual marriage repudiates the notion of marriage being directed toward reproduction. Biological and legal parenthood would be separated. This ignores the fact that there are marriages between people unable to have children. It also ignores reality, in that women are able to become pregnant through donor insemination and *in vitro* fertilization, without the legal parent necessarily being the biological one.

A final and frequent argument is that a child needs both a father figure and a mother figure. Moreover, there is said to be a risk of the child becoming homosexual. This reveals reliance on the "role model" of how homosexuality is acquired and how strongly heterosexuality is considered the desirable norm.

Among homophile circles too, the reaction has not always been positive. By allowing homosexual marriage, a homosexual relationship is made into a copy of the traditional heterosexual two-person relationship. At the same time and increasingly frequently, it is argued that individual choice should not be limited; everyone should be free to choose whether or not to marry.

Both those who agree and those who disagree with homosexual marriage continue the debate very much within the conceptual framework of traditional relationships. This ignores the point that increasing numbers of both heterosexual and homosexual people remain, whether or not of their own choosing, uncoupled. For years the COC refused to take as its starting point for its policy and activities the idea of a two-person relationship, preferring to promote individualism as an ideal and as a basis for legislation. Abolition of the inequalities between married and unmarried couples on the basis of their gender may still leave in place inequalities between single people and couples. Single people must pay tax and insurance geared to requirements they themselves do not need, notably pensions for spouses who survive them and state funded education for children.

MANDATORY AIDS TESTING FOR HOMOSEXUAL MEN (AND LESBIANS)

In the medical sector, but also in the business community, the prevention of AIDS has resulted in a policy that has led to a form of indirect discrimination against men who have homosexual contacts. A debate, originating in the homophile movement, has been going on since the first half of the 1980s on the very restrictive admission policy of blood banks (Hendriks & Markenstein, 1992). Donors were made to sign a declaration that they had had no current homosexual relations. Later, their policy was further tightened so that "men who since 1980 have had sexual relations with another man" were considered to be "persons having risk-bearing relations" (Letter from the Board for Blood Transfusion, 1988). Within the homophile movement this criterion is considered much too broad. Even strictly monogamous men and homosexual men without homosexual contacts are asked not to give blood. The homophile movement has been pleading, still in vain, for setting the period of exclusion back to 6 months — the "open window" period during which medical opinion considers that infection with HIV remains latent and not detectable on testing.

Another controversial issue is the acceptance policy of private insurers. It is permissible to require a candidate for insurance of over 200,000 Dutch guilders (NLG) ($US120,000) or disability insurance over NLG 40,000 to take an HIV test. Moreover, an insurance company may prescribe an HIV test upon medical indications. The fact that someone is homosexual is in itself not a medical indication. The application forms of many companies contain the question: "Has your blood ever been tested for HIV and if so, what were the results?" Since the applicant has to declare that he has answered all questions in good faith, he must furnish the correct information. An indirect attempt is also made to find out about any possible HIV status by asking for the name and sex of one's partner in life. Since the real reason for rejecting a candidate for insurance is difficult to discover, demonstrating unequal treatment is not an easy task. However, it is clear that homosexual men have to face more obstacles in taking out insurance than the members of most other sections of the population, including lesbians.

ALTERNATIVE REPRODUCTIVE TECHNIQUES

Artificial insemination or *in vitro* fertilization (Hendriks & Markenstein, 1992) are sometimes chosen by lesbians who want to have a baby. A number of academic and "ordinary" hospitals use these methods for lesbians, but others reserve them exclusively for heterosexual couples. Discussion focuses on arguments that alternative reproductive possibilities are to be considered strictly medical treatment, for which a medical need is required, or that the interests of children are best served by having a father and a mother. These arguments ignore the fact that many lesbians simply would not want to go to bed with a man and are therefore dependent on alternative reproductive techniques. Furthermore, very many children, because of divorce or other reasons, grow up in single-parent families.

Conclusion

The Netherlands is regarded as one of the most tolerant countries with regard to homosexuality. Consensus is almost absolute that homosexuals must be able to live as they themselves wish. This is not to say that everyone wishes to be confronted with their lifestyle. This tolerance has increased dramatically over the past 25 years. Until the beginning of the 1970s, the law still criminalized homosexual contacts under certain circumstances. Now the legislation is of an entirely different nature. Unequal treatment of homosexuals can be addressed through both civil and criminal law. But the legislation has not gone all the way. Laws on marriage, adoption, and pensions continue to discriminate against homosexuals. Marriage between homosexual and lesbian couples is an issue of heated public and parliamentary debate, but the decision on legislation has been deferred for the time being pending the findings of a committee. The Dutch have a reputation for gaining time by appointing committees.

References

Boogaart, H. van den, & Stolk, B. van Potenrammers. (1992). Vandalisme tegen mensen. In J. Fiselier & F. Strijbosch (Eds.), *Cultuur en Dekict* (pp. 57–70). Den Haag, The Netherlands: Vuga.

Dobbeling, M., & T. Koenders, P. (1985). *Het topje van de ijsberg.* Utrecht, The Netherlands: Publikatiereeks Homostudies.

Haveman, R., & Moerings, M. (1992). Dehomogeniteit van het strafrecht. In M. Moerings & A. Matijssen (Eds.), *Homoseksualiteit en recht* (pp. 39–62). Arnhem, The Netherlands: Gouda Quint.

Hendriks, A., & Markenstein, L. (1992). Recht als medicijn. In M. Moerings & A. Mattijssen (Eds.), *Homoseksualiteit en recht.* (pp. 185–214). Arnhem, Gouda Quint.

Schedler, P. E. (1992) *Buitenstaanders binnenshuis, vrouwen en homo's in organisaties.* Leiden, The Netherlands: Rijksuniversiteit Leiden, DSWO Press.

Sengers, W. J.(1971). *Gewoon hetzelfde: een visie op vragen rond de homofilie.* Bussum, The Netherlands: Brand.

Sociaal en Cultureel Planbureau Rijswijk. (1992). *Sociaal en cultureel rapport 1992.* Den Haag, The Netherlands: Vuga.

Stolk, B. van. (1991). *Eigenwaarde als groepsbelang, sociologische studies naar de dynamiek van zelfwaardering.* Bohn, The Netherlands: Stafleu van Loghum.

Tuijl, P. van, & Arts, J. (1987). *Geweld en homoseksualiteit.* Eindhoven, The Netherlands: Gemeente.

Veen, E. van der, & Dercksen, A. (1990). *Onderzoeksverslag I; een analyse van antihomoseksueel en antilesbisch geweld 1974–1989,* Utrecht, The Netherlands: Centrum Antidiscriminatie Homoseksualiteit.

Waaldijk, K. (1992). Zó niet getrouwd: hetero-huwelijk en bovenwettelijk discriminatieverbod. In M. Moerings & A. Mattijssen (Eds.), *Homoseksualiteit en recht.* (pp. 63–96). Arnhem, The Netherlands: Gouda Quint.

Warmerdam, H. (1991). Guerrillero's tegen normaliteit. De radicale homobeweging in Nederland 1975–1980. In I. C. Meijer, J. W. Duyvendak, & M. P. N. van Kerkhof (Eds.), *Over normaal gesproken.* (pp. 102–112). Amsterdam: Schorer.

20

Supposed Origins of Homosexuality and Implications for Social Control

Donald J. West

Definition and Measurement

Little has been said thus far in this volume about sexual science, although research into the origins and frequency of homosexual behavior has relevance to social policy. The positions taken up in political debate are often based on presumptions about matters on which pro or con evidence is available, for example, on the extent to which homosexual desires are innate or learned, immutable or modifiable (Green, 1988). To moral absolutists such considerations may seem irrelevant, but they should not be ignored by those with practical responsibility for determining social control policy.

The first requirement of research is to be clear about what is being investigated, so operational definitions are essential. Homosexual acts are easy to specify, but what is meant by a homosexual, a homosexual orientation or a homosexual identity is less certain (Gonsiorek & Weinrich, 1991; McWhirter, Sanders, & Reinish, 1991). A simple count of the frequency and type of sexual acts is not enough. For most people the directions of desire, fantasy, and behavior are congruent, but not everyone's sexual practice corresponds to their real desires. Marriage may be entered into for reasons of status, and (especially in prisons and other closed institutions) individuals can be persuaded, bribed, or coerced into taking part in acts against their usual inclination. Sexual habits can change over time, and some individuals, especially bisexuals, may identify themselves as straight or gay for predominantly social reasons. Sell and Petrulio (1995) recommend assessing heterosexual and homosexual attractions and behaviors as four separate variables. For most purposes, however, it is convenient to classify sexual orientation as homosexual, bisexual, or heterosexual on the basis of the direction of sexual desire — whether erotic feelings and physiological sex arousal occur mostly in response to the same sex, to both sexes, or to the opposite sex. As Kinsey and colleagues (1948, 1953) were the first to show, such a classification fits well for the majority of persons, at least in the Western world, and most do not change their orientation once mature adulthood has been reached. Contributors to this volume seem to have tacitly adopted the gay/lesbian/bisexual divisions as understandable and sufficient for their purposes.

Gender discordant behavior and temperament or cross-dressing interests are not relevant to this basic classification. Such features occur among a minority of male and female homosexuals, but they also occur among the heterosexually oriented. Male homosexuality is still wrongly equated with effeminacy in many parts of the world. Even some male

DONALD J. WEST • Institute of Criminology, University of Cambridge, Cambridge CB3 9DT, England, United Kingdom.

Sociolegal Control of Homosexuality, edited by West and Green, Plenum Press, New York, 1997.   313

transsexuals, who think of themselves as "trapped in a body of the wrong sex," are not pri-marily homosexual, being more concerned with performing the social role of women than with having sex with other men. In the rather rare cases of physical intersexuality, labelling as homosexual or otherwise becomes academic when the person's sex is ambiguous.

Insofar as American and European surveys provide a guide, recent research suggests that people with a clear and permanent homosexual orientation are fewer than Kinsey supposed, 4 percent rather than 10 percent among males and a half that among females (Diamond, 1993; Laumann et al., 1994; Wellings, Field, Johnson, & Wadsworth, 1994). Some surveys suggest that the hard core of men with a clear-cut homosexual orientation is of similar size in some widely differing cultures (Whitam & Mathy, 1986). The number of bisexuals is less certain. They are less visible, having fewer organizations and community facilities than gays and lesbians. Many lead outwardly conventional heterosexual lifestyles and may class themselves as heterosexuals despite wanting and having considerable and continuing homosexual experiences.

The literature on lesbianism in historical times is considerable (Faderman, 1991), but modern research into patterns of sexual feeling and behavior among women has lagged far behind studies of male homosexuality. Sexual orientation may be classifiable in the same way as for males, but the divisions are less clear-cut. Many male homosexuals have at some time had heterosexual experience, but in contrast to their ready arousability in homosexual situations, these early contacts, if not complete failures through impotence, prove unsatis-fying. Women, however, sometimes have a more prolonged bisexual or even heterosexual period before settling into permanent lesbian relationships. Long periods of varying balance between their homosexual and heterosexual relationships, or changes in later life from heterosexual marriage to homosexual partnerships, occur in women more than in men. Emphasis on emotional satisfaction in sexual relationships is a particular feature of lesbianism. Among bisexuals, a pattern of serial monogamy appears more common in women, as an ongoing relationship with a man is followed by one with a woman, or vice versa. Within the bisexual population women find greater sensitivity and emotional intimacy in same-sex contacts, whereas men enjoy less intimacy but more vigorous erotic stimulation with males (Weinberg, Williams, & Pryor, 1994).

The development of a homosexual orientation is undoubtedly governed by a multi-plicity of interacting factors that differ in their relative importance from one person to another. In some cases homosexual fantasy and feeling develop very early and initial homo-sexual contacts may be actively sought out rather than incidentally encountered. In the days when Western psychiatrists applied heroic measures to convert male homosexuals they were met with scant success. A sense of homosexual identity is often so ingrained that change seems inconceivable. On the other hand, changes in orientation do sometimes occur and immutability is not invariable.

BIOLOGICAL EXPLANATIONS

Because biological influences are thought (sometimes wrongly) to produce unmodi-fiable effects, they have often been cited as support for the contention that homosexuals have a recognizable and unalterable "condition" for which they are in no way responsible. The search for physical differences between homosexuals and heterosexuals has gone on ever since the first sexologists began in the nineteenth century to discuss disapproved sexual interests in terms of medical pathology. As with past attempts to identify physical peculiarities in criminals, these efforts have in the past so often produced false leads that a certain skepticism is justified until findings are repeatedly confirmed.

The physical processes of differential sex development are gradually being unravelled. Initially the fetus is sexually neutral, possessing both Mullerian and Wolffian ducts, the potential precursors of the female and male internal genital organs. Which develops and which regresses depends on the presence or absence of a recently identified gene on the Y chromosome that triggers development along the path that eventually produces a male. Along the way the developing male testes first produce an anti-Mullerian hormone, which promotes regression of the female structures to vestigial remnants, and later the hormone testosterone, which promotes the development of the Wolffian duct and indirectly (as long as the facilitating enzyme 5-alpha-reductase is present) causes the prostate and male external genitalia to develop. These diverging male and female developments involve the production of different hormone mixtures that may so affect the developing brain that males and females are born with different sized nuclei in certain regions, particularly in the hypothalamus.

It has been shown that in animals certain nuclei are linked to mating behavior and that experimental interference at these centers can provoke cross-sex behaviors. A number of investigators, of whom LeVay (1993) is the most often quoted, believe that they have found that the average size of certain anatomical structures differ between the brains of homosexual and heterosexual males. The corpus callosum (Allen & Gorski, 1992), the supra chiasmatic nucleus of the hypothalamus (Swaab, Gooren, & Hofman, 1995), the interstitial nucleus of the anterior hypothalamus 3 (LeVay, 1993), and the degree of laterality of brain function (Reite, Sheeder, Richardson, & Teale, 1995) have all been implicated. Some of these studies are open to criticism on methodological grounds, including small samples, use of untypical cases, flaws in measurement, and conflicting claims (Byne, 1995). One can only await the outcome of further research.

Although direct evidence is as yet unattainable, the implication from such research is that a potential for homosexual or heterosexual arousal is somehow programmed into the brain during fetal development and that an anomalous program may be implanted if the normal course of development goes wrong. That this may happen in animals has been shown by exposing the brain to artificial sex hormone levels at critical phases of development. When the animal matures, although its circulating hormones are then quite normal, it displays sex reversal behaviors as a result of the changes in its brain. This provides a theoretical model of causation of human homosexuality through hormone anomalies during fetal development. The effects might be brought about by disorders in the mother, such as diabetes, during her pregnancy. The theory explains how it can be that levels of circulating male or female hormones in the blood of adult homosexuals appear normal.

Most of the research on biological factors has dealt with males, but there is some evidence that hormonal influences can contribute to lesbianism. In the inherited condition congenital adrenal hyperplasia, the overactive adrenal gland produces an excess of male hormone during fetal development. The effect on female babies is that they are born with an enlarged clitoris looking like a penis; unless treated with cortisone, further masculinization occurs as these girls develop. The incidence of boyish behavior and interests in these girls—and of lesbian inclinations—as they mature is reportedly high, presumably due to a masculinizing effect of the abnormal hormone level on their brains during a critical phase of development (Money, 1988).

If homosexual orientation could be shown to be linked with some measurable physical characteristic, that would lend greater plausibility to biological causation. The simplistic notion that the male homosexual physique deviates toward a feminine configuration has not stood the test of systematic measurement (Evans, 1972). The impression probably came from the exaggerated mannerisms and dress styles (e.g., "butch" lesbian and male "queen") deliberately assumed and worn as a badge of identity by some members of the Western gay and lesbian subculture.

Evidence for some hereditary predisposition to homosexuality, at least among male homosexuals, is quite strong. Families with numerous homosexual members have been reported, but this could be due to upbringing or influences in the family environment. Studies of twins raised together have regularly shown a significantly higher concordance rate for homosexuality between identical than between nonidentical pairs, though by no means the 100 percent concordance that was at one time suggested (Bailey & Pillard, 1991). Most of the reports concern males, although a similar effect has now been found among lesbians (Bailey, Pillard, Neale, & Agyei, 1993). The fact that identical twins do not always have the same sexual orientation is not unexpected and does not negate the importance of inheritance. Many factors affect the likelihood of a difference on a particular gene producing a noticeable effect (Turner, 1994). For example, gross differences in development may occur if the twins have unequal access to the maternal circulation during pregnancy. The splitting of the fertilized egg to produce two individuals occurs after a number of cell divisions, and subtle differences in the gene components of some or all of the cells of an individual twin may result.

More direct evidence that male homosexuality may sometimes be linked to an identifiable gene peculiarity has been produced by Hamer (1994). He sampled families in which there was more than one homosexual brother and found that in a high proportion of cases, though not in all, the gay brothers carried the same marker on the long arm of the female (X) sex chromosome, which males inherit from their mothers. The work has been challenged and one attempted independent replication has failed to confirm the findings. There is, however, collateral support from a quite different observation, namely, that there is an imbalance in the sex ratio among the maternal ancestors of male homosexuals, with more maternal aunts than maternal uncles (Turner, 1995). Given that gene abnormalities on the X chromosome are known to produce a high incidence of abortion of male fetuses, this fits in with Hamer's contention that some male homosexuals carry a peculiarity on the X chromosome inherited through the female line. However, as researchers point out (Hamer & Copeland, 1994), a statistical relationship does not mean a direct cause, and the association with a peculiarity on the X chromosome is likely to be much less close among homosexuals in the general population than in the highly selected families, each with two gay sons, that were the subjects in these studies.

Another observation that points to a biological influence, first put forward by Lang (1940), is an imbalance in the sex ratio of the siblings of male homosexuals. On average, compared with heterosexual men, samples of male homosexuals have an excess of brothers. One explanation, so far entirely hypothetical, is that some mothers develop an increasing immune reaction to the Y chromosome in their successive male fetuses and that the antibodies they produce have an effect on the sex differentiation of the brain of their offspring such as to favor the development of homosexual orientation.

More research into the biology of homosexuality is needed, but it is not without complications. Scientists who become involved in such work risk having their findings exaggerated and sensationalized in the media. One risk is of premature social action based on unwarranted extrapolations from research findings. For instance, in Germany dubious brain surgery has been used to control homosexual pedophilia (West, 1977), and upon first publication of Hamer's work suggestions were made that potential homosexuals, like potential sufferers from cystic fibrosis or Down syndrome, should be identified at the fetal stage and aborted.

ENVIRONMENTAL CAUSES

Regardless of any possible innate predisposition, it is likely that environmental pressures and learning experiences may affect the development of sexual orientation. Influenced by Freudian psychoanalytic theories, mental health professionals once widely believed that upbringing in early childhood and the nature of the emotional bonds between the child and his or her parents were crucial. Freud suggested that an unresolved Oedipus complex (manifest in males by close attachment to mother and indifference or hostility to father) leads to anxiety about heterosexual temptations, because these are linked to guilt-ridden incestuous feelings. Substitute sexual outlets, notably homosexuality, then become less anxiety provoking. Despite the popularity of the notion consistent with this theory that male homosexuals tend to be mother-bound and often alienated from their fathers, some major surveys have failed to find such a pattern in the generality of cases (Bell, Weinberg, & Hammersmith, 1981). In any event, this constellation could be a consequence rather than a cause. Paternal rejection might occur because a boy is not conforming to a masculine ideal. Mothers may form closer ties with sons who don't spend time with girlfriends. Another expectation from Freudian theory, that homosexuals should feel panic at the idea of heterosexual contact, seems not to be borne out by experience. Lack of interest in the opposite sex rather than determined avoidance appears a more common characteristic. Lesbians, in particular, may engage in heterosexual intercourse for other than erotic desire (e.g., to achieve marital status or to become a mother).

Markedly effeminate boys often become adult homosexuals (Green, 1987). It is often assumed that the same underlying biological predisposition is responsible for both the cross-gender characteristics and the homosexual orientation in such cases, but alternative explanations are possible. Ever since the pioneering work of Benedict and Mead early in this century, it has become clear that gender roles, and some of the interests and attitudes that go with them, are to a considerable extent culturally determined and not a necessary or universal consequence of biological differences between males and females. Individuals discontented with the roles expected of them–the sensitive, artistic male of delicate physique who shuns rough-and-tumble sports and macho interests, for instance, or the assertive female who wants to dominate in a man's world — may be predisposed to develop homosexuality. For poeple with such temperaments, a homosexual orientation could be a secondary development, a reaction to finding themselves more at home in a homosexual subculture where displays of cross-gender characteristics are acceptable.

The extreme form of gender rejection classed as transsexuality, in which a seemingly physically normal male or female exhibits a strong need to be accepted as a member of the opposite sex, to the extent of demanding major surgery to change the genitals, can often be accompanied by homosexual behavior, but this can sometimes be more an assertion of cross-gender identity than a primary aim. The relevance of this relatively rare condition to homosexuality in general is unclear.

The "seduction theory" of homosexuality suggests that sexually excitable young people whose earliest experiences are with members of their own sex acquire a lasting preference for that form of gratification. If they masturbate subsequently to thoughts of homosexual contact that will further reinforce the direction of the desire first instilled by the actions of the seducer (McGuire, Carlisle, & Young, 1965). There is not much evidence for this idea. Homosexual males, more often than heterosexuals, recall having had sexual experiences with men when they were boys, but this could be because they have more reason to remember such incidents or because at the time they were already receptive to being approached. Heterosexual men who remember similar approaches generally report having found them disconcerting rather than seductive (West & Woodhouse, 1990). Most boys who have had a fond but sexualized relationship over a period of years with a devoted pedophile nevertheless develop customary heterosexual interests at adolescence (Brongersma, 1987; Wilson, 1981). In the days of sex-segregated male boarding schools adolescent boys were liable to have more sex contacts with each other than with girls. In his study of traditional British boarding schools for socially privileged boys, Hickson (1995) concluded that the minority of pupils who became homosexual men did not blame this on their experiences at school, many having been aware from an early age that their homosexual feelings were unusually intense and that they lacked their companions' desire for heterosexual experimentation. Indeed, in this situation, just because of their susceptibilities, some developing homosexuals tended to avoid the cruder homosexual antics of the boisterous heterosexual majority (Grosskurth, 1984).

Anthropological studies of the practices of homosexual initiation of boys, which were once prevalent in South Pacific tribal societies as well as in other parts of the world, prove that youthful homosexual acts usually do not lead to homosexuality in adulthood. The Sambia of New Guinea (Herdt, 1981) provide a striking example. Gender roles for men and women were sharply differentiated. All young boys underwent an initiation ceremony followed by segregation in an all-male compound together with older boys already past their first initiation. There they were required regularly to fellate the older boys and when they themselves reached the required age a younger cohort fellated them. Only after passing through these phases of homoerotic development were they instructed in heterosexual intercourse, allocated a wife and, following further ceremonies, awarded adult status. Homosexual activity was not permitted after a final ceremony marking the birth of the first child, although a few men did continue covert homosexual contacts along with their marital relations (Herdt, 1994). Underlying the system was the belief that the ingestion of semen promoted masculinity and fertility.

It would be foolish to suggest that sexual experiences can have no effect. Sexual tastes can indeed be learned, as exemplified by individuals developing over time new interests in varied sexual positions, use of sex toys, and novel means of stimulation. There is evidence also that addiction to unusual means of obtaining sexual arousal, so-called kinky sex or paraphilia, such as use of enemas or wanting to be tied up, caned on the buttocks, or ordered about and humiliated, can sometimes be traced back to childhood experiences (Money, 1988).

Conditioning treatments used by some clinical psychologists, although out of fashion for the purpose of converting homosexuals to heterosexuals, would not work at all were not sexual arousal patterns to some extent modifiable (Gunn & Taylor, 1993; Hawton, 1993). In principle, the method consists of showing the patient erotic slides or videos of various kinds, encouraging a sexual response to socially appropriate targets (e.g., opposite-sex adults), but delivering an electric shock or other aversive stimulus when the subject becomes excited by a homosexual target. The technique is most often applied to men. An instrument attached to the penis, the penile plethysmograph, registers any erectile swelling, so that the shocks can be given at the correct moment. Patients can be trained to carry out conditioning exercises in fantasy, imagining forbidden sexual temptations and then imagining the unpleasant consequences that may follow. These methods are nowadays most often applied to pedophiles in attempts to diminish their sexual attraction to children. Experience suggests that changes in the age of maximal attraction rather than a radical shift of gender preference are more likely to occur. Short-term measurable decreases in homosexual responsiveness and some development of heterosexual interest were often reported, but they tended to be temporary and could have been brought about by extraneous influences, such as the therapists' instructions or the clients' expectation (O'Donohue & Plaud, 1994). Effectiveness was rarely tested by systematic, long-term follow-up of behavior and feelings. A shift toward heterosexual behavior was more feasible in subjects with previous bisexual experience. Attempts at radical conversion of persons of exclusive homosexual orientation were more likely to bring about anxiety, inhibition, and confusion about any sexual outlet.

The weight of evidence is against the belief that conditioning, or for that matter any form of psychotherapy, psychoanalysis, or religious instruction, is generally effective in converting homosexuals (Haldeman, 1991; Silverstein, 1991). The most ambitious attempt to validate the effectiveness of psychoanalysis was reported by Bieber and colleagues (1962). Though sometimes cited as positive, the outcome was not really favorable. Apart from the dubiously subjective assessment of change, only a minority of those who underwent long-term treatment (300 or more hours) were classed as having made a significant shift toward heterosexuality, and most of these subjects had been bisexual at the outset.

One important reason for regarding all these approaches as ethically dubious is that, in the past, they were so often applied to unhappy, vulnerable people coerced into cooperation by social pressures, such as threat of imprisonment or family rejection, rather than from a real dissatisfaction with their sexuality. When therapy failed it was the patient who was blamed for lack of adequate motivation or unwillingness to forego the "secondary gain," that is, the sexual pleasure, derived from his homosexuality.

The sociologist McIntosh (1968) pioneered the idea that a homosexual orientation is not a condition intrinsic to the individual, but rather a social role available in Western society but nonexistent in some other cultures. Anthropological observations show that the circumstances in which homosexual behavior occurs, the ages of those involved, the types of sex acts performed, the emotional meaning to the participants, whether the behavior is socially accepted, and whether it is linked with cross-gender attributes or lack of heterosexual interest are all features that vary according to differing cultural imperatives. From this it is argued that homosexuality is a social construction, not a biological variant.

An alternative view, while recognizing that cultural tradition imposes expectations and limits on sexual behavior, contends that this does not mean an absence of innate potentials. The relatively modern cultural belief in the innocent asexuality of children does not mean that Western children are biologically different from children in societies where their sexual play is unrestricted. Weinrich and Williams (1991) argue that, notwithstanding the varying forms of homosexual behavior in the ancient world (Dynes & Donaldson, 1992) and in tribal societies (Herdt, 1994), it is still possible to recognize, within the confines of rigid social systems, indications of homosexual orientation as it is understood in the West.

In some cultures where contrasting roles for men and women were firmly prescribed and homosexual behavior was condemned, exceptions were made for certain individuals who were allowed to adopt the dress and habits of the opposite sex. Among the North American Indians, men, and sometimes women, who wanted to change their place in society went through ceremonies that awarded them the recognized and respected status of *berdache*. Not only could they then dress and behave differently, but male *berdaches* could also live with a (presumably) heterosexual man and have sexual relations with him in the guise of a wife. This was the ideal, although in some cases the transformation was less complete, the clothing adopted being distinctive without being a precise gender reversal and some heterosexual activity continuing (Roscoe, 1994). *Berdaches* were often credited with magical powers, especially among Siberian tribes, in which they could become Shamans and act as healers and diviners. In modern China, where sex change surgery has recently been legitimized, gender reversal, especially in theatrical contexts, seems to arouse less hostility than simple homosexuality.

Viewed from a Western standpoint, these systems might be regarded as institutionalized outlets for homosexual individuals, but particularly for persons with cross-gender as well as homosexual yearnings. Indeed, in the case of the Hijras of India, a male religious caste, the devotees are more like what would be classed in the West as transsexuals. They not only appear as women and earn a living by theatrical performances dressed in drag, but also submit to castration to assert their female status. Unlike the *berdaches*, their social standing is low (Nanda, 1990).

Historic records of homosexual practices in different civilizations are also sometimes cited in support of the idea that Western concepts of sexual orientation are products of a particular culture. The state-regulated systems of pederasty in ancient Greece might suggest that male homosexuality at that time was limited to man–boy relationships of a primarily educational and secondarily erotic nature. The system was meant to guide young males toward adult responsibilities, including marriage, not to produce permanent homosexuals. However, as Weinrich and Williams (1991) point out, other forms of homosexual behavior, relationships between adults and patronage of homosexual brothels, for example, were known and commented upon, usually adversely. The involvement of prepubertal children was never a part of the Greek system, and coercion was taboo. Consensual anal penetration by the older partner was expected, but far from leading to effeminacy, such relationships were made use of in military training to produce loyalty among soldiers of the Spartan and Theban armies. The famous Theban "sacred band of lovers" was credited with remarkable military prowess and heroism, finally allowing themselves to be massacred rather than surrender. A similar system operated among the warrior samurai of Japan (Watanabe & Iwata, 1989).

The ancient Romans are popularly thought to have been permissive toward homosexuality, since a series of emperors were blatantly bisexual and a number of writers made open reference to homosexual activities, sometimes involving themselves. However, other writers were highly condemnatory, attributing such habits to the corrupting influence of the Greeks. Summing up the evidence from records of numerous moral controversies about homosexuality, MacMullen (1992) concludes that a minority of Romans preferred sex with other males and another minority was bisexual, but their proportions among the population were probably no different than that among the Greeks.

In modern times, in some South American countries for example, only those men who display effeminate mannerisms and allow anal penetration are identified and despised as homosexuals. The assertively masculine man, especially if he is married, can make use of known homosexuals, ostensibly using them as substitutes for a woman, without attracting the label homosexual.

IMPLICATIONS FOR PUBLIC POLICY

Science cannot yet produce unequivocal answers to many of the questions that exercise politicians or excite moral debate. Research points to manifestations of homosexuality being the outcome of ongoing interplay between a multiplicity of factors, some genetic, some environmental, the latter including the environment of the developing fetus as well as upbringing, family situation, social and legal climate, and culturally permitted outlets. It appears likely that the direction of sexual impulses in some individuals is largely a matter of innate, biological predisposition, whereas in others the kind of sexual experiences to which they are exposed is more influential. There appears to be in many contrasting societies a hard core of homosexuals whose behavior is not altered by even the most draconian sanctions. The causes may well be different for homosexuals whose general behavior conforms to what is expected of their sex than for those who do not comply with gender expectations in either social behavior or heterosexual performance.

Empirical information is available relevant to some of the reasons advanced for supposing it to be in the interests of the community to try to suppress homosexuality. For example, empirical research does not support the once popular belief that a homosexual orientation is necessarily linked with character weakness, a view promulgated by some exponents of psychoanalytic theory. Psychological tests of personality, once they came to be applied to gays and lesbians who were not clients of penal or mental health agencies, failed to demonstrate the generalized inferiority that was expected (West, 1977). The supposed connection between male homosexuality, abuse of intoxicants, and prostitution were less likely to be due to inherent character disorder than to the nature of the urban subculture to which homosexuals tended to gravitate as a consequence of barriers to their full integration into mainstream society.

Homosexuals are said to be more likely to have a stronger sexual interest in children than heterosexuals do, but this is contradicted by evidence from surveys using the plethysmograph to test degree of arousal toward different age groups among homosexual and heterosexual men (Freund, 1981). However, if homosexual men have no particular liability to pedophilia, some other explanation must be found for the fact that there is a higher proportion of boys among children reported to have had sexual encounters with men outside the family circle than would be expected from the proportion of homosexual men in the community. Research with the plethysmograph again provides some evidence. Among pedophiles, who comprise a much smaller minority among the male population than do homosexuals, age is the important factor, gender being a less crucial determinant of sexual arousal than it is for the generality of either homosexual or heterosexual men (Freund & Kuban, 1993). That being so, the readier availability of unchaperoned young boys and their less cautious attitude toward suggestions from older males may contribute further to their being preferentially singled out by pedophiles. The proportion of males among adolescents involved in sexual offenses committed with or against them by adults is not a reliable indicator of the relative incidence of attraction to minors among heterosexual and homosexual men. It may simply reflect the higher "age of consent" some jurisdictions impose on homosexual contacts or the greater public reaction and prosecution risk when the adolescent has been involved in homosexual acts.

On the vexed question of whether homosexual "preference" is a matter of personal choice, and hence something for which the individual can be held morally responsible, the available evidence suggests that there is no universal rule. The many unsuccessful attempts at conversion therapy, even with subjects earnestly wanting to change, and the persistence in many cases of homosexual urges despite great social disadvantage or liability to severe punishment, suggests that for some at least change is not an option. On the other hand, the existence of bisexuals, the fact that deprivation of heterosexual contacts promotes homosexual behavior, and the fact that many males and even more females with a preference for their own sex can and do engage in heterosexual relations all point to some individuals having a greater facility than others for flexibility.

REASONS FOR DISAPPROVAL

Reasons for the great public concern about homosexuality, amounting sometimes to passionate denunciation, are not immediately obvious. Like any group displaying atypical habits, homosexuals risk prejudicial stereotyping or active scapegoating. It reinforces loyalty to the dominant group to scorn nonconformists. Religious or political dissidents are especially vulnerable because they challenge generally accepted assumptions and social arrangements that are especially dear to authorities interested in maintaining the status quo. Their supposed dangerousness is often imaginary or wildly exaggerated. Even such innocuous people as epileptics and the left-handed have at times been feared and reviled, but usually there is some faint substance to popular prejudice.

Attitudes are rooted in traditions, some of which have their origins in circumstances no longer applicable or long forgotten. In primitive societies, chronically at war with their neighbors and suffering from a high rate of infant mortality, keeping up numbers was essential and nonprocreative sexuality could be seen as a threat to survival. In societies so organized that a woman's economic and social viability depended on having a man's support, any reluctance to play the role of husband could cause chaos. Circumstances pertaining at the time of the ancient Israelites, whose writings, via Judeo-Christian religious teachings, have influenced Western thought so greatly, may have been responsible for the condemnatory passages in the Old Testament. Some authorities (Bailey, 1955; Helminiak, 1994; Vasey, 1995) suggest that the biblical prohibitions were mostly concerned about links between homosexual practices and the heretical beliefs and sexual ceremonies of rival tribal religions (a thought oddly reminiscent of the more recent linkage between "reds," "spies," and "queers"). The continuing force of these prohibitions needs further explanation, however, as other biblical directives — those relating to diet, witchcraft, money lending, and menstruation, for example — no longer bother most people.

To this day some societies remain organized around the assumption that life's sole purpose is marriage and carrying the family into the next generation. Against such a background, acceptance of a community of permanently single, homosexually oriented people is difficult. Likewise, in strong macho cultures, where gender roles are sharply demarcated and men dominate economically, socially, and sexually, disapproval is directed more at the effeminate or sexually submissive male whose behavior challenges the ideology of male supremacy than at the homosexual per se.

When dictatorial regimes hold sway, nonconformity of any sort is considered dangerous, sexuality is strictly regulated, and homosexuals are likely to be condemned. Such was the case in Russia under Stalin and Germany under Hitler and such is the case in places like China and Iran, as the relevant chapters in this volume have described. Another example is Cuba. Following the revolution of 1959, when Castro took over and the country became dependent economically on the Soviet Union, homosexuality became politicized and denounced as a vice attributable to the decadent influence of the once-dominant West. Homosexuals were lumped together with dissidents and bohemians as suitable candidates for reeducation in punitive camps or for imprisonment for *peligrosidad*, a vaguely worded law against the socially dangerous "invoked against gamblers, drunkards, vagrants, prostitutes and other 'dangerous' elements, but its chief targets [were] homosexuals" (Young, 1981, p. 52). The notorious mass exodus to the United States in 1980 consisted of an odd mixture of victims of this harsh levelling down: the wealthy, political activists, social misfits, ex-prisoners, and a quota of identified homosexuals.

While condemnation of sexual nonconformity has characterized some dictatorships of both the right- and left-wing varieties, ostensibly democratic societies also were often criticized by the early gay liberation movement for seeking to control sexual life in the interests of the established pecking order. Bob McCubbin (1993), a typical exponent of what he calls the "Marxist view," argued that the development of technology brought with it a socioeconomic hierarchy dominated by men, with women treated as chattel, chained to maternal and home duties. Sexual freedom for women became incompatible with the patriarchal monogamous family and homosexual sons became an impediment to the continuation of the prized patriarchal lineage (McCubbin, 1993). The development of nations organized on monopoly–capitalist lines encouraged the subjugation of the working masses to the needs of mass production and the pursuit of imperialist wars. Propaganda that helped to divide and rule the workers aided the process of exploitation. For example, "The German Nazi regime made full use of homophobia as well as racism, sexism and national chauvinism in its efforts to destroy all resistance to capitalist rule and imperial adventures" (McCubbin, 1993, p. 69).

Whatever one may think of the heuristic value of such global interpretations, they enabled the Western gay liberation movement to claim common cause with the left-wing supporters of movements against racial and gender discrimination. The alliance was fragile and in some respects counterproductive. Feminists, in particular, became embarrassed by the prominence of lesbians among their pioneers. Supposed links with left-wing politics made gays more unpopular than ever among the more conservatively inclined. Opponents are thus able to link gays' defiance of conservative sexual morality with a decline in family values and an "anything goes" philosophy that undermines order in society.

Even in democratic countries gays have had a struggle to combat traditionally hostile views supported by conservative media. They form too small a minority to be able, themselves, to have much effect on voting trends; they depend on the support of sympathizers. The politicization of gay issues polarizes opinion and ensures publicity for extreme views. Despite evidence to the contrary, a reputation for child molestation and seduction still clings to homosexuals, enhanced by the extraordinary rise in concern internationally about child sexual abuse and about "sex tourism" that targets children.

Male homosexual promiscuity is a real phenomenon that attracts disapproval. Before the AIDS epidemic, men used to, and in some places still do, congregate in steam baths or the dark rooms found at some gay bars and cinemas for semipublic orgies. Promiscuity and anal sex habits were the prime cause of the high incidence of syphilis and other sexually transmitted diseases among urban gay males before the era of 'safe sex.' Promiscuity was also responsible for HIV infection establishing itself so quickly once it started among homosexual communities.

In countries where they are free to do so, gays sometimes behave publicly in ways calculated to offend. For example, Gay Pride parades, although intended to advertise the strength of the gay and lesbian community, tend to attract a disproportionate number of individuals whose outlandishly provocative dress and demeanor give an impression of decadence. The most obvious "gay scene" is a commercialized sex market: fashion stores, specialized sex shops, and crowded bars where most clients are looking for a partner for the night and only the young and physically attractive are truly welcome. Older, less presentable or less "clubbable" gays may resort to public toilets or after-dark cruising grounds for what often turns out to be on-the-spot sex with any stranger they can find. Gay contact magazines are filled with advertisements for sadomasochistic and fetishistic activity. Male homosexual prostitution flourishes and among the devotees of the bars and discos alcohol and drug problems abound. Although the literature and arguments of some (not all) gay activists pay homage to the ideal of a faithful, lasting, one-to-one love and sex relationship, analogous to the romantic heterosexual ideal, the reality seems very different. Lesbians are less open to criticism for their sexual style since, true to their female gender, they seem less promiscuously inclined, more disposed to lasting love relationships, and unsupportive of same-sex prostitution.

The impression conveyed by some of the public manifestations of male homosexual habits that, like the "undeserving poor," they are an immoral and irresponsible lot unworthy of support is not justified. Whether for cultural or biological reasons the fact is that men are generally more promiscuously inclined than women and male homosexuals have less reason for restraint than family men with responsibilities for children. Moreover, their sexual development is different. The homosexual male adolescent lacks experience in or the need for heterosexual courtship rituals. His first sexual contacts are likely to be illegal because of age and conducted secretly in circumstances not conducive to an ongoing relationship. In the absence of social supports for young same-sex lovers, young gays leave the parental home to look for others of their kind. They naturally gravitate to the urban gay scene. There intermale contacts are primarily sexual and swiftly accomplished, little different from an encounter with a prostitute, with nothing of the bodily modesty or social conventions of heterosexual "dating" and no thought to the establishment of common interests. Small wonder, then, that many gay relationships begun this way appear to be, on heterosexual standards, shallow and unstable. All too often a lifestyle develops in which daily living is divorced from a secret sexual nightlife of brief encounters. As for the prevalence of "fist fucking" and other exotic sexual activities, which are viewed disapprovingly by heterosexuals, these may be accounted for in part by the absence of the option of vaginal intercourse and in part by the tendency of men, whose sexual relations are essentially a matter of physical release, to seek more and more novel forms of stimulation to avoid boredom.

These aspects of uninhibited sexuality may offend the sensibilities of even very liberal societies, but they are not typical of large numbers of homosexually oriented individuals whose relationships, social obstacles notwithstanding, are as permanent and emotionally fulfilling as most heterosexual marriages. Moreover, apart from the link between bisexuality and the spread of AIDS, promiscuous homosexual behavior does no obvious damage to nonparticipants and some of the more "perverse" forms of sexual activity actually carry less health risks than penetrative sex.

Reasoned argument is never likely to overcome altogether a natural antipathy toward a minority whose deepest feelings and intimate habits are different from those of the majority. Considering how much of ordinary socializing, especially among the disco-dancing, party-going young, is geared to heterosexual requirements, it is easy to see the potentially alienating effects of a homosexual orientation. It means, at the least, that an important part of life experience cannot be so readily shared when persons of the same sex have a different sexual orientation. The unease described by some childless couples in their contacts with happy parents has something of the same quality of reserve and feeling of ultimate isolation that causes many homosexuals to socialize mostly with others similarly placed. Whether this sense of a special identity leads to personal satisfaction or to poor self-esteem depends upon both individual susceptibility and the prevailing social climate.

REFERENCES

Allen, L. S., & Gorski, R. A. (1992). Sexual orientation and the size of the anterior commissure in the human brain. *Proceedings of the National Academy of Science, US, 89,* 7199–7202.
Bailey, D. S. (1955). *Homosexuality and the Western Christian tradition.* London: Longmans.
Bailey, J. M., & Pillard, R. C. (1991). A genetic study of male sexual orientation. *Archives of General Psychiatry, 48,* 1089–1096.
Bailey, J. M., Pillard, R. C., Neale, M. C., & Agyei, Y. (1993). Hereditable factors influence sexual orientation in women. *Archives of General Psychiatry, 50,* 217-223.
Bell, A. P., Weinberg, M. S., & Hammersmith, S. K. (1981). *Sexual preference: Its development in men and women.* London: Mitchell Beazley.
Bieber, I., Dain, H. J., Dince, P. R., Drellich, M. G., Grand, H. G., Gundlach, R. H., Kremer, M. W., Rifkin, A. H, Wilbur, C. B., & Bieber, T. B. (1962). *Homosexuality: A psychoanalytic study.* New York: Basic Books
Brongersma, E. (1987). *Loving boys: A multidisciplinary study of sexual relations between adult and minor males.* New York: Global Academic.
Byne, W. (1995). Science and belief: Psychobiological research on sexual orientation. In J. P. DeCecco & D. Allen (Eds.), *Sex, cells and same sex desire: The biology of sexual preference.* (pp. 303–344). Binghamton, NY: Harrington Park Press.
Diamond, M. (1993). Homosexuality and bisexuality in different populations. *Archives of Sexual Behavior, 22,* 291–310.
Dörner, G. (1976). *Hormones and brain differentiation.* Amsterdam: Elsevier.
Dynes, W. R., & Donaldson, S. (Eds.). (1992). *Homosexuality in the ancient world.* New York: Garland.

Evans, R. B. (1972). Physical and biochemical characteristics of homosexual men. *Journal of Consulting and Clinical Psychology, 39,* 140–147.

Faderman, F. (1981). *Surpassing the love of men: Romantic friendship and love between women from the Renaissance to the present.* New York: Wm. Morrow.

Freund, K. (1981). Assessment in paedophilia. In M. Cook & K. Howells (Eds.), *Adult sexual interest in children.* (pp. 139–179). London: Academic Press.

Freund, K., & Kuban, M. (1993). Deficient erotic gender differentiation in pedophilia: A follow up. *Archives of Sexual Behavior, 22,* 619–628.

Gonsiorek, J. C., & Weinrich, J. D. (1991). *Homosexuality: Research implications for public policy.* Newbury Park, CA: Sage.

Green, R. (1987). *The "sissy boy syndrome" and the development of homosexuality.* New Haven, CT: Yale University Press.

Green, R. (1988). The immutability of (homo)sexual orientation: Behavioral science implications for a constitutional (legal) analysis. *Journal of Psychiatry and Law, 16,* 537–575.

Grosskurth, P. (Ed.). (1984). *The memoirs of John Addington Symonds.* London: Hutchinson.

Gunn, J., & Taylor, P. T. (Eds.). (1993). *Forensic psychiatry: Clinical, legal and ethical issues.* Oxford: Butterworth-Heinemann.

Haldeman, D. A. (1991). Sexual orientation conversion therapy for gay men and lesbians: A scientific examination. In J. C. Gonsiorek & J. D. Weinrich (Eds.), *Homosexuality: Research implications for public policy.* (pp. 149–160). Newbury Park, CA: Sage.

Hamer, D. H., & Copeland, P. (1994). *The Science of desire: The search for the gay gene and the biology of behavior.* New York: Simon & Schuster.

Hawton, K. (1983). Behavioural approaches to the management of sexual deviations. *British Journal of Psychiatry, 143,* 248–255.

Helminiak, D. A. (1994). *What the bible really says about homosexuality.* San Francisco: Alamo Square Press.

Herdt, G. H. (1981). *Guardians of the flute: Idioms of masculinity.* London: McGraw-Hill.

Herdt, G. H. (Ed.). (1994). *Third sex, third gender: Beyond sexual dimorphism in culture and history.* New York: Zone Books.

Hickson, A. (1995). *The poisoned bowl: Sex, repression and the public school system.* London: Constable.

Kinsey, A. C., Pomeroy, W. B., & Martin, C. E. (1948). *Sexual behavior in the human male.* Philadelphia: Saunders.

Kinsey, A. C., Pomeroy, W. B., Martin, C. E., & Gebhard, P. H. (1953). *Sexual behavior in the human female.* Philadelphia: Saunders.

Lang, T. (1994). Studies in the genetic determination of homosexuality. *Journal of Nervous and Mental Disease, 92,* 55–64.

Laumann, E. O., Gaymon, J. H., Michael, R. T., & Michaels, S. (1994). *The social organization of sexuality: Sexual practices in the United States.* Chicago: University of Chicago Press.

LeVay, S. (1993). *The sexual brain.* Cambridge, MA: MIT Press.

McCubbin, R. (1993). *The roots of lesbian and gay oppression: A marxist view.* (3rd ed.). New York: World View Publishers.

McGuire, R. J., Carlisle, J. M., & Young, B. G. (1965). Sexual deviations as conditioned behaviour. *Behaviour Research and Therapy, 2,* 185–190.

McIntosh, M. (1968). The homosexual role. *Social Problems, 16,* 182–192.

MacMullen, R. (1992). Roman attitudes to Greek love. In W. R. Dynes & S. Donaldson (Eds.), *Homosexuality in the ancient world.* New York: Garland.

McWhirter, D. P., Sanders, S. A., & Reinish, J. M. (Eds.), *Homosexuality/heterosexuality: Concepts of sexual orientation.* Oxford: Oxford University Press.

Money, J. (1988). *Gay, straight and in-between.* New York: Oxford University Press.

Nanda, S. (1990). *Neither man nor woman: The Hijras of India.* Belmont, CA: Wadsworth.

O'Donahue, W., & Plaud, J. J. (1994). The conditioning of human sexual arousal. *Archives of Sexual Behavior, 23,* 321–344.

Reite, M., Sheeder, J., Richardson, D., & Teale, P. (1995). Cerebral laterality in homosexual males. *Archives of Sexual Behavior, 24,* 585–593.

Robson, R. (1992). *Lesbian (out)law: Survival under the rule of law.* NY: Firebrand Books.

Roscoe, W. (1994). How to become a berdache: Towards a unified analysis of gender diversity. In G. H. Herdt (Ed.), *Third sex, third gender*. (pp. 329–372). New York: Zone Books.

Sell, R. L., & Petrulio, C. (1995). Sampling homosexuals, bisexuals, gays and lesbians for public health research: A review of the literature from 1990–1992. *Journal of Homosexuality, 30*(4), 31–47.

Silverstein, C. (1991). Psychological and medical treatments of homosexuality. In J. C. Gonsiorek & J. D. Weinrich (Eds.), *Homosexuality: Research implications for public policies*. Newbury Park, CA: Sage.

Swaab, D. F., Gooren, L. J. G., & Hofman, M. A. (1995). Brain research, gender and sexual orientation. In J. P. De Cecco & A. A. Parker (Eds.), *Sex, cells and same sex desire*. (pp. 283–302). Binghamton, NY: Harrington Park Press.

Turner, W. J. (1994). Comments on discordant monozygotic twinning in homosexuality. *Archives of Sexual Behavior, 23*, 115–119.

Turner, W. J. (1995). Homosexuality, type 1: an Xq28 phenomenon. *Archives of Sexual Behavior, 24*, 109–134.

Vasey, M. (1995). *Strangers and friends: A new exploration of homosexuality and the bible*. London: Hodder and Stoughton.

Watanabe, T., & Iwata, J. (1989). *The love of the samurai: A thousand years of Japanese homosexuality*. London: Gay Men's Press.

Weinberg, M. S., Williams, C. J., & Pryor, D. W. (1994). *Dual attraction: Understanding bisexuality*. Oxford: Oxford University Press.

Weinrich, J. D., & Williams, W. L. (1991). Strange customs, familiar lives: Homosexualities in other cultures. In J. C. Gonsiorek & J. D. Weinrich (Eds.), *Homosexuality: Research implications for public policy* (pp. 44–59). Newbury Park, CA: Sage.

Wellings, K., Field, J., Johnson, A. M., & Wadsworth, J. (1994). *Sexual behaviour in Britain*. London: Penguin.

West, D. J. (1977). *Homosexuality re-examined*. London: Duckworth.

West, D. J., & Woodhouse, T. P. (1990). Sexual encounters between boys and adults. In C. K. Li, D. J. West, & T. P. Woodhouse (Eds.), *Children's sexual encounters with adults* (pp. 3–137). London: Duckworth.

Whitam, F. L., & Mathy, R. M. (1986). *Male homosexuality in four societies: Brazil, Guatemala, the Philippines and the United States*. New York: Praeger.

Wilson, P. (1981). *The man they called a monster: Sexual experiences between men and boys*. North Ryde, New South Wales: Cassell.

Young, A. (1981). *Gays under the Cuban Revolution*. San Francisco: Grey Fox.

Conclusion

DONALD J. WEST AND RICHARD GREEN

These contributions from widely differing parts of the world reveal the enormous contrasts that exist between places where detected homosexual behavior attracts severe, sometimes capital, punishment and places where many people look upon it as a legitimate form of sexual expression to be regulated no differently from heterosexual behavior. Whereas in one nation (the United States) civil law is increasingly concerned with regulating an otherwise permitted form of sex (e.g., unwanted homosexual overtures in the workplace), in other places (China, Islam) those engaging in homosexual behavior under any circumstances face criminal conviction and lengthy prison sentences.

The chapter on Islam and the work of Amnesty International (1994) shows that the rise of Islamic Fundamentalism, a movement very different from the gentler forms of classical Islamic teaching, poses an increasing threat to the life and liberty of homosexuals in many parts of the world. Even in smaller countries like Yemen and Mauritania, homosexual behavior has become an offense punishable by death. There are reports, difficult to substantiate, of the whipping and even stoning to death of lesbians in Iran. Certainly, lesbians in that country risk persecution from male relatives and enjoy no support from native feminist groups (Rosenbloom, 1995). According to a press release (Deutsche Presse Agentur, August 24, 1994) Egypt's Grand Mufti was said to have issued a *fatwa* [proclamation] urging the killing of any homosexuals participating in the United Nations Conference on Population held in Cairo. In September 1995, at the United Nations conference on the Status of Women held in Bejing, the inclusion of sexual orientation was successfully excluded from an antidiscrimination resolution through the opposition of a majority of Muslim countries, including Algeria, Bangladesh, Egypt, Iran, Jordan, Kuwait, Libya, Sudan, Syria, United Arab Emirates, and Yemen. These are instances of modern intransigence. Homosexual relations were once part of respected military tradition in Ottoman Turkey (Murray, 1987), and, until recently, homosexual prostitution was allowed to flourish in Morocco (Landau, 1952; West, 1992).

The ruthless persecution to which persons professing or practicing homosexuality are subjected by some state authorities is starkly revealed in the pleas of refugees seeking political asylum away from their native lands. Countries like the United States, Canada, Australia, New Zealand, Norway, and Sweden have each acknowledged the legitimacy, under United Nations rules, of claims to refugee status by applicants who, as a consequence of their homosexuality, have a "well-founded fear of being persecuted for reasons of membership of a particular social group or political opinion." Clear evidence of actual

DONALD J. WEST • Institute of Criminology, University of Cambridge, Cambridge CB3 9DT, England, United Kingdom.   RICHARD GREEN • Institute of Criminology, University of Cambridge, Cambridge CB3 9DT, England, United Kingdom; and Gender Identity Clinic, Charing Cross Hospital, London W6 8RF, England, United Kingdom.

Sociolegal Control of Homosexuality, edited by West and Green, Plenum Press, New York, 1997.

"persecution" is required. In 1992, the Canadian Refugee Board rejected an application from a Brazilian student who reported harassment from strangers, humiliating treatment by police, and fear of death squads known to target gays with impunity. The panel rejected as unconfirmed evidence from the homophile *Grupo de Bahia* that many gays are killed in organized attacks. They noted the acceptance of transvestic displays in Brazil and the known homosexuality of some accepted public entertainers. Apparently they failed to realize that such phenomena are not necessarily incompatible. According to Mott (1995), the Brazilian Generals' dictatorship of the 1970s tolerated flamboyantly transvestic homosexuality, yet "cruel homophobia" remains strong and it is common to hear sentiments like "fags must be killed" or "I'd prefer my son dead than queer." Indeed, many killers of gays escape punishment by claiming they acted to protect their (sexual) honor, and more such murders would be known about if ashamed relatives did not manage to "convince the press not to include scandalous details." In Colombia, beatings and killings of young, homeless people are seen as necessary "social cleansing," Church and popular press are hostile to homosexuality, and young male prostitutes are at grave risk of being murdered by gangs paid by local merchants who want the streets cleared (Ordoñez, 1993).

The Canadian Refugee Board granted asylum in 1994 for the first time to a Chinese man who had been beaten up by police at home. They heard expert testimony on his behalf from Vincent Yang of Simon Fraser University to the effect that Chinese police have discretion to use the ill-defined crime of *liumang-zui* [hooliganism] to send homosexuals to a labor re-education camp for 2 years. The expert found the applicant's story of having been forced to fellate a policeman under threat of being jailed entirely credible. Refugees are sometimes hampered in their applications by fear of reprisals against their family and friends if they name their contacts in an attempt to establish that they are homosexuals. Before being granted asylum by the Australian authorities in February 1994, one Iranian applicant spent 2 years in a detention camp until he finally convinced them of his homosexuality by reluctantly telephoning his imprisoned homosexual lover's family to confirm his claim.

Our examination of documents concerning applications from homosexual refugees [a collection of which has been made available by the International Gay and Lesbian Human Rights Commission in San Francisco (1995)] shows that homosexuality is often used as a convenient charge to bring against individuals who are open or covert political dissidents. A well-known example was the execution in Iran in 1992 of the prominent surgeon and Sunni Moslem activist Dr. Ali Mozaffarian. He was charged with spying for the United States and Iraq, coupled with adultery and sodomy. His taped "confessions" were broadcast on television (Amnesty International, 1994).

Freedom to pursue homosexual relationships may seem of less importance in countries where more extreme abuses, such as arbitrary arrest and torture, are prevalent. That grossly oppressive conditions can persist in the modern world is due in part to the ability of governments to deny any official recognition of what occurs.

Recent experiences of one of the authors (Green) reflect the continuing phenomena of denial and censorship. He was informed at a medical meeting in China that theirs is a nation without homosexuals — in a population of over 1 billion! Upon his receipt of a medal from the Polish Academy of Sexology in Warsaw after the overthrow of the communist regime, his address to the academy noted with concern the continued oppression, largely religion based, of Polish homosexuals. When he later received the videotape of the lecture, that segment of the talk was missing.

In the face of advancing media technology and the advent of the global village it is becoming more difficult to insulate any nation from foreign information and influence. Ever more international travel, foreign press, satellite television, and the Internet all deliver an increasingly universal message. This has fostered a relaxation of traditionally restrictive attitudes and has stimulated the development of incipient homophile movements in some very hostile environments. According to Amnesty International (1994), "Lesbians and gay men are organizing throughout Asia and the Pacific" (p. 38). They name activist groups from Malaysia, Philippines, Indonesia, Singapore, Thailand, and India.

The chapter on Singapore compares the relative quiescence of that state with the development of homophile activism elsewhere in Asia, but activist groups are often small and struggling hard against entrenched tradition. For example, in 1992, Nicaragua passed a law (art. 204) providing 1–3 years imprisonment for anyone who induces, promotes, propagandizes, or practices in a scandalous form sexual intercourse between persons of the same sex. Gays protested, but an appeal to the Supreme Court contending that the law was unconstitutional was dismissed in March 1994.

In India, homophile groups are emerging, but Hindu culture remains hostile, and the law on "unnatural offences," derived from British colonial rule (art. 377), prescribes long imprisonment for "whoever voluntarily has carnal intercourse against the order of nature with any man, woman or animal." This law has even been invoked against a female-to-male transsexual on the grounds that his relations with his wife were actually lesbian and therefore criminal (Rosenbloom, 1995). Notwithstanding explicit sexuality in Hindu art — in the Kama Sutra and the Konark temples — individuals have little freedom of action outside the all-powerful Hindu family. The strength of tradition is exemplified in arranged marriages, the dowry system, and strictly differentiated gender roles, all of which generate a strong preference by parents for boy children and are the cause of a significant excess of surviving males in the population. Although cities like Delhi and Bombay have many male prostitutes, there is great reluctance to admit the existence of exclusive gays. Indian homophobia "is not so much rooted in fear of breaking sensual and sexual taboos, but with the threat to the traditional order of life — an order centered on the patrilineal heritage of the family" (Matteson, 1991, p. 63). Much the same comment might have been made about Japanese society.

The otherwise tragic AIDS pandemic, in nations where it has been concentrated among homosexually active males, has had one positive impact — namely, to oblige reluctant governments and individuals (as in Bolivia) to acknowledge the existence of a homosexual subculture. In nations where gay individuals and groups were dispersed, AIDS has united them against the common enemy and enabled them, under the umbrella of public health projects, to secure some social support and funding. Despite moral denunciations, AIDS has not generated the mass backlash against male homosexuals that might have been feared. In the United States, where hundreds of thousands have been blighted, gay men have not become the new lepers.

The rationales for social control of homosexuality are varied. They include a duty to reproduce, pronouncements of religious doctrine, and moral beliefs in one "natural" form of sexual expression. Rooted in these philosophies, public opinion does not immediately follow changes in official policy. Although Russia decriminalized homosexual behavior, a substantial minority of the populace favors "liquidation" of homosexuals. Within even the most tolerant of countries, some sections of the population, particularly members of the stricter Roman Catholic and fundamentalist Protestant or orthodox Jewish groups, are unhappy with what they regard as a falling away from moral standards. The conflict is particularly evident in parts of Eastern Europe, where political pressure to conform to Western European systems conflicts with long-established traditions of dislike for sexual nonconformity. In Poland, for example, a constitutional committee charged with drafting terms for the new constitution ran into difficulty when, in April 1995, it introduced a human rights clause (par. 2, art. 2) that included "sexual orientation" among the categories of persons who should not be discriminated against. The clause, strongly opposed by the Catholic Church, has caused divisions among politicians and may well not come into force.

Romania is a particularly striking example of a hostile tradition (in this case encouraged by political parties such as the Socialist Workers as well as by the Catholic Church), preventing the passage of decriminalizing legislation that had been urged upon the government by the Council of Europe. A poll taken in March 1995 showed equal public resentment of gays and lesbians, with 53 percent believing that lesbians should not be accepted into society (Baciu, Cimpeanu, & Nicora, 1995). In November 1995 the Chamber of Deputies voted down a mild amendment to Article 200 of the penal code limiting punishment of 1–5 years imprisonment for homosexual or lesbian acts only to acts committed "in public or which cause public scandal." Since the latter condition had been previously ruled to include an act becoming known to two or more persons who disapprove of it, this would still have left wide discretion for prosecution. The often devastating effect upon individuals of such continuing hostility from powerful authority is exemplified by the case of the then 18-year-old Romanian Ciprian Cocu and his 22-year-old partner Marian Mutascu described in the chapter on Europe (Amnesty International, 1995).

In the Western world the psychiatric profession has been a major player in the social and legal control of homosexuality. Until 20 years ago, homosexuals were by definition mentally ill according to the American Psychiatric Association. In the United States and elsewhere many hundreds of patients (usually male) underwent extensive therapies to reorientate their sexual drive. Through the combined influences of poor success rates, consumer boycott, and a changing professional milieu, including the recent abandonment by the World Health Organization of its medical diagnosis of homosexuality, this labeling and these treatments are nearly gone. In the United Kingdom, the activist organization OutRage wants compensation for damage done to gay patients by such treatments, which still continue in China and Russia. It is no small irony, and perhaps a metaphor, that the most enduring and strident American psychoanalytic proponent of the illness model of homosexuality should have a son who is a gay activist attorney in the U.S. president's administration.

That South Africa, following the admission of its black majority into government, put into its new constitution a specific protection for its citizens against sexual orientation discrimination suggests a spillover of concern from the worldwide power struggle of oppressed groups generally. In the United States, the "gay liberation" movement sought to claim common ground with those subject to racial discrimination. Recently, a combination of xenophobia, racism, and homophobia has re-emerged in the official propaganda of Iran and Zimbabwe, which identifies homosexuality as a phenomenon of decadence spread by American culture and by white colonialists. This seems ironic in view of the way white travelers of the last century stigmatized Asian and African cultures for their toleration of homosexual pederasts and cross-dressers. African views unfavorable to whites may well have their roots in the days when European homosexual expatriates took up residence in exotic places for the sake of easy sexual contacts with the natives or, more recently, when fast travel enabled gay (and heterosexual) tourists to have brief adventures in the highly commercialized facilities in "sexopolises" like Rio, Saõ Paulo, Acapulco, Bangkok, or Manila (Bleys, 1993).

Criminal law, civil law, and public acceptance tend to change at different rates. In the United States, where the chief topics of public debate and the issues most frequently before today's courts concern the finer points of civil rights and discrimination against self-identified gays and lesbians, it seems paradoxical that all homosexual acts remain criminalized, at least theoretically, in a large part of the country. There the political opponents of criminal law reform are powerful enough to block any change, though not powerful enough to insist upon general enforcement. While South African law now prohibits "discrimination," it still criminalizes homosexual behavior, although, in view of the speed of change in that country, this anomaly may be rectified soon. In some countries, notably in Latin America, as the chapter on Bolivia illustrates, identified homosexuals are little tolerated, although the criminal law may be silent on the issue of homosexuality and by implication seem permissive. In reality, in response to popular disapproval, persons identified as homosexuals are dealt with quite harshly through arbitrary police action, sometimes outside the law, sometimes making use of elastic legislation stretched to snare homosexuals. Although the criminalization of homosexual behavior has been rightly blamed for encouraging blackmail and extortion, public disapproval, with or without the backing of the law, is equally instrumental.

The United Nations and the European Union support the "human right" not to be discriminated against on grounds of sexual orientation, although the former, in particular, has a poor reputation for enforcement of its directives. As the chapter on European International Control has described, the Council of Europe is more forthright in its directives and more successful in having them introduced into state law, but this may be due largely to the more liberal tradition in this respect of most European countries, many of them inheritors of the secular-inspired Napoleonic Code. Germany and Britain, like the United States, have been more inclined than most to resist liberal legal trends, while simultaneously tolerating pockets of publicly obvious homosexual activity in their larger cities.

Great contrasts in attitudes toward homosexuality are observable not only between such widely separated cultures as Japan, India, the Islamic World, and Latin America, but also between the contiguous nations of Europe and even between the different states in America. Traditionally, Great Britain has been considered unduly sensitive on sexual issues, whereas France and Italy have been more accepting. The French tradition of realism in its classic fiction, including analytic accounts of homosexual relationships, was established a century ago. England has hardly any writers to compare in this regard with Colette, Gide, Proust, or Genet. In England, E.M. Forster felt obliged to leave his one overtly homosexual novel to be published posthumously. Furthermore, France's strictly secular politics and its adherence to the Napoleonic Code have favored a less emotional and more pragmatic approach to sexual matters. In France, a prominent politician with a mistress causes no excitement; in Britain it is scandal and occasion for resignation.

Despite all the signs of a seemingly unstoppable progression of liberal law and philosophy regarding homosexuality in nearly all Western industrial nations, some double standards remain. Tolerance of public displays of romantic (not sexual) expression differs for same-sex and mixed-sex couples. New Zealand, in spite of its antidiscrimination stance, demands a longer period of association before a foreign member of a same-sex couple, as opposed to a heterosexual couple, is granted residency rights (Chauvel, 1994). In many nations, some of which otherwise appear to accommodate homosexuality, the age at which a person can legally consent to sexual interaction continues to discriminate. Youth, it is claimed, need protection from corruption (read homosexuality). With no empirical support, preventing early and midadolescent contact is seen as preventing the development of a homosexual orientation.

Public anxiety about child sex abuse has caused homosexual activists to distance themselves from campaigns about the sexual rights of young people old enough to know when they want to have contact with an older person of either sex. A Dutch psychologist (Sandfort, 1987) has suggested that, on the contrary, gay organizations should be more sympathetic toward pedophile concerns and should recognize and oppose unnecessary oppression of youthful homosexuality.

It is clear that substantial sections of the population of democratic countries still resist acceptance of homosexuality. For generations parents in Western nations have been taught by the pop psychology press that they have brought about their child's (usually son's) homosexuality. Supposedly, seductive mothers and abdicating fathers are most at fault. The consequent guilt feelings have caused parents to scorn their homosexual offspring. This casting out has served as a model for the larger community and may be one reason for the high rate of attempted suicides among young homosexuals upon a realization that they are part of a despised minority that risks rejection by families and friends (Remafedi, 1994). It may be that popularization of the biological origins of sexual orientation, over which parents have no control, will foster less rejection. But belief in biological causation can cut both ways. If homosexual expression were seen as a minority pattern of brain organization and thus likened to left-handedness (also previously the target of derision and efforts to change), social condemnation might lessen. However, biological determinants of unwanted traits are increasingly being intercepted with prenatal and postnatal interventions. If a biological predisposition to homosexuality became identifiable, calls for termination of pregnancies or for gene splicing might begin.

Even in the Netherlands, renowned as a leader of the liberal approach to sexuality, it appears that hate crimes against homosexuals still occur. Where such crimes are the work of extremist right-wing organizations like the neo-Nazis, other minorities are targeted, Jews and immigrants especially. The insecurity of the perpetrators, many of whom come from a powerless, uneducated underclass and have a need to find some way to assert themselves, may sometimes be a more potent force than the issue of homosexuality itself. However, men who specifically target gays may have a particular need to display a super macho, super heterosexual stance in the face of haunting doubts about their own sexuality. The fact that "gay bashing" is a gang activity indicates such individuals can easily find others of like mind.

The persistence of anti-gay sentiment is also reflected in the ambivalence of Western legislators, the long delays in passing legal reforms, and the convoluted and legalistic arguments used to oppose antidiscrimination measures. This is well illustrated in the many conflicting decisions taken in various state jurisdictions in America, the reluctance of the U.S. Supreme Court to accept the right of privacy against criminalization of private consensual homosexual behavior, and the recent split on matters of discrimination in the Canadian Supreme Court. Yet another reflection of public attitudes toward homosexuality is evidenced by the total absence of any openly homosexual person among the world's leaders.

Homosexual communities are affected by changes in political power. The chapter on Germany shows how the treatment of homosexuals changed over the years with successive changes of government, and the chapter on Russia shows how sudden changes of power can create uncertainty. Politicization brings homosexual issues to the fore and can promote change, but it can also give voice to extremist groups. When the balance of power between major parties is precarious, extremists can exert an influence disproportionate to their numbers. This is particularly evident in regard to emotive issues of sexual rights when homosexuality tends to be linked with other subjects of disapproval, such as abortion, teen pregnancy, sexually transmitted diseases, child sex abuse and abandoned marriages. The influence of a few far-right Christian politicians and "family values" groups in the United States serves as an example. When particular political parties become identified with a pro or con stance toward homosexual rights, this can result in legislation becoming dependent on the fortunes of the party concerned, which are in turn governed by economic and other factors far removed from homosexual concerns. Politicization of homosexual issues can sometimes backfire, as appears to have happened in Zimbabwe, where the president's extremist stance stimulated protest and forced the concerns of the gay community onto the public stage.

Redefining traditional definitions of "family" are probably prerequisite for fuller integration of homosexuals and their relationships into society. The increasing acceptance of cohabitation and childbearing by unmarried heterosexual couples and the tentative acceptance of mothers in lesbian relationships signal that at least some societies may in time incorporate further alternatives to the traditional family.

Within nations where opinions remain ambivalent about the acceptability of gay lifestyles, a gay subculture nevertheless operates openly in regional pockets of freedom. The Castro Street neighborhood in San Francisco and the gay "village" in Manchester, England, have been mentioned. In Germany where, as in the United States, states have differing traditions, in many places trendy gay bars and cafés the envy of the straight world are allowed to flourish; in some places commercially run gay orgy clubs advertise publicly and obviously without official intervention. Yet, in Halle, Germany, in June 1996, 160 armed policemen raided a gay bar and arrested and strip-searched 70 customers, leaving three injured.

In spite of contrary examples, the dominant world trend, especially among Western nations, seems to be toward tolerance, if not full integration, of gays and lesbians. Legal challenges to various forms of discrimination are happening so frequently that any account of them must soon appear out of date. In the United Kingdom, for example, at the time of this writing, decisions are awaited from the European Court of Human Rights on issues of gays in the military, differential age of consent, and gay partners' rights to benefits enjoyed by the spouses of employees. The refusal until recently of the United Kingdom to incorporate the European Convention into its domestic law has encouraged such challenges. Despite pockets of resistance (such as the delay by the Australian state of Tasmania in changing the law making homosexual behavior a criminal offense), most liberal, democratic countries are now preoccupied with issues of civil discrimination rather than with criminalizing homosexual acts. In New Zealand, for example, where criminal sanctions against consensual homosexual conduct between males over 16 ceased with the passing of the Homosexual Law Reform Act of 1986, discrimination on grounds of sexual orientation has been prohibited since the passing of the Human Rights Act in 1988. In 1994 verbal harrassment by fellow workers when an employee's homosexuality became known was pronounced illegal by an Employment Tribunal in Wellington (Stuart, 1995). Israel, which decriminalized homosexual acts in 1988, has made it illegal to discriminate on grounds of sexual orientation. Even Belarus is reported to have lifted its total ban on homosexuality under Article 119.1, although there has been little, if any, official publicity about it. In 1995 the Japanese Society of Psychiatry and Neurology fell into line with the World Health Organization in removing homosexuality from its list of mental disorders. But perhaps the most important recent change is the successful incorporation, though not without some stiff resistance, of the principle of nondiscrimination on grounds of sexual orientation into the constitutions of Canada and South Africa.

Prospects of further increases in accommodation, if not integration, of homosexual status and conduct come from trends and demographics of public opinion polls. The older generations are the more rejecting. Time is not on their side.

REFERENCES

Amnesty International. (1994). *Breaking the silence: Human rights violations based on sexual orientation.* New York: Author.
Amnesty International. (1995). *Romania: Broken commitments to human rights.* London: Author.
Baciu, I., Cimpeanu, V., & Nicora, M. (1995). Romania. In R. Rosenbloom (Ed.), *Unspoken rules: Sexual orientation and women's human rights.* (pp. 161–170). San Francisco: International Gay and Lesbian Human Rights Commission.
Bleys, P. (1993). Homosexual exile: The sexuality of the imaginary paradise, 1800–1980. In R. Mendès Leite (Ed.), *Gay studies from the French cultures.* (pp. 165–182). Binghamton, NY: Harrington Park Press.
Chauvel, C. (1994). New Zealand's unlawful immigration policy. *Australasian Gay and Lesbian Law Journal, 4,* 73–84.
International Gay and Lesbian Human Rights Commission. (1995). *The International Tribunal on Human Rights Violations against Sexual Minorities* (October 17th 1995, New York City). San Francisco: Author.
Landau, R. (1952). *Moroccan journal.* London: Robert Hale.
Matteson, D. R. (1991). Invisible minority. *Empathy, 3*(1), 58–65.
Mott, L. (1995). The gay movement and human rights in Brazil. In S. O. Murray (Ed.), *Latin American male homosexualities.* (pp. 221–230). Albuquerque: University of New Mexico Press.
Murray, S. O. (1987). Ottoman Turkey. In S. O. Murray (Ed.), *Cultural diversity and homosexualities.* (pp. 220–227) New York: Irvington.
Ordoñez, J. P. (1995). *No human being is disposable: Social cleansing, human rights, and sexual orientation in Colombia.* San Francisco: International Gay and Lesbian Human Rights Commission.
Remafedi, G. (Ed.). (1994). *Death by denial: Studies of suicide in gay and lesbian teenagers.* Boston: Alyson.
Rosenbloom, R. (Ed.). (1995). *Unspoken rules: Sexual orientation and women's human rights.* San Francisco: International Gay and Lesbian Human Rights Commission.
Sandfort, T. (1987). Pedophilia and the gay movement. In A. X. van Naerssen (Ed.), *Gay life in Dutch society.* (pp. 89–110). Binghamton, NY: Harrington Park Press
Stuart, B. (1995). The works' outing: The New Zealand workplace harassment case of *L v M Ltd. Australasian Gay and Lesbian Law Journal, 5,* 86–92.
West, D. J. (1992). *Homosexual prostitution.* New York: Haworth Press.

Index